returned on or before
ned below

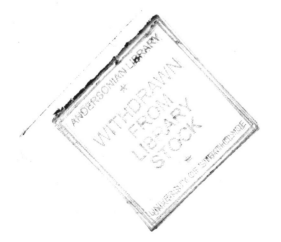

Pathophysiology and Therapeutics of Myocardial Ischemia

Monographs of the Physiological Society of Philadelphia

Volume 1

IMMUNOPHARMACOLOGY
Proceedings of the Conference on Immunopharmacology,
Philadelphia, January 27-28, 1975
Marvin E. Roşenthale and Herbert C. Mansmann, Jr., Editors

Volume 2

NEW ANTIHYPERTENSIVE DRUGS
Proceedings of the A.N. Richards Symposium,
King of Prussia, Pennsylvania, May 19-20, 1975
Alexander Scriabine and Charles S. Sweet, Editors

Volume 3

PROSTAGLANDINS IN HEMATOLOGY
Proceedings of the International Symposium on Prostaglandins in Hematology
Philadelphia, March 4-5, 1976
M.J. Silver, J.B. Smith, and J.J. Kocsis, Editors

Volume 4

PATHOPHYSIOLOGY AND THERAPEUTICS OF MYOCARDIAL ISCHEMIA
Proceedings of the A.N. Richards Symposium,
Philadelphia, May 6-7, 1976
Allan M. Lefer, Gerald J. Kelliher, and Michael J. Rovetto, Editors

Pathophysiology and Therapeutics of Myocardial Ischemia

Proceedings of the A.N. Richards Symposium
Philadelphia, May 6-7, 1976

Edited by

Allan M. Lefer, Ph.D.
Jefferson Medical College
Thomas Jefferson University

Gerald J. Kelliher, Ph.D.
Medical College of Pennsylvania

and

Michael J. Rovetto, Ph.D.
Jefferson Medical College
Thomas Jefferson University

S P Books Division of
SPECTRUM PUBLICATIONS, INC.
New York

SPECTRUM PUBLICATIONS, INC.
175-20 Wexford Terrace, Jamaica, N.Y. 11432

Library of Congress Cataloging in Publication Data

Richards (A. N.) Symposium, 18th, Philadelphia, 1976.
   Pathophysiology and therapeutics of myocardial
ischemia.

   (Monographs of the Physiological Society of Philadel-
phia ; 4)
   Bibliography: p.
   Includes index.
   1. Coronary heart disease--Congresses. 2. Heart--
Infarction--Congresses. I. Lefer, Allan M.
II. Kelliher, Gerald J. III. Rovetto, Michael J.
IV. Title. V. Series: Physiological Society of
Philadelphia. Monographs of the Physiological Society
of Philadelphia ; 4.
RC685.C6R5   1976   616.1'23   77-5072
ISBN 0-89335-020-6

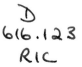

Contributors

CLYDE BARLOW, Ph.D.
Department of Biochemistry and
  Biophysics
Johnson Research Foundation
University of Pennsylvania
Philadelphia, Pennsylvania

ANDREW B. BEASLEY, Sc.D.
Department of Pharmacology
Medical College of Pennsylvania
Philadelphia, Pennsylvania

ALAN BINDER, M.D.
Department of Medicine
Division of Cardiology
North Shore University Hospital
Manhasset, New York

NORMAN BRACHFELD, M.D.
Division of Cardiology
The New York Hospital
Cornell Medical Center
New York, New York

EUGENE BRAUNWALD, M.D.
Department of Medicine
Harvard Medical School and Peter
  Bent Brigham Hospital
Boston, Massachusettes

BRITTON CHANCE, Ph.D.
Department of Biochemistry and
  Biophysics
Johnson Research Foundation
University of Pennsylvania
Philadelphia, Pennsylvania

GILBERT DELEEUW, B.A.
Department of Biochemistry and
  Biophysics
Johnson Research Foundation
University of Pennsylvania
Philadelphia, Pennsylvania

LEONARD DREIFUS, M.D.
Department of Medicine
Jefferson Medical College and
  Lankenau Hospital
Philadelphia, Pennsylvania

NABIL EL-SHERIF, M.D.
Division of Cardiology
Veteran's Administration Hospital
University of Miami
School of Medicine
Miami, Florida

MARIO FEOLA, M.D.
Department of Surgery
Division of Cardiothoracic Surgery
Jefferson Medical College
Philadelphia, Pennsylvania

ARTHUR C. FOX, M.D.
Department of Medicine
Division of Rheumatology and
  Cardiology
New York University
School of Medicine
New York, New York

DORIS GENNARO, B.S.
Department of Medicine
Division of Rheumatology and
  Cardiology
New York University
School of Medicine
New York, New York

THOMAS M. GLENN, Ph.D.
Department of Pharmacology
University of South Alabama
School of Medicine
Mobile, Alabama

ROY D. GOLDFARB, Ph.D.
Department of Physiology
Albany Medical College
Albany, New York

STEPHEN GULOTTA, M.D.
Department of Medicine
Division of Cardiology
North Shore University Hospital
Manhasset, New York

HAL K. HAWKINS, M.D., Ph.D.
Department of Pathology
Duke University Medical Center
Durham, North Carolina

MARY L. HILLS, B.S.
Department of Pathology
Duke University Medical Center
Durham, North Carolina

SYLVIA HOFFSTEIN, Ph.D.
Department of Medicine
Division of Rheumatology and
  Cardiology
New York University
School of Medicine
New York, New York

JANE A. IDELL-WENGER, Ph.D.
Department of Physiology
Milton S. Hershey Medical College
  of Pennsylvania State University
Hershey, Pennsylvania

ROBERT B. JENNINGS, M.D.
Department of Pathology
Duke University Medical Center
Durham, North Carolina

RACE KAO, Ph.D.
Department of Physiology
Milton S. Hershey Medical College
  of Pennsylvania State University
Hershey, Pennsylvania

GERALD J. KELLIHER, Ph.D.
Department of Pharmacology
Medical College of Pennsylvania
Philadelphia, Pennsylvania

CLAIRE LATHERS, Ph.D.
Department of Pharmacology
Medical College of Pennsylvania
Philadelphia, Pennsylvania

RALPH LAZZARA, M.D.
Division of Cardiology
Veteran's Administration Hospital
University of Miami
School of Medicine
Miami, Florida

ROBERT J. LEE, Ph.D.
Department of Pharmacology
Squibb Institute for Medical
Research
Princeton, New Jersey

ALLAN M. LEFER, Ph.D.
Department of Physiology
Jefferson Medical College
Philadelphia, Pennsylvania

PETER R. MAROKO, M.D.
Department of Medicine
Harvard Medical College
Boston, Massachusetts

A. GARRETT MILLER, B.S.
Department of Pharmacology
University of South Alabama
College of Medicine
Mobile, Alabama

HOWARD E. MORGAN, M.D.
Department of Physiology
Milton S. Hershey Medical College
of Pennsylvania State University
Hershey, Pennsylvania

JOHN MORRISON, M.D.
Department of Medicine
Cornell Medical Center
New York, New York

SYED JAMAL MUSTAFA, Ph.D.
Department of Pharmacology
University of South Alabama
College of Medicine
Mobile, Alabama

JAMES R. NEELY, Ph.D.
Department of Physiology
Milton S. Hershey Medical College
of Pennsylvania State University
Hershey, Pennsylvania

SATOSHI OGAWA, M.D.
Department of Medicine
Lankenau Hospital
Philadelphia, Pennsylvania

TAKESHI OGAWA, M.D.
Department of Cardiology
Cedars-Sinai Medical Center
Los Angeles, California

MINORU OKUDA, M.D.
Department of Medicine
Defense Medical College
Saitaima Prefecture, Japan

MARY JANE OSMICK, B.S.
Department of Medicine
Lankenau Hospital
Philadelphia, Pennsylvania

ROY PIZZARELLO, M.D.
Department of Medicine
Division of Cardiology
North Shore University Hospital
Manhasset, New York

D. EUGENE RANNELS, JR.,
Ph.D.
Department of Physiology
Milton S. Hershey Medical College
of Pennsylvania State University
Hershey, Pennsylvania

LAWRENCE REDUTO, M.D.
Department of Medicine
Division of Cardiology
North Shore University Hospital
Manhasset, New York

TERRELL RICH, Ph.D.
Department of Biochemistry and
Biophysics
Johnson Research Foundation
University of Pennsylvania
Philadelphia, Pennsylvania

JAY ROBERTS, Ph.D.
Department of Pharmacology
Medical College of Pennsylvania
Philadelphia, Pennsylvania

ROBERT ROBERTS, M.D.
Cardiovascular Division
Washington University
School of Medicine
St. Louis, Missouri

CONTRIBUTORS

HAROLD B. ROSE Sc.D.
Department of Cardiology
Cedars-Sinai Medical Center
Los Angeles, California

MICHAEL J. ROVETTO, Ph.D.
Department of Physiology
Jefferson Medical College
Philadelphia, Pennsylvania

BENJAMIN J. SCHERLAG, Ph.D.
Division of Cardiology
Veteran's Administration Hospital
University of Miami
School of Medicine
Miami, Florida

EARL SHRAGO, M.D.
Departments of Medicine and
   Nutritional Sciences
University of Wisconsin
Madison, Wisconsin

BURTON E. SOBEL, M.D.
Cardiovascular Division
Washington University
School of Medicine
St. Louis, Missouri

JOSEPH F. SPEAR, Ph.D.
Department of Animal Biology
School of Veterinary Medicine
University of Pennsylvania
Philadelphia, Pennsylvania

CHARLES STEENBERGEN, B.S.
Department of Biochemistry and
   Biophysics
Johnson Research Foundation
University of Pennsylvania
Philadelphia, Pennsylvania

HEI SOOK SUL, Ph.D.
Departments of Medicine and
   Nutritional Sciences
University of Wisconsin
Madison, Wisconsin

TERUO TAKANO, M.D.
Department of Cardiology
Cedars-Sinai Medical Center
Los Angeles, California

RAYMOND C. TRUEX, Ph.D.
Department of Anatomy
Temple University
School of Medicine
Philadelphia, Pennsylvania

JOHN K. VYDEN, M.B.
Department of Cardiology
Cedars-Sinai Medical Center
Los Angeles, California

YOSHIO WATANABE, M.D.
Department of Medicine
Lankenau Hospital
Philadelphia, Pennsylvania

GERALD WEISSMANN, M.D.
Department of Medicine
Division of Rheumatology and
   Cardiology
New York University
School of Medicine
New York, New York

LESLIE WIENER, M.D.
Department of Medicine
Division of Cardiology
Jefferson Medical College
Philadelphia, Pennsylvania

JOHN R. WILLIAMSON, Ph.D.
Department of Biochemistry and
   Biophysics
Johnson Research Foundation
University of Pennsylvania
Philadelphia, Pennsylvania

Preface

Each May, the Physiological Society of Philadelphia holds a symposium in honor of A. N. Richards on a topic of current interest to the biomedical community of the Philadelphia area. This year, as part of the Bicentennial of the United States, the Society elected to hold the symposium on the topic of Myocardial Ischemia. It was felt that this topic would be of interest to physiologists, pharmacologists, cardiologists, surgeons and a wide variety of other basic scientists and clinicians. The topic itself is of great interest to the biomedical community, since it has been the subject of intensive investigation in recent years. Moreover, this effort has proven to be extremely fruitful in providing a greater understanding of the pathophysiologic mechanisms involved in myocardial ischemia leading to the development of myocardial infarction. This knowledge has also resulted in a concerted effort to prevent or retard these deleterious processes. In this regard, application of existing knowledge to this problem has met with definite success in a number of cases. These developments, although encouraging to many in this field, are nevertheless preliminary and represent only a superficial achievement. Much more work is required to interrelate these modest successes and to be able to develop a more complete understanding of the processes involved in myocardial ischemia, myocardial infarction, cardiogenic shock, and cardiac arrhythmias related to these events.

The purposes of this symposium were, therefore, to relate the cardiac electrophysiology, the metabolism of the heart, and the subcellular and hemodynamic alterations to the pharmacology of modifying the ischemic process. This volume contains the proceedings of the symposium held in Philadelphia on May 6-7, 1976. It represents a diversity of findings and opinion and is intended to stimulate the thinking of both the scholar in the field and the interested student.

ALLAN M. LEFER
GERALD J. KELLIHER
MICHAEL J. ROVETTO

CONTENTS

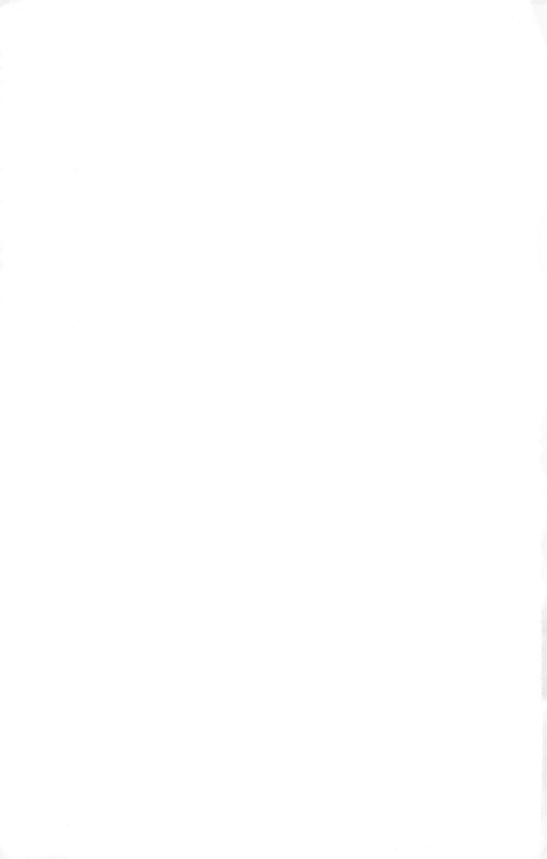

Part I

CARDIAC ELECTROPHYSIOLOGY IN MYOCARDIAL ISCHEMIA

1

Anatomy of Cardiac Conduction System with Related Blood Supply and Autonomic Innervation

RAYMOND C. TRUEX

INTRODUCTION

It is most appropriate that a scientific discussion of myocardial ischemia should begin with a survey of the basic morphologic substrates. Indeed the conduction system, coronary circulation, cardiac innervation and contractile muscle cells are integral units that are intimately involved in an ischemic episode. The clinical importance of myocardial ischemia has long attracted the research interests of many disciplines and a formidable body of literature has accumulated. Many pertinent papers related to myocardial failure and infarction were incorporated recently into one volume that could serve equally well as a source book for the present conference on ischemia (Braunwald, 1974). However, the failure to include a discussion of the conduction system in that volume was regrettable, for the ventricular subendocardium is in great jeopardy during transient and sustained cardiac ischemia or infarction (Bell and Fox, 1974; Neill et al., 1975; Willerson et al., 1975; Horowitz et al., 1976). Let us recall briefly the structure, organization and distribution of components within this unique cellular system.

3

SINOATRIAL NODE AND ATRIAL MYOCARDIUM

The sinoatrial node (SAN) is a slender, elongated mass of pacemaker tissue located in the sulcus terminalis at the junction of the superior vena cava and right atrium (Copenhaver and Truex, 1952; Truex et al., 1967; James, 1961a). This tissue mass consists of small nodal cells, transitional cells and a lesser number of large angular "P cells" believed by some to represent the pacemaker elements (James et al., 1966). This network of heterogeneous anastomosing muscle cells is embedded in a matrix of collagen fibers that increases with age (Lev, 1954; Sims, 1972). It is pertinent to note that the superior portion of the SAN is the only segment of the conduction system located within the epicardium—the other atrial and ventricular components are in the subendocardium (Fig. 1). Location, collagen matrix and arterial blood supply are pertinent factors that help explain structural alterations of the human SAN, associated with pericarditis and a host of other diseases (Hudson, 1960; Kaplan et al., 1973; Greenwood et al., 1975; Engel et al., 1975).

In man and other mammals, the network of nodal cells usually surrounds a discrete nodal artery which serves as a useful landmark to the epicardial location of the SAN. In the majority of human hearts, the SAN artery arises from the initial segment of the right coronary artery (Fig. 2). Less frequently, the SAN is supplied by the right intermediate atrial artery as it is in the canine heart, from branches of the left coronary artery, or from both of these sources. As indicated in Fig. 1, the SAN is tapered superiorly and inferiorly as small nodal and transitional cells become continuous with larger muscle cells of the right atrium (Truex, 1976a). On the myocardial surface between these two tapered ends, the SAN also has multiple cellular anastomoses with atrial myocardial cells. Such zones of anastomoses between SAN and adjacent atrial myocardium are believed by some investigators to correspond with the origins of three discrete atrial internodal pathways composed of larger specialized cells (James, 1963; Wagner et al., 1966; Merideth and Titus, 1968; James and Sherf, 1971). Large atrial cells are scattered throughout both the atria and the interatrial septum (Truex, 1966, 1974). Some large cells may indeed be present in the bundles of atrial muscle cells that converge to join the superior and endocardial surfaces of the atrioventricular node (AVN; 5 in Fig. 1). The thicker muscle bundles that diverge from the periphery of

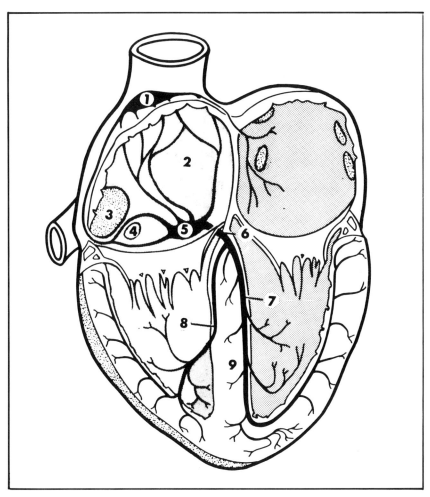

1 Diagram of cardiac conduction system components and their intracardiac relationships. The fossa ovalis (2), opening of the inferior vena cava (3) and ostium of the coronary sinus (4) are important right atrial landmarks used to locate the sinoatrial (1) and atrioventricular (5) nodes. Note the subendocardial relations of the AV bundle (6), left bundle branch (7) and right bundle branch (8) to the muscular interventricular septum (9).

the SAN can be seen to have close relationships to the interatrial septum, fossa ovalis, inferior vena cava and ostium of the coronary sinus. Such bundles of atrial muscle may provide preferential routes for propagation of the cardiac action potential between the SAN and the atrioventricular node (AVN). There is also ample evidence that such bands of atrial muscle continue to conduct even in the presence of hyperkalemia. The positions of these atrial muscle bands (Fig. 1) indicate how they may be interrupted inadvertently during surgical repairs of interatrial septal defects and correction of other cardiac malformations (Holsinger et al., 1968; Isaacson et al., 1972). If several atrial muscle bundles were interrupted low in the interatrial septum as they converged upon the AVN, one might reasonably anticipate an alteration in the atrial conduction interval. For a more detailed review of preferential atrial conduction, the reader is referred to the recent paper by Janse and Anderson (1974).

ATRIOVENTRICULAR NODE AND ATRIOVENTRICULAR BUNDLE

These junctional segments of the conduction system are extremely vulnerable to surgical and vascular injuries which may result in a variety of conduction abnormalities (5 and 6 in Fig. 1). The structure of the human AVN has been presented in several detailed studies (Copenhaver and Truex, 1952; James, 1961b; Truex and Smythe, 1965, 1967; Truex, 1970). Converging bands of atrial cells form the approaches of the AVN as they join its superior, posterior and endocardial surfaces (Hecht et al., 1973). The compact part of the node has the shape of a tennis racquet. It is a thin, broad sheet of small anastomosing cells that coalesce and become continuous to form the atrioventricular bundle (AVB or bundle of His) or racquet handle (6 in Fig. 1). Few large atrial cells penetrate any distance into the AVN and these rapidly blend with the network of small nodal cells. Around the coronary sinus, in the atrial septum and among the approaches of the AVN are clusters of parasympathetic ganglion cells, numerous small beaded autonomic and sensory nerve fibers, and one or more arteries and veins. The vagal neural structures adjacent to the AVN, as well as the nodal cells, display large stores of the enzyme, acetylcholinesterase. It is not surprising that the latticed superior and endocardial surfaces of the AVN are presumed to represent the region of greatest delay in AV conduction.

The AV bundle of some mammals (ungulates, cetacea) is composed of large characteristic Purkinje cells. In man, the AVB contains an admixture of anastomosing large and small nodal muscle cells, as it courses through the right fibrous trigone and comes to lie at the junction of the membranous and muscular interventricular septum (IVS). A large number of sensory and thin beaded visceral motor nerve fibers accompany this fascicle across the AV junction. Some authors diagrammed compartments within the proximal AVB, whereby cellular fascicles or subdivisions become insulated and separated from each other by connective tissue septa (Sherf and James, 1969). Thus, an isolated subdivision of the AVB could contain the cells destined for one bundle branch, or another fascicle might contain cells that conduct to a discrete part of the ventricular septum. This concept provided an explanation for preferential longitudinal depolarization in the AV bundle, as described by the authors. However, this organizational concept is not compatible with either the cellular anastomoses observed within the AVB and bundle branches (Truex, 1973, 1974) or the point to point physiological stimulation experiments with the AVB and bundle branches (Lazzara et al., 1973).

Several features that pertain to the location of the AVB are worthy of emphasis, for in normal hearts it provides the sole connection between atrial and ventricular myocardium (Fig. 1). First, the bundle traverses the junctional zone of both the embryonic and adult cardiac chambers. During septation, this junctional zone becomes closed by mesodermal tissues derived from several different regions of the heart (e.g., endocardial cushions, conal ridges, conoventricular flange, and interventricular septum). Hence, during developmental closure of the IVS, the AV bundle or its major branches may be partly or completely incarcerated in dense scar tissues when the anulus is malformed (e.g., congenital heart block). Secondly, malformations of the AV junction and septum also permit embryonic muscle connections to persist in newborn and adult hearts (accessory AV bundles of Kent, and anomalous atrio-His bypass tracts). Such anomalous muscular AV connections are often associated with pre-excitation and troublesome supraventricular tachycardia. Later in life, if cardiac function is compromised by vascular lesions, ischemia, infarction, or myocardial fibrosis, the anomalous tracts may initiate or participate in intractable supraventricular arrhythmias, or initiate a sudden lethal ventricular rhythm.

One remaining point concerns the arterial blood supply of this junctional area, whereby the proximal AVB receives terminal twigs of the AV nodal artery and is also supplied by the first and second perforating branches of the anterior interventricular artery (Truex, 1963, 1973; Frink and James, 1973). It should also be recalled that numerous small veins drain the top of the IVS and then accompany the AVB in its course across the AV junction (Truex and Schwartz, 1951; Truex, 1970). This vascular complex may account for the frequent occurrences of ischemia, fibrosis, calcification and hemorrhage in and along the course of the AV bundle.

The terminal left and right bundle branches of the AVB can be identified by anatomical methods, as they course distally in the subendocardium of the IVS (7, 8, 9 in Fig. 1). The long narrow right bundle branch is usually composed of small Purkinje cells and gives rise to secondary branches only as it approaches or crosses the anterior papillary muscle of the right ventricle. The anterior and posterior fascicles of the left bundle branch have larger Purkinje cells, particularly in the more distal regions of the ventricle. As shown in Fig. 1, the bundle branches proceed distally toward the apex of their respective ventricles and then ascend toward the base of the heart. It should be noted that Purkinje cells of the bundle branches leave the endocardium and blend with the contractile ventricular muscle cells, as they course toward the epicardium. The anterior and posterior fascicles of the left bundle branch (7 in Fig. 2) may be involved separately, together, or in conjunction with a lesion of the right bundle branch (bifascicular and trifascicular blocks). Fibrotic lesions in the endocardium are often secondary to ischemia, arterial disease, or occlusion. Functionally, this unique system of modified cardiac muscle has slow conduction velocities in the small cells of the SA and AV nodes. There is more rapid conduction of the action potential by the large Purkinje cells of the AVB and bundle branches (Truex, 1972). Conduction velocity is again slower in the ventricular myocardium. It is not surprising that conduction delay, block, or re-entry commonly occur at junctional zones along this specialized system of cells. Since the structural and functional integrity of the conduction system and contractile myocardium are dependent upon a viable blood supply, the distribution of the coronary vessels is presented next.

CORONARY CIRCULATION

The origin of the left and right coronary arteries from the aorta and their distribution on the anterior surface of the heart are shown diagrammatically in Fig. 2. The left coronary artery gives origin to the great anastomotic ramus, then promptly divides into two major subdivisions—the circumflex and anterior interventricular arteries. These two vessels and their branches supply the left atrium, walls of the left ventricle, anterior two-thirds of the muscular IVS, and the adjacent anterior wall of the right ventricle. Medium-sized penetrating vessels arise from the deep surface of branches of the left coronary artery and plunge directly into the ventricular myocardium. These small intramural arteries give off numerous arterial twigs, as they continue through the myocardium *en route* to their terminal distribution in endocardial structures. This vascular arrangement in the left ventricle accounts in part for the vulnerability of the endocardium to ischemia and fibrosis. It explains also the frequency with which fibrous plaques are observed in the distributions of the left bundle branch.

Small intracardiac collaterals have been demonstrated in the subendocardium and myocardium of mammalian hearts, including that of man (Baroldi et al., 1956; Fulton, 1965; Schaper, 1971; Levin, 1974; Frick et al., 1976). Most of the collateral arterioles have a luminal diameter between 20 and 60 μm. These collateral channels provide interconnecting routes between the left and right coronary arteries (intercoronary anastomoses), as well as between smaller branches of the same major artery (intracoronary anastomoses). The number and location of existing coronary collaterals is variable from specimen to specimen, and is believed to be congenitally determined. The functional role of such collateral channels is obvious in human left ventricle function, the prevention of ischemia, reduction of infarct size, and during coronary artery spasm (Oliva et al., 1973; Maseri et al., 1975; Chahine et al., 1975; Mehta et al., 1976). The recent data of Frick et al. (1976) is of particular interest for it showed that, in some patients with verified ischemic heart disease, the collateral circulation reacted to ischemia which resulted from atrial pacing by enhancement to the collateral coronary flow. However, the functional significance of this response remained obscure.

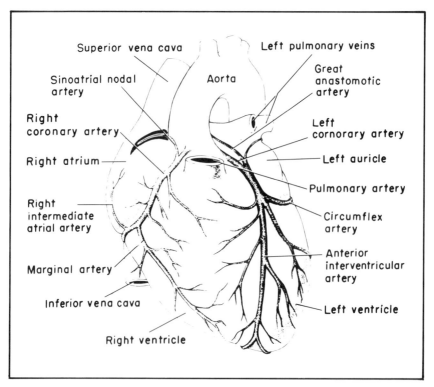

Superior vena cava

Sinoatrial nodal artery

Right coronary artery

Right atrium

Right intermediate atrial artery

Marginal artery

Inferior vena cava

Right ventricle

Aorta

Left pulmonary veins

Great anastomotic artery

Left cornorary artery

Left auricle

Pulmonary artery

Circumflex artery

Anterior interventricular artery

Left ventricle

2 Arteries on anterior surface of the heart. Note origins and branches of the left and right coronary arteries. Blackened area on terminal part of the SA nodal artery indicates position of SAN in the sulcus terminalis of the right atrium.

The anterior ventricular branches of the right coronary artery arise from the side of the parent vessel. Secondary and tertiary branches then penetrate and supply muscle cells of the thinner right ventricle myocardium. This mode of branching provides a "feathery pattern" to injection casts of the right coronary artery. Two small tenuous branches of the right coronary artery merit special emphasis, for they provide blood supply to the SA and AV nodal pacemaker tissues (Figs. 2 and 3). In both diagrams, the thin shape and location of these nodal masses are indicated as black areas astride the respective nodal artery. The lumen of one or both of the nodal arteries may be markedly reduced by vascular disease and calcification (James, 1968; James and Schatz, 1969; Kennel et al.,

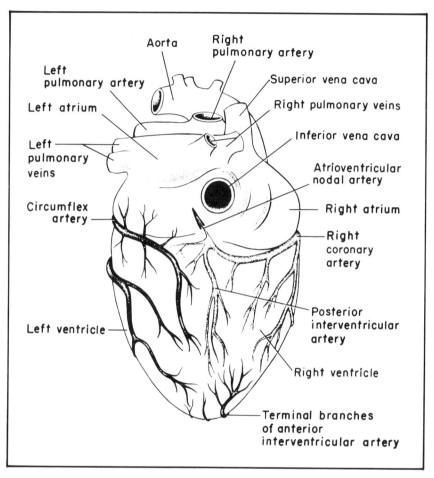

3 Arteries on posterior surface of the heart. In most human hearts, the AV node artery and posterior interventricular artery are branches derived from the right coronary artery. Black area on terminal part of nodal artery indicates relations of AV node to AV sulcus and inferior vena cava.

1973; Becker and van Mantgem, 1975). Coronary angiographers have observed various degrees of bradycardia and other hemodynamic changes induced by dye injections into normal, abnormal, and obstructed coronary arteries. The cardiac slowing was believed to be the result of two factors—namely, ischemic effect of the dye upon pacemaker cells (White et al., 1976), or a reflex vagal slowing of the node. Recent angiographic studies by Frank et al. (1975) validated this belief by correlating the bradycardia response in different patients with the variable patterns in their blood supply to the SA and AV nodes. They observed that selective infusion of atropine into the appropriate right or left coronary arteries prevented the reflex vagal suppression of the sinus pacemaker cells. More details on the functional role of the cardiac nerves are presented later in this communication.

The early literature contains many references related to the "predominant coronary artery." Such predominance was determined solely on the basis of which artery supplied the junctional zone on the posterior surface of the heart, where all four chambers and the two septa meet (i.e., crux of the heart). The coronary artery that supplies this zone normally makes a sharp U-shaped bend and gives off the AV nodal artery before it descends as the posterior interventricular artery (Fig. 3). In most human hearts, the right coronary artery gives origin to both the SA and AV nodal arteries, as well as to the blood supply to the IVS and posterior surfaces of both ventricles (James, 1961c; Truex, 1963). Although the right was said to be the predominant coronary artery, when both arteries are present, the left coronary is of dominant size and supplies most of the crucial left ventricular myocardium. The arterial distributions of left and right coronary arteries (Figs. 2 and 3) thus provide a distribution pattern whereby ischemia, infarction, necrosis, fibrosis, calcification, aneurysms and antemortem cardiac dysfunctions can often be correlated with the pathology observed at necropsy. A simple, consistent histological stain procedure to demonstrate early myocardial ischemia would be highly desirable. The recent histochemical technique of Lie et al. (1971, 1972) has produced neither reliable nor consistent results in this laboratory. The positivity or fuchsinorrhagic staining of presumed ischemic heart cells is markedly enhanced by the time interval, as well as by slight agitation of the slides during immersion in the fuchsin solution. On the other hand, shorter or longer intervals, plus agitation in the picric acid solution, completely eliminated fuchsinorrhagic staining and produced false-positive and false-negative ischemic responses. Similar equivocal and unreliable results have been reported by other investigators (van Reempts et al., 1976). There is indeed an established time course between vascular myocardial insult and pathologic sequellae—particularly when viewed at the ultrastructural level. However, the identification of the very early ischemic changes at the light microscope level must await the development of an infallible microscopic method. Can reflex neural mechanisms induce spasm in the coronary vascular bed and thereby induce myocardial ischemia and angina? For a better appreciation to this query and a host of interrelated questions, we next consider some basic concepts of the neural and humoral mechanisms that participate in the regulation of the circulatory system.

CARDIAC INNERVATION

Bundles of sensory and visceral motor nerve fibers from spinal dorsal root ganglia, the vagus nerves and the ganglionated sympathetic chain form complex patterns as they converge upon the great vessels at the base and posterior surfaces of the heart (Fig. 4). The pattern of the cardiac nerves varies from one animal species to another, and the nerve bundles are usually an admixture of sensory and motor axons from two or more sources. On rare occasions, a single cardiac nerve may consist only of sensory nerve fibers, or another nerve may contain pure vagal or only sympathetic motor axons. This intimate intermingling of extrinsic and intrinsic visceral afferent and efferent axons explains the difficulty encountered when attempts were made to unravel autonomic cardiac innervation by the use of anatomical and physiological methods. Hence, the complex distribution of axons, variations in methods, and individual interpretations of the research data obtained, all account for the many conflicting statements on cardiac innervation that appear in the literature. An extensive review of the central and peripheral autonomic pathways to the heart is beyond the scope of this paper. Such reviews and monographs have been published elsewhere and the reader is referred to them for more detailed information (Mitchell, 1956; von Euler, 1959; Uvnäs, 1960; Rushmer, 1962; Smith, 1965; James, 1967; Korner, 1971; Truex, 1973; Higgins et al., 1973; Öberg, 1976).

In the early embryo, the heart begins to beat synchronously prior to the ingrowth of nerve axons and before intrinsic ganglion cells appear. Later in development, the central and peripheral autonomic neural elements establish pathways that secondarily come to help regulate the intrinsic myogenic activities of the heart (Phillips et al., 1964; Navaratnam, 1965a, 1965b; Wekstein, 1965; Adolph, 1967; Schwieler et al., 1970; Gootman et al., 1972; Nuwayhid et al., 1975; Walker, 1975). Sensory and preganglionic vagal axons appear to reach the heart early in gestation (Garrey and

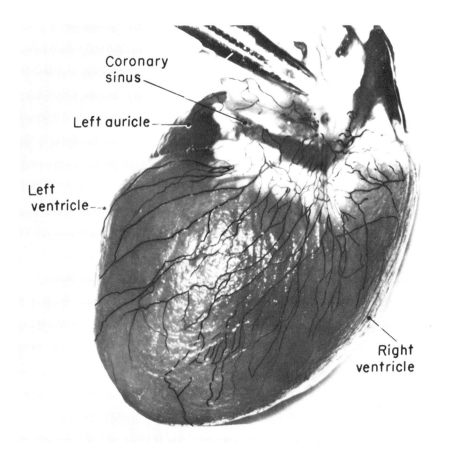

Coronary
sinus

Left auricle

Left
ventricle

Right
ventricle

4   Nerve bundles on posterior epicardial surface of ferret heart, stained by acetylcholinesterase (AChE) method of Bojsen-Moller and Tranum-Jensen (1971a). Small dark round areas (arrow) are clusters of AChE-positive ganglion cells. Note the number of cholinergic nerve bundles that are distributed to the ventricles.

Townsend, 1948; Smith, 1970, 1971). The enzyme acetylcholinesterase (Fig. 4), as well as intensely fluorescent cells and a few postganglionic adrenergic axons have been observed also in embryos of several species (Ignarro and Shideman, 1968; Lipp and Rudolph, 1972; Anderson, 1972; Dail and Palmer, 1973; Anderson et al., 1974; Partanen and Korkala, 1974). Early physiological and anatomical studies on neonate canine hearts indicated that autonomic regulation of cardiac pacemaker tissues was still incomplete at birth (Truex et al., 1955). These observations have recently been repeated and confirmed in subsequent studies of newborn puppies and in a series of newborn miniature swine (Truex, 1976b). Vagal innervation of the heart does precede the appearance of adrenergic nerves. However, both the parasympathetic and sympathetic neural mechanisms do not appear to be fully mature in most laboratory mammals on the day of birth.

Cardiac innervation differs from that of skeletal muscle cells in several interesting ways. For example, there are no highly differentiated or encapsulated sensory and motor endings in the heart similar to those that occur in skeletal muscles (e.g., neuromuscular spindle, Golgi-tendon organ, and motor-end plates). The epicardium contains bundles of nerve fibers and clusters of acetylcholinesterase-positive ganglion cells (Fig. 4). These ganglionic masses are most numerous on the posterior surfaces of the atria and cavae, around the ostium of the coronary sinus, between the ascending aorta and pulmonary arteries, and adjacent to the coronary arteries within the AV sulci We have observed an occasional cluster of ganglion cells, as well as isolated postganglionic cells distal to the AV junction, in several animal species (rat, ferret, dog, monkey, pig, calf, whale, and man). Such ventricular ganglion cells were most frequently seen in association with the AV bundle and rarely in the proximal bundle branches. Ganglion cells have been observed also in the ventricular epicardium, along the branches of the right and left coronary arteries. Lastly, it should be noted that the contractile myocardial cells can survive and continue to function after all the extrinsic cardiac nerves are severed, as in denervation experiments or as occurs following cardiac transplantation (Long et al., 1958; Cooper et al., 1961; Donald et al., 1964). It will be recalled that skeletal muscle cells rapidly undergo degenerative changes and develop denervation hypersensitivity to acetylcholine if their neurotrophic connections are interrupted. Unlike skeletal muscle, the cardiac cells cannot undergo mitosis to replace lost cells, yet they can survive in the absence of all sensory and motor axons. The reason for this curious finding lies in the fact that the heart does not increase or decrease its contractile force by adding or subtracting muscle motor units as occurs in skeletal muscle. Magnitude of the cardiac contractile response is regulated, instead, by muscle-cell length at the time of activation, as a direct result of end-diastolic volume and the attendant filling pressure (i.e., muscle length and the tension applied).

It should not be assumed from the above that the profuse

sensory and motor networks present in the epicardium (Fig. 4), myocardium and endocardium are not essential to normal cardiac function. Indeed, the axons constitute a neural servomechanism that monitors beat-by-beat the heart rate, atrial tensions, atrial contraction and arterial pressures. Reflex neural alterations of heart rate normally perform adjustments in cardiac output under routine non-stressful circumstances. When these sensory and motor axons are severed, both the contractile cardiac muscle and cells of the conduction system survive. However, the cardiac metabolism of the surviving cells does differ from that of the normally innervated cells. After complete cardiac autonomic blockade, the mean resting human heart rate was reported to be 111 beats per minute (Leon et al., 1970). The denervated and transplanted human heart has a fixed rate at rest that approximates 90 to 100 beats per minute (Shaver et al., 1969; Scheuer et al., 1969; Beck et al., 1969). A reappearance of sinus arrhythmia several months later is indicative of parasympathetic axonal regrowth (Thames et al., 1969).

Sensory axons from a wide variety of cardiac receptors travel centrally in the cardiac nerves *en route* to cells of origin in either the dorsal root or vagal ganglia. Visceral afferent fibers from both the atria and ventricles accompany sympathetic visceral motor axons through the sympathetic trunk ganglia and rami to reach the upper four thoracic dorsal root ganglia (Malliani et al., 1972; Fowlis et al., 1974; Gillis et al., 1974; Coote, 1975; Gupta, 1975; Malliani, 1975; Kostreva et al., 1975; Uchida, 1975). Other atrial, septal, ventricular, aortic and carotid visceral afferent axons ascend in the vagus nerves to terminate centrally in the pressor and depressor areas (vasomotor centers) of the medulla (Higgins et al., 1973; Paintal, 1973; Korner, 1971; Simon and Riedel, 1975; Koizumi et al., 1975; Thorén, 1976; Recordati et al., 1976).

The course and central connections of these sensory axons are indicated in Fig. 5. Visceral afferent fibers from the lungs, bronchi and trachea follow similar axonal routes to the spinal cord and medulla. In this diagram, descending polysynaptic central autonomic pathways interconnect limbic areas of the cerebral cortex with hypothalamus, tegmentum and reticular formation neurons of the brain stem (Calaresu and Thomas, 1975; Hilton, 1975; Korner and Uther, 1975; Trzebski et al., 1975). Similarly, ascending multisynaptic tracts (not shown) provide visceral inputs into each level of the central nervous system (CNS). Impulse traffic in both the ascending and descending tracts is either facilitated or inhibited by the mediation of appropriate neurotransmitter substances.

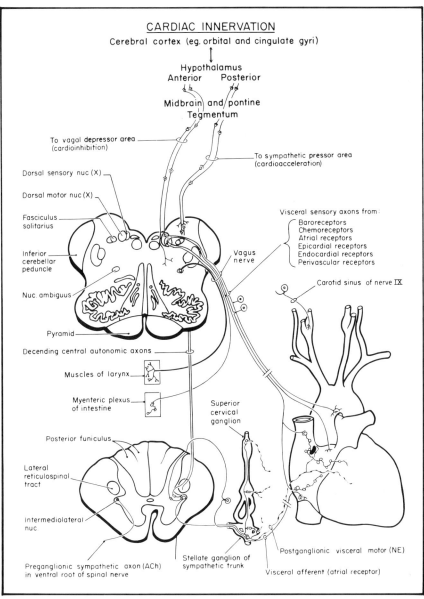

CARDIAC INNERVATION

Cerebral cortex (eg. orbital and cingulate gyri)

Hypothalamus
Anterior   Posterior

Midbrain and pontine
Tegmentum

To vagal depressor area
(cardioinhibition)

To sympathetic pressor area
(cardioacceleration)

Dorsal sensory nuc (X)

Dorsal motor nuc (X)

Fasciculus
solitarius

Inferior
cerebellar
peduncle

Nuc. ambiguus

Pyramid

Descending central autonomic axons

Muscles of larynx

Myenteric plexus
of intestine

Posterior funiculus

Lateral
reticulospinal
tract

Intermediolateral
nuc.

Preganglionic sympathetic axon (ACh)
in ventral root of spinal nerve

Vagus
nerve

Visceral sensory axons from:
Baroreceptors
Chemoreceptors
Atrial receptors
Epicardial receptors
Endocardial receptors
Perivascular receptors

Carotid sinus of nerve IX

Superior
cervical
ganglion

Stellate ganglion of
sympathetic trunk

Postganglionic visceral motor (NE)

Visceral afferent (atrial receptor)

5   Diagram of central (CNS) and peripheral autonomic pathways involved in cardiac innervation. Note that visceral afferent fibers follow sympathetic axons to reach the thoracic spinal cord. Other afferents are components of the vagus and glossopharyngeal nerves en route to the vasomotor areas of the medulla. Visceral efferent neurons of the parasympathetic system are cholinergic (ACh), as are the preganglionic sympathetic axons. Note that postganglionic sympathetic neurons and their axons have norepinephrine (NE) as the neurotransmitter substance.

Through such pathways, a variety of normal and abnormal stimuli from higher centers in the human brain can dramatically alter both the medulla and spinal cord centers that regulate the peripheral circulation (Katz, 1967; Abildskov, 1975; Ibrahim, 1975; Klutzow et al., 1975; Young et al., 1975). For example, intracranial hemorrhage, pressure or tumors may induce a precipitous fall in blood pressure and bradycardia with wide deep T-waves in the electrocardiogram. Psychic or emotional stress, as well as stimulation of the sympathetic nerves, can initiate intense overactivity of the sympathetic outflow to the heart. Results of such procedures lead to electrical instability of the heart, with changes in cardiac rate, arterial pressure, the P-T and Q-T intervals of the electrocardiogram and even ventricular fibrillation (James et al., 1973; Schwartz and Malliani, 1975; Frank and Friedberg, 1976; Lown et al., 1976; Lown and Verrier, 1976).

INTRACARDIAC PARASYMPATHETIC AXONS

It will be noted in Fig. 5 that only two preganglionic vagal axons are shown to end upon two postganglionic cells in the right atrium. Both pre- and postganglionic vagus axons have beaded varicosities and release the neurotransmitter substance acetylcholine (ACh). Thousands of beaded vagal preganglionic axons traverse the atrial tissues to end on the soma and dendrites of innumerable postganglionic neurons. The postganglionic axons follow longer or shorter courses in the interstices between cells of the SA and AV nodes, to bundles of contractile atrial muscle cells, and along the AV bundle and its major branches (Bojsen-Moller and Tranum-Jensen, 1971a, 1971b). Each of the varicosities along a postganglionic vagal axon contains clear round vesicles of ACh when properly fixed specimens are observed with the electron microscope (van der Zypen et al., 1974; Tranum-Jensen, 1975, 1976). Such beaded axons can be demonstrated in preparations stained by several histological methods, such as silver, methylene blue, or histochemical localization of the enzyme, acetylcholinesterase (AChE). However, no study has demonstrated specialized terminal motor endings on either the myocardial or conduction system cells. Thus, the strands of vagal visceral motor axons lie within interstitial spaces, in close proximity to nodal, atrial, Purkinje, transitional and ventricle muscle cells (Fig. 6). As a consequence of a nerve action potential, quanta of ACh are released and this transmitter,

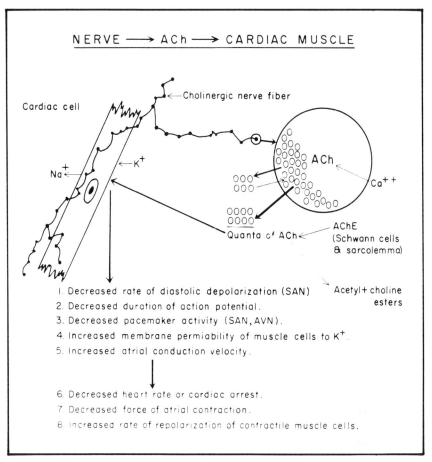

NERVE ⟶ ACh ⟶ CARDIAC MUSCLE

Cardiac cell

←—Cholinergic nerve fiber

ACh

Na⁺

K⁺

Ca⁺⁺

Quanta of ACh

AChE
(Schwann cells
& sarcolemma)

Acetyl + choline
esters

1. Decreased rate of diastolic depolarization (SAN)
2. Decreased duration of action potential.
3. Decreased pacemaker activity (SAN, AVN).
4. Increased membrane permiability of muscle cells to K⁺.
5. Increased atrial conduction velocity.

6. Decreased heart rate or cardiac arrest.
7. Decreased force of atrial contraction.
8. Increased rate of repolarization of contractile muscle cells.

6   Diagram of acetylcholine (ACh) vesicles in an enlarged varicosity of a beaded postganglionic parasympathetic axon in cardiac muscle. Fate and action of the liberated ACh is indicated by arrows. The enzyme, acetylcholinesterase (AChE), located in Schwann cells and along the sarcolemma can rapidly hydrolize ACh into acetyl and choline esters. Action potentials along vagal axons liberate ACh which, in turn, acts for a brief time interval on receptor sites of the postsynaptic membranes of cardiac muscle cells. Resultant chemical and physical changes in muscle cells induce the functional cardiac changes listed in word schema.

in turn, activates appropriate receptor sites on the postsynaptic muscle membranes. The ACh receptor transduces the binding of ACh into an increase in cation permeability of the muscle membrane, especially for the influx of potassium ions. These ionic alterations of postsynaptic membrane permeability are essential chemical events in the processes of depolarization, repolarization and conduction of the cardiac action potential. The ACh shift of cations and changes in muscle membrane properties normally results in decreased pacemaker activity in nodal cells, a decrease in heart rate and a decrease in force of atrial contraction. Action of ACh also appears to enhance the rate of atrial muscle repolarization. As indicated in Fig. 6, both the Schwann cells and sarcolemma contain the enzyme, AChE. This enzyme, after a short time interval, inactivates the liberated but unused intercellular ACh into its acetyl and choline esters. It is not surprising that the greatest amounts of AChE and the enzyme, choline acetyltransferase, are present in the atrial tissues (Mommaerts et al., 1953; Carbonell, 1956; James and Spence, 1966; Ehinger et al., 1968; Hirano and Ogawa, 1969; Ekström, 1970). It is also well known that atropine sulfate, in adequate doses, blocks the muscle-membrane receptor site for ACh and thereby prevents vagally-induced cardiac events. As a consequence of atropine blockade, sympathetic neural activity upon the heart becomes unopposed, as expressed by cardio-acceleration, enhanced activity of pacemaker cells and increased conduction velocity (Fig. 7). More details of these pharmacological mechanisms will be presented later in this volume.

INTRACARDIAC SYMPATHETIC AXONS

As shown in Fig. 5, the preganglionic sympathetic axons arise in the intermediolateral cell column of the thoracic spinal cord. These thinly myelinated cholinergic axons leave the cord mostly in spinal ventral roots T_{1-4} and enter the sympathetic trunk via white communicating rami. Each cholinergic preganglionic fiber terminates synaptically upon a large number of postganglionic cells located in one or more of the sympathetic ganglia. The postganglionic neurons and their beaded non-myelinated axons contain granular vesicles of norepinephrine (NE). Bundles of such adrenergic postganglionic axons join the vagus and cardiac nerves to reach the blood vessels, cells of the conduction system, and contractile cells of the atrial and ventricular myocardium. Only one fine branching

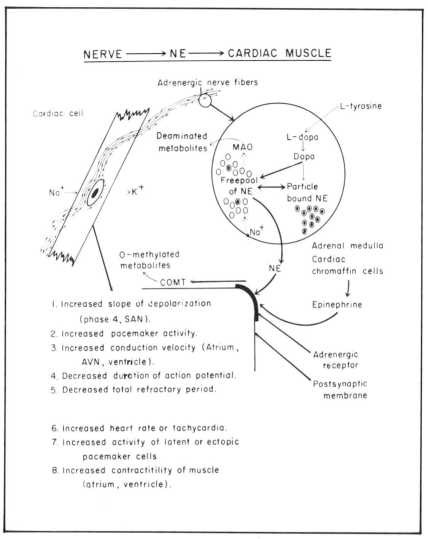

NERVE ──────→ NE ──────→ CARDIAC MUSCLE

Adrenergic nerve fibers

L-tyrosine

Cardiac cell

Deaminated
metabolites

MAO

L-dopa
↓
Dopa

Freepool
of NE ←──────→ Particle
bound NE

Na⁺

K⁺

Na⁺

O-methylated
metabolites

NE

Adrenal medulla
Cardiac
chromaffin cells

COMT ←

1. Increased slope of depolarization
   (phase 4, SAN).
2. Increased pacemaker activity.
3. Increased conduction velocity (Atrium,
   AVN, ventricle).
4. Decreased duration of action potential.
5. Decreased total refractory period.

Epinephrine

Adrenergic
receptor

Postsynaptic
membrane

6. Increased heart rate or tachycardia.
7. Increased activity of latent or ectopic
   pacemaker cells
8. Increased contractility of muscle
   (atrium, ventricle).

7 Diagram of the norepinephrine (NE) vesicles in the fine beaded
varicosities of postganglionic sympathetic axons. Precursors in the
synthesis of NE and the fate of the unbound NE vesicles are
indicated by arrows. Action potentials along sympathetic axons
liberate NE which, in turn, acts at beta adrenergic receptor sites
on the postsynaptic membranes of cardiac muscle cells. Resultant
chemical and physical changes in muscle cells induce the functional
cardiac changes listed in word schema.
COMT = carboxy -o-methyl transferase; MAO = monoamine oxidase.

adrenergic sympathetic axon was included in Fig. 5 in order to avoid confusion. However, unbelievably fine plexuses of beaded adrenergic axons are visualized in all layers of each region of the heart when cardiac tissue is observed after appropriate fluorescence microscopic techniques (Falck et al., 1962; Dahlström, 1965; Jacobowitz et al., 1967; Eränkö, 1967; Ehinger et al., 1968; Fuxe and Jonsson, 1973).

The chemical precursors and NE synthesis, as well as the fate of liberated NE, are indicated schematically in Fig. 7. The cellular activities initiated by NE and epinephrine upon receptor sites of the postsynaptic muscle membrane are included in summary form only, for such pharmacological reactions are topics to be presented later in this volume. It should be noted that chromaffin and dopamine cells have both been observed within mammalian hearts and such cells may be a source of endogenous catecholamines (Trinci, 1907; Truex, 1950; Jacobowitz, 1967; Ehinger et al., 1968; Dail and Palmer, 1973). Recently, the chromaffin cells have been found to receive cholinergic innervation via the vague nerves (Jacobowitz et al., 1967; Vassalle et al., 1970). Although not included in Figs. 5 and 7, it should be emphasized that these fine adrenergic axons are actually distributed to two effectors or cardiac sympathomimetic receptor sites. Sympathetic axon terminals and their transmitter substances distributed to smooth muscle receptors of the coronary vessels are arbitrarily designated as "alpha receptors," since their vasoconstrictor responses are least reactive to isoproterenol (Ahlquist, 1948). The peripheral vasoconstrictor responses classified as "alpha" have different chemical blocking agents, and the roles of such agents in myocardial ischemia and hypoxia are pertinent to the subjects discussed in this volume. However, cardiac excitation with increased heart rate and contractility, along with vasodilation, are found to be highly responsive to circulating isoproterenol and such responses are believed to occur at the "beta receptors." Only cardiac responses induced by activation of beta muscle receptors are shown in Fig. 7. Chemical agents that block the beta receptor sites, such as propranolol, practolol, or sotalol HCl, result in a slowed heart rate, decreased myocardial contractility, lessened oxygen need, and reduced activity in latent ectopic pacemaker cells.

Many factors participate in the regulation of myocardial work and support cardiac metabolic needs. The pulmonary and myocardial circulations ,the autonomic nerves and their transmitter substances and, lastly, an intact cardiac conduction system are all essential factors. They are the substrates that form the woof and the warp of the semantic entities so simply identified as myocardial ischemia, myocardial infarction, and angina pectoris. In reading this volume, it will be necessary to recall pertinent details about the conduction, circulation and innervation substrates. In the process, it will be essential to also interrelate these three important factors, for "we cannot consider one without the others."

ACKNOWLEDGMENTS

This project has been supported by N.I.H. grant HL-07047.

The author expresses his sincere appreciation to Mrs. Deborah Marino for her valued research assistance and meticulous care in preparation of the manuscript. He is indebted to Mrs. Marino, Ms. Karen Rogers and Ms. Beth Young for their technical assistance; and to Ms. Crystel Passauer for the medical art.

REFERENCES

Abildskov, J. A.: The nervous system and cardiac arrhythmias. *Circulation* 51 and 52 (Suppl. III): 116-119 (1975).

Adolph, E. F.: Ranges of heart rates and their regulations at various ages (rat). *Am. J. Physiol.* 212:595-602 (1967).

Ahlquist, R. P.: Study of adrenotropic receptors. *Am. J. Physiol.* 153:586-600 (1948).

Anderson, R. H.: The disposition and innervation of atrioventricular ring specialized tissue in rats and rabbits. *J. Anat.* 113:197-211 (1972).

Anderson, R. H., Davies, M. J., and Becker, A. E.: Atrioventricular ring specialized tissue in the normal heart. *Eur. J. Cardiol.* 2:219-230 (1974).

Baroldi, G., Manteri, O., and Scomazzoni, G.: The collaterals of the coronary arteries in normal and pathologic hearts. *Circ. Res.* 4:223-229 (1956).

Beck, W., Barnard, C. N., and Schrire, V.: Heart rate after cardiac transplantation. *Circulation* 40:437-445 (1969).

Becker, A. E., and van Mantgem, J.: The coronary arteries in Marfan's syndrome. *Am. J. Cardiol.* 36:315-321 (1975).

Bell, J. R., and Fox, A. C.: Pathogenesis of subendocardial ischemia. *Am. J. Med. Sci.* 268:2-13 (1974).

Bojsen-Møller, F., and Tranum-Jensen, J.: Whole-mount demonstration of cholinesterase-containing nerves in the right atrial wall, nodal tissue, and atrioventricular bundle of the pig heart. *J. Anat.* 108:375-386 (1971a).

Bojsen-Møller, F., and Tranum-Jensen, J.: On nerves and nerve endings in the conducting system of the moderator band (septomarginal trabecula). *J. Anat.* 108:387-395 (1971b).

Braunwald, E. (Ed.): *The Myocardium: Failure and Infarction.* HP Publishing Co., Inc., New York (1974), pp. 409.

Calaresu, F. R., and Thomas, M. R.: Electrophysiological connections in the brain stem involved in cardiovascular regulation. *Brain Res.* 87:335-338 (1975).

Carbonell, L. M.: Esterases of the conductive system of the heart. *J.Histochem. Cytochem.* 4:87-95 (1956).

Chahine, R. A., Raizner, A. E., Ishimori, T., Luchi, R. J., and McIntosh, H. D.: The incidence and clinical implications of coronary artery spasm. *Circulation* 52:972-978 (1975).

Cooper, T., Gilbert, J. W., Bloodwell, R. D., and Crout, J. R.: Chronic cardiac denervation by regional neural ablation: Description of the operation, verification of the denervation and its effects on myocardial catecholamines. *Circ. Res.* 9:275-281 (1961).

Coote, J. H.: Physiological significance of somatic afferent pathways from skeletal muscle and joints with reflex effects on the heart and circulation. *Brain Res.* 87:139-144 (1975).

Copenhaver, W. M., and Truex, R. C.: Histology of the atrial portion of the cardiac conduction system in man and other mammals. *Anat. Rec.* 114: 601-626 (1952).

Dahlström, A.: Observations on the accumulation of noradrenaline in the proximal and distal parts of peripheral adrenergic nerves after compression. *J. Anat.* 99:667-690 (1965).

Dail, W. G., Jr., and Palmer, G. C.: Localization and correlation of catecholamine-containing cells with adenyl cyclase and phosphodiesterase activities in the human fetal heart. *Anat. Rec.* 177:265-288 (1973).

Donald, D. E., Milburn, S. E., and Shepherd, J. T.: Effect of cardiac denervation on the maximal capacity for exercise in the racing greyhound. *J. Appl. Physiol.* 19:849-852 (1964).

Ehinger, B., Falck, B., Persson, H., and Sporrong, B.: Adrenergic and cholinesterase-containing neurons of the heart. Histochemie 16: 197-205 (1968).

Ekström, J.: Distribution of choline acetyltransferase in the hearts of mammals. *Acta Physiol. Scand.* 80:73-78 (1970).

Engel, T. R., Meister, S. G., Feitosa, G. S., Fischer, H. A., and Frankl, W. S.: Appraisal of sinus node artery disease. *Circulation* 52:286-291 (1975).

Eränkö, O.: Histochemistry of nervous tissues: Catecholamines and cholinesterases. *Ann. Rev. Pharmacol.* 7:203-222 (1967).

Falck, B., Hillarp, N. Å., Thieme, G., and Torp, A.: Fluorescence of catecholamines and related compounds condensed with formaldehyde. *J. Histochem. Cytochem.* 10:348-354 (1962).

Fowlis, R. A. F., Sang, C. T. M., Lundy, P. M., Ahuja, S. P., and Colhoun, H.: Experimental coronary artery ligation in conscious dogs six months after bilateral cardiac sympathectomy. *Am. Heart J.* 88:748-757 (1974).

Frank, J. P., and Friedberg, D. Z.: Syncope with prolonged QT interval. *Am. J. Dis. Child.* 130:320-322 (1976).

Frick, M. H., Valle, M., Korhola, O., Riihimäki, E., and Wiljassalo, M.: Analysis of coronary collaterals in ischemic heart disease by angiography during pacing induced ischemia. *Br. Heart J.* 38:186-189 (1976).

Frink, R. J., and James T. N.: Normal blood supply to the human His bundle and proximal bundle branches. *Circulation* 47:8-18 (1973).

Frink, R. J., Merrick, B., and Lowe, H. M.: Mechanism of the bradycardia during coronary angiography. *Am. J. Cardiol.* 35:17-22 (1975).

Fulton, W. F. M.: *The Coronary Arteries*. Charles C. Thomas Co. Springfield, Ill. (1965), pp. 354.

Fuxe, K., and Jonsson, G.: The histochemical fluorescence method for the demonstration of catecholamines. *J. Histochem. Cytochem.* 21:293-311 (1973).

Garrey, W. E., and Townsend, S. E.: Neural responses and reactions of the heart of a human embryo. *Am. J. Physiol.* 152:219-224 (1948).

Gillis, R. A., Pearle, D. A., and Hoekman, T.: Failure of beta-adrenergic receptor blockade to prevent arrhythmias induced by sympathetic nerve stimulation. *Science* 185:70-72 (1974).

Gootman, N., Gootman, P. M., Buckley, N. M., Cohen, M. I., Levine, M., and Speilberg, R.: Central vasomotor regulation in the newborn piglet Sus scrofa. *Am. J. Physiol.* 222:994-999 (1972).

Greenwood, R. D., Rosenthal, A., Sloss, L. J., LaCorte, M., and Nadas, S. A.: Sick sinus syndrome after surgery for congenital heart disease. *Circulation* 52:208-213 (1975).

Gupta, P. D.: Spinal autonomic afferents in elicitation of tachycardia in volume infusion in the dog. *Am. J. Physiol.* 229:303-308 (1975).

Hecht, H. H., Kossmann, C. E., Childers, R. W., Langendorf, R., Lev, M., Rosen, K. M., Pruitt, R. D., Truex, R. C., Uhley, H. N., and Watt, T. B., Jr.: Atrioventricular and intraventricular conduction. *Am. J. Cardiol.* 31: 232-244 (1973).

Higgins, C. B., Vatner, S. F., and Braunwald, E.: Parasympathetic control of the heart. *Pharmacol. Rev.* 25:119-155 (1973).

Hilton, S. M.: Ways of viewing the central nervous control of the circulation —old and new. *Brain Res.* 87:213-219 (1975).

Hirano, H., and Ogawa, K.: Ultracytochemical demonstration of cholinesterase activity in the atrium of the guinea pig. *Histochemie* 17:49-56 (1969).

Holsinger, J. W., Jr., Wallace, A. G., and Sealy, W. C.: The identification and surgical significance of the atrial internodal conduction tracts. *Ann. Surg.* 167:447-453 (1968).

Horowitz, L. N., Spear, J. F., and Moore, E. N.: Subendocardial origin of ventricular arrhythmias in 24-hour-old experimental myocardial infarction. *Circulation* 53:56-63 (1976).

Hudson, R. E.: The human pacemaker and its pathology. *Br. Med. J.* 22: 153-167 (1960).

Ibrahim, M. M.: Localization of lesion in patients with idiopathic orthostatic hypotension. *Br. Heart J.* 37:868-872 (1975).

Ignarro, L. J., and Shideman, F. E.: Appearance and concentrations of catecholamines and their biosynthesis in the embryonic and developing chick. *J. Pharmacol. Exp. Ther.* 159:38-48 (1968).

Isaacson, R., Titus, J. L., Merideth, J., Feldt, R. H., and McGoon, D. C.: Apparent interruption of atrial conduction pathways after surgical repair of transposition of great arteries. *Am. J. Cardiol.* 30:533-535 (1972).

Jacobowitz, D.: Histochemical studies of the relationship of chromaffin cells and adrenergic nerve fibers to the cardiac ganglia of several species. *J. Pharmacol. Exp. Ther.* 158:227-240 (1967).

Jacobowitz, D., Cooper, T., and Barner, H. B.: Histochemical and chemical studies of the localization of adrenergic and cholinergic nerves in normal and denervated cat hearts. *Circ. Res.* 20:289-298 (1967).

James, T. N.: Anatomy of the human sinus node. *Anat. Rec.* 141:109-141 (1961a).

James, T. N.: Morphology of the human atrioventricular node with remarks pertinent to its electrophysiology. *Am. Heart J.* 62:756-771 (1961b).

James, T. N.: *Anatomy of the Coronary Arteries.* Paul B. Hoeber, Inc. Medical Division of Harper & Brothers, New York (1961c), pp. 211.

James, T. N.: The connecting pathways between the sinus node and A-V node and between the right and the left atrium in the human heart. *Am. Heart J.* 66:498-508 (1963).

James, T. N.: Cardiac innervation: Anatomic and pharmacologic relations. *Bull. N.Y. Acad. Med.* 43:1041-1086 (1967).

James, T. N.: The coronary circulation and conduction system in acute myocardial infarction. *Prog. Cardiovasc. Dis.* 10:410-449 (1968).

James, T. N., and Schatz, I. J.: Pathology of cardiac conduction system in Marfan's syndrome. *Arch. Intern. Med.* 114:339-343 (1969).

James, T. N., and Sherf, L.: Specialized tissues and preferential conduction in the atria of the heart. *Am. J. Cardiol.* 28:414-427 (1971).

James, T. N., Sherf, L., Fine, G., and Morales, A. R.: Comparative ultrastructure of the sinus node in man and dog. *Circulation* 34:139-163 (1966).

James, T. N., and Spence, C. A.: Distribution of cholinesterase within the sinus node and AV node of the human heart. *Anat. Rec.* 155:151-161 (1966).

James, T. N., Urthaler, F., and Isobe, J. H.: Neurogenic influence on the atrial repolarization (P-T$_p$) segment. *Am. J. Cardiol.* 32:799-807 (1973).

Janse, M. J., and Anderson, R. H.: Specialized internodal atrial pathways—fact or fiction? *Eur. J. Cardiol.* 2:117-136 (1974).

Kaplan, B. M., Langendorf, R., Lev, M., and Pick, A.: Tachycardia-bradycardia syndrome (so-called "Sick Sinus Syndrome"). *Am. J. Cardiol.* 31:497-508 (1973).

Katz, R. L.: Clinical experience with neurogenic cardiac arrhythmias. *Bull. N.Y. Acad. Med.* 43:1106-1118 (1967).

Kennel, A. J., Titus, J. L., McCallister, B. D., and Pruitt, R. D.: The vasculature of the atrioventricular conduction system in heart block. *Am. Heart J.* 85:593-600 (1973).

Klutzow, F. W., Earle, K. M., and Webster, D. D.: Disorders of autonomic function (Dysautonomias). *Milit. Med.* 140:338-344 (1975).

Koizumi, K., Ishikawa, T., Nishino, H., and Brooks, C. McC.: Cardiac and autonomic system reactions to stretch of the atria. *Brain Res.* 87:247-261 (1975).

Korner, P. I.: Integrative neural cardiovascular control. *Physiol. Rev.* 51:312-367 (1971).

Korner, P. I., and Uther, J. B.: Reflex autonomic control of heart rate and peripheral blood flow. *Brain Res.* 87:293-303 (1975).

Kostreva, D. R., Zuperku, E. J., Purtock, R. V., Coon, R. L., and Kampine, J. P.: Sympathetic afferent nerve activity of right heart origin. *Am. J. Physiol.* 229:911-915 (1975).

Lazzara, R., Yeh, B. K., and Samet, P.: Functional transverse interconnections within the His bundle and the bundle branches. *Circ. Res.* 32:509-515 (1973).

Leon, D. F., Shaver, J. A., and Leonard, J. L.: Reflex heart rate control in man. *Am. Heart J.* 80:729-739 (1970).

Lev, M.: Ageing changes in the human sinoatrial node. *J. Gerontol.* 9:1-9 (1954).

Levin, D. C.: Pathways and functional significance of the coronary collateral circulation. *Circulation* 50:831-837 (1974).

Lie, J. T., Holley, K. E., Kampa, W. R., and Titus, J. L.: New histochemical method for morphologic diagnosis of early stages of myocardial ischemia. *Mayo Clin. Proc.* 46:319-327 (1971).

Lie, J. T., Holley, K. E., and Titus, J. L.: Fuchsinorrhagia—a new histochemical indication of inapparent early myocardial ischemia. *Lab. Med.* 3(3): 37-40 (1972).

Lipp, J. M., and Rudolph, A. M.: Sympathetic nerve development in the rat and guinea-pig heart. *Biol. Neonate* 21:76-82 (1972).

Long, D. M., Truex, R. C., Friedmann, K. R., Olsen, A. K., and Phillips, S. J.: Heart rate of dogs following autonomic denervation. *Anat. Rec.* 130:73-89 (1958).

Lown, B., Temte, J. V., Reich, P., Gaughan, C., Regestein, Q., and Hai, H.: Basis for recurring ventricular fibrillation in the absence of coronary heart disease and its management. *N. Engl. J. Med.* 294:623-629 (1976).

Lown, B., and Verrier, R. L.: Neural activity and ventricular fibrillation. *N. Engl. J. Med.* 294:1165-1170 (1976).

Malliani, A., Lombardi, F., Pagani, M. Recordati, G., and Schwartz, P. J.: Spinal cardiovascular reflexes. *Brain Res.* 87:239-246 (1975).

Malliani, A., Peterson, D. F., Bishop, V. S., and Brown, A.M.: Spinal sympathetic cardiocardiac reflexes. *Circ. Res.* 30:158-166 (1972).

Maseri, A., Mimmo, R., Chierchia, S., Marchesi, C., Pesola, A., and L'Abbate, A.: Coronary artery spasm as a cause of acute myocardial ischemia in man. *Chest* 68:625-633 (1975).

Mehta, J., Aintablian, A., and Hamby, R. I.: Coronary artery spasm. *N.Y. State J. Med.* 76:447-449 (1976).

Merideth, J., and Titus, J. L.: The anatomic atrial connections between sinus and AV node. *Circulation* 37:566-579 (1968).

Mitchell, G. A. G.: *Cardiovascular Innervation.* E. and S. Livingstone, London (1956), pp. 196-225.

Mommaerts, W. F. H. M., Khairallah, P. A., and Dickens, M. F.: Acetylcholinesterase in the conductive tissue of the heart. *Circ. Res.* 1:460-465 (1953).

Navaratman, V.: Development of the nerve supply to the human heart. *Br. Heart J.* 27:640-650 (1965a).

Navaratman, V.: The ontogenesis of cholinesterase activity within the heart and cardiac ganglia in man, rat, rabbit and guinea pig. *J. Anat.* 99:459-467 (1965b).

Neill, W. A., Oxendine, J., Phelps, N., and Anderson, R. P.: Subendocardial ischemia provoked by tachycardia in conscious dogs with coronary stenosis. *Am. J. Cardiol.* 35:30-36 (1975).

Nuwayhid, B., Brinkman, C. R., III, Bevan, J. A., and Assali, N. S.: Development of autonomic control of fetal circulation. *Am. J. Physiol.* 228:337-344 (1975).

Öberg, B.: Overall cardiovascular regulation. *Annu. Rev. Physiol.* 38:537-570 (1976).

Oliva, P. B., Potts, D. E., and Pluss, R. G.: Coronary arterial spasm in Prinzmetal angina. Documentation by coronary arteriography. *N. Engl. J. Med.* 288:745-790 (1973).

Paintal, A. S.: Vagal sensory receptors and their reflex effects. *Physiol. Rev.* 53:159-227 (1973).

Partanen, S., and Korkala, O.: Catecholamines in human fetal heart. *Separ. Experientia* 30:798-799 (1974).

Phillips, S. J., Agate, F. J., Jr., Silverman, W. A., and Steiner, P.: Autonomic cardiac reactivity in premature infants. *Biol. Neonate* 6:225-249 (1964).

Recordati, G., Lombardi, F., Bishop, V. S., and Malliani, A.: Mechanical stimuli exciting type A atrial vagal receptors in the cat. *Circ. Res.* 38: 397-403 (1976).

Rushmer, R. F.: Effects of nerve stimulation and hormones on the heart: The role of the heart in general circulatory regulation. In *Handbook of Physiology*, Sect. 2, Vol. 1, *Circulation*, W. F. Hamilton, ed. Williams and Wilkins, Baltimore (1962), pp. 533-550.

Schaper, W.: *The Collateral Circulation of the Heart*. D. A. K. Black, ed. American Elsevier Publishing Co., Inc., New York (1971), pp. 5-16.

Scheuer, J., Shaver, J. A. Harris, B. C., Leonard, J. L., and Bahnson, H. T.: Electrocardiographic findings in cardiac transplantation. *Circulation* 40: 289-296 (1969).

Schwartz, P. J., and Malliani, A.: Electrical alternation of the T-wave: Clinical and experimental evidence of its relationship with the sympathetic nervous system and with the long Q-T syndrome. *Am. Heart J.* 89:45-50 (1975).

Schwieler, G. H., Douglas, J. S., and Bouhuys, A.: Postnatal development of autonomic efferent innervation in the rabbit. *Am. J. Physiol.* 219:391-397 (1970).

Shaver, J. A., Leon, D. A., Gray, S., III, Leonard, J. L., and Bahnson, H. T.: Hemodynamic observations after cardiac transplantation. *N. Engl. J. Med.* 281:822-827 (1969).

Sherf, L., and James, T. N.: A new electrocardiographic concept: Synchronized sinoventricular conduction. *Dis. Chest* 55:127-140 (1969).

Simon, E., and Riedel, W.: Diversity of regional sympathetic outflow in integrative cardiovascular control; patterns and mechanisms. *Brain Res.* 87: 323-333 (1975).

Sims, B. A.: Pathogenesis of atrial arrhythmias. *Br. Heart J.* 34:336-340 (1972).

Smith, O. A., Jr.: Anatomy of central neural pathways mediating cardiovascular functions. In *Nervous Control of the Heart*, W. C. Randall, ed. Williams and Wilkins Co., Baltimore (1965), pp. 34-53.

Smith, R. B.: The development of the intrinsic innervation of the human heart between the 10 and 70 mm stages. *J. Anat.* 107:271-279 (1970).

Smith, R. B.: Intrinsic innervation of the human heart in foetuses between 70 mm and 420 mm crown-rump length. *Acta Anat.* (Basel) 78:200-209 (1971).

Thames, M. D., Kontos, H. A., and Lower, R. R.: Sinus arrhythmia in dogs after cardiac transplantation. *Am. J. Cardiol.* 24:54-58 (1969).

Thorén, P. N.: Atrial receptors with nommedullated vagal afferents in the cat. *Circ. Res.* 38:357-362 (1976).

Tranum-Jensen, J.: The ultrastructure of the sensory end-organs (baroreceptors) in the atrial endocardium of young mini-pigs. *J. Anat.* 119:255-275 (1975).

Tranum-Jensen, J.: The fine structure of the atrial and atrioventricular (AV) junctional specialized tissues of the rabbit heart. In *The Conduction System of the Heart: Structure, Function and Clinical Implications*, H. J. J. Wellens, K. I. Lie, and M. J. Janse, eds. H. E. Sternfert Kroese B. V.-Lieden, The Netherlands (1976), pp. 55-81.

Trinci, G.: Cellule cromaffini e "Mastzellen" nella regione cardiaca dei mammiferi. *Mem. Reale Accad. Sci. Ist. Bologna* 4:191-205 (1907).

Truex, R. C.: Chromaffin tissue of the sympathetic ganglia and heart. *Anat. Rec.* 108:687-698 (1950).

Truex, R. C.: The distribution of the human coronary arteries. In *Coronary Heart Disease*, W. Likoff and J. H. Moyer, eds. Grune and Stratton, New York (1963), pp. 4-10.

Truex, R. C.: Anatomical considerations of the human atrioventricular junction. In *Mechanisms and Therapy of Cardiac Arrhythmias*. L. S. Dreifus and W. Likoff, eds. Grune and Stratton, New York (1966), pp. 333-340.

Truex, R. C.: Anatomy related to atrioventricular block. *Cardiovasc. Clin.* 2: 1-22 (1970).

Truex, R. C.: Myocardial cell diameters in primate hearts. *Am. J. Anat.* 135: 269-280 (1972).

Truex, R. C.: Anatomy of the specialized tissues of the heart. In *Cardiac Arrhythmias*, L. S. Dreifus and W. Likoff, eds. Grune and Stratton, New York (1973), pp. 1-12.

Truex, R. C.: Structural basis of atrial and ventricular conduction. *Cardiovasc. Clin.* 6:1-24 (1974).

Truex, R. C.: The sinoatrial node and its connections with the atrial tissues. In *The Conduction System of the Heart: Structure, Function and Clinical Implications*, H. J. J. Wellens, K. I. Lie, and M. J. Janse, eds. H. E. Sternfert Kroese, B. V.-Lieden, The Netherlands (1976a), pp. 209-226.

Truex, R. C.: Cardiac innervation of the newborn miniature swine. *Anat. Rec.* 184:549 (1976b).

Truex, R. C., and Schwartz, M. J.: Venous system of the myocardium with special reference to the conduction system. *Circulation* 4:881-889 (1951).

Truex, R. C., Scott, J. C., and Smythe, M. Q.: Effect of vagus nerves on heart rate of young dogs: An anatomic-physiologic study. *Anat. Rec.* 123:201-225 (1955).

Truex, R. C., and Smythe, M. Q.: Recent observations on the human cardiac conduction system, with special considerations of the atrioventricular node and bundle. In *Electrophysiology of the Heart*, B. Taccardi and G. Marchetti, eds. Pergamon Press, New York (1965), pp. 177-198.

Truex, R. C., and Smythe, M. Q.: Reconstruction of the human atrioventricular node. *Anat. Rec.* 158:11-19 (1967).

Truex, R. C., Smythe, M. Q., and Taylor, M. J.: Reconstruction of the human sinoatrial node. *Anat. Rec.* 159:371-378 (1967).

Trzebski, A., Lipski, J., Majcherczyk, S., Szulczyk, P., and Chruscielewski, L.: Central organization and interaction of the carotid baroreceptor and chemoreceptor sympathetic reflex. *Brain Res.* 87:227-237 (1975).

Uchida, Y.: Afferent aortic nerve fibers with their pathways in cardiac sympathetic nerves. *Am. J. Physiol.* 228:990-995 (1975).

Uvnäs, B.: Central cardiovascular control. In *Handbook of Physiology*, Sect. 1, Vol. 2. *Neurophysiology*, J. Field, ed. Williams and Wilkins, Baltimore (1960), pp. 1131-1162.

van der Zypen, E., Hasselhorst, G., Merz, R., and Fillinger, H.: Histochemische und elektronenmikroskopische Untersuchungen an den intramuralen Ganglien des Herzens bei Mensch und Ratte. *Acta Anat.* (Basel) 88:161-187 (1974).

van Reempts, J., Borgers, M., and Reneman, R. S.: Early myocardial ischemia: Evaluation of the histochemical haematoxylin—basic fuchsin—picric acid (HBFP) staining technique. *Cardiovasc. Res.* 10:262-267 (1976).

Vassalle, M., Mandel, W. J., and Holder, M. S.: Catecholamine stores under vagal control. *Am. J. Physiol.* 218:115-123 (1970).

von Euler, U. S.: Autonomic neuroeffector transmission. In *Handbook of Physiology*, Sect. 1, Vol. 1, *Neurophysiology*, J. Field, ed. Williams and Wilkins, Baltimore (1959), pp. 215-237.

Wagner, M. L., Lazzara, R., Weiss, R. M., and Hoffman, B. F.: Specialized conducting fibers in the interatrial band. *Circ. Res.* 18:502-518 (1966).

Walker, D.: Functional development of the autonomic innervation of the human fetal heart. *Biol. Neonate* 25:31-43 (1975).

Wekstein, D. R.: Heart rate of the preweanling rat and its autonomic control. *Am. J. Physiol.* 208:1259-1262 (1965).

White, C. W., Eckberg, D. L., Inasaka, T., and Abboud, F. M.: Effects of angiographic contrast media on sino-atrial nodal function. *Cardiovasc. Res.* 10:214-223 (1976).

Willerson, J. T., Parkey, R. W., Bonte, F. J., Meyer, S. L., and Stokely, E. M.: Acute subendocardial myocardial infarction in patients. Its detection by technetium 99-m stannous pyrophosphate myocardial scintigrams. *Circulation* 51:436-441 (1975).

Young, R. R., Asbury, A. K., Corbett, J. L., and Davis, R. D.: Pure pandysautonomia with recovery description and discussion of diagnostic criteria. *Brain* 98:613-636 (1975).

Pathophysiology and Therapeutics of Myocardial Ischemia

2

Patterns of Ventricular Activation During Ventricular Arrhythmias 24 Hours Following Experimental Myocardial Infarction

JOSEPH F. SPEAR

INTRODUCTION

In 1950, Harris described an experimental technique for studying arrhythmias induced by acute myocardial infarction. Within 2 to 5 min following acute ligation of a major portion of the left anterior descending (LAD) coronary artery, an initial stage of ventricular arrhythmias appears. This stage is associated with the occurrence of spontaneous ventricular fibrillation. The initial arrhythmias subside within about 30 min following the ligation and 4 to 8 hr later a second period of ventricular ectopic activity appears. The ventricular arrhythmia peaks in 15 to 30 hr and persists for approximately 72 hr. Electrophysiological studies from several laboratories have verified that the subendocardial Purkinje system overlying the infarcted ventricular muscle survives (Friedman et al., 1973; Lazzara et al., 1973; Friedman et al., 1975). It has been suggested that the ventricular arrhythmias which occur 24 hours following acute coronary ligation originate in the surviv-

31

ing subendocardial Purkinje network (Friedman et al., 1973; Scherlag et al., 1974; Horowitz et al., 1976). Arrhythmias similar to those associated with left anterior descending coronary ligation also occur following acute ligation of the anterior septal artery in the dog (Lumb et al., 1959). In addition, since this anterior septal infarct involves the proximal specialized ventricular conducting system, atrioventricular (AV) conduction disturbances occur acutely (Lumb et al., 1959; El-Sherif et al., 1974).

The present report describes studies carried out in our laboratory, comparing the electrophysiological characteristic of ventricular activation during arrhythmias which occur 24 hr following either a left anterior descending coronary artery occlusion or an anterior septal coronary artery occlusion. In the former experimental system, the area of infarction involves the anterior free wall of the left ventricle, as well as the left anterior inferior septum and associated peripheral Purkinje system. On the other hand, the septal artery occlusion produces an infarction which, while restricted to the septum, involves not only parts of the peripheral Purkinje system but also the His bundle, and right and left bundle branch systems.

METHODS

The experiments were carried out on 24 healthy mongrel dogs, weighing between 10 and 18 kg and anesthetized with sodium pentobarbital (30 mg/kg, i.v.). Two series of experiments were performed. In one series, after the animals were anesthetized and their chests opened through a small left lateral thoracotomy, the left anterior descending coronary artery was occluded by the two-stage procedure described by Harris (1950). The ligation was located approximately 1 cm from the origin of the main left coronary artery and did not involve the circumflex or anterior septal arteries. Following the ligation, the animals' chests were closed and they were allowed to recover. In a second series of animals, the anterior septal coronary artery was selectively occluded after its location by blunt dissection. These animals were also allowed to recover.

Twenty-four hours following the initial procedure, the animals were reanesthetized with either morphine or diazepam and sodium pentobarbital. Upon the induction of anesthesia, the animals were ventilated, using a positive-pressure room air ventilator, and the chests were reopened in the fifth left intercostal space. The heart was suspended in a pericardial sling to provide the exposure for the electrophysiological studies. In addition, a catheter was inserted in the right femoral or internal jugular veins to allow supplementary doses of anesthetic to be given. Standard electrocardiographic leads were continuously monitored. The arrhythmias were initially studied utilizing epicardial mapping techniques which have been previously described (Horowitz et al., 1976; Kastor et al., 1972). The technique involves inserting a bipolar plunge-type electrode into non-infarcted ventricular muscle. This fixed electrode serves as a reference point for the mapping procedure. A hand-held bipolar roving electrode is then moved through predetermined points along the epicardial surfaces of right and left ventricle. The time of activation of these epicardial points, relative to the fixed reference activation time, allows us to construct epicardial activation maps defining the sequence and direction of activation.

In addition, electrical activity within the specialized ventricular conduction system, as well as atrial and ventricular myocardium and ventricular septum, were recorded using plunge-type bipolar electrodes. We were able, therefore, to correlate epicardial activation with conduction within the ventricular septum, His bundle, bundle branches, and Purkinje systems.

In the series of animals in which the anterior septal artery was occluded, the extent of myocardial infarction was not always apparent on the surfaces of the septum. In these studies, we delineated the extent of myocardial damage by utilizing the vital stain nitro blue tetrazolium, according to the technique of Nachlas and Shnitka (1963).

RESULTS

In all animals which had undergone either left anterior descending coronary artery ligation or anterior septal ligation, ventricular tachycardia competing with sinus rhythm was present at 24 hr following coronary ligation. Upon reanesthesia and crushing of the sinus node to eliminate supraventricular competition with the ventricular tachycardia, stable ventricular rhythms established themselves. According to electrocardiographic criteria, these rhythms were usually of the monofocal type or of two competing foci. Table 1 shows the characteristic spontaneous rates of the stable ventricular rhythms which occurred following either left anterior descending coronary occlusion or septal artery occlusion, and

Table 1. Spontaneous rates of ectopic ventricular rhythms

A-V DISSOCIATION (beats/min.)	L.A.D. OCCLUSION (beats/min.)	ANTERIOR SEPTAL OCCLUSION (beats/min.)
49.2 ± 8.4	196 ± 19.5	133 ± 35.9

compares these with the normal ventricular automaticity which is demonstrated during AV dissociation induced by electrocautery of the bundle of His (Spear and Moore, 1973). The mean spontaneous rates for the rhythms following LAD occlusion and anterior septal artery occlusion were 196 beats/min and 133 beats/min, respectively. These values were significantly above the 49 beats/min, which was the spontaneous rate of ventricular escape pacemakers exhibiting normal automaticity.

VENTRICULAR ACTIVATION DURING RHYTHMS INDUCED BY LAD OCCLUSION

In a previously published study from our laboratory (Horowitz et al., 1976), basically two types of rhythm were observed following LAD occlusion. In all cases, epicardial mapping disclosed the origin of epicardial breakthrough to be on the left ventricle, at the margins of the infarcted myocardium. In one type of rhythm, producing a primarily qS pattern in the electrocardiogram, the early epicardial breakthrough was inferior and posterior along the border of the infarct. In the second type of rhythm, producing primarily monophasic R-wave or qR pattern, the earliest area of epicardial breakthrough was located on the anterior-superior border of the infarct. Fig. 1 shows typical electrocardiographic recordings and epicardial maps, comparing these two types of rhythm which occur 24 hr following LAD occlusion. In Fig. 1A, the electrocardiographic tracing of the tachycardia exhibits a stable monofocal ventricular rhythm of the rS variety. Above, the epicardial map indicates that the early area of epicardial breakthrough was along the inferior and posterior border of the infarct and produced early activation of the left ventricle. Right ventricular activation

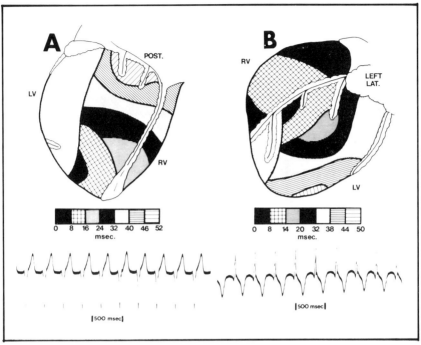

1 The ventricular epicardial activation sequences and the corresponding electrocardiograms in an animal during two episodes of ventricular tachycardia, 24 hours following occlusion of the left anterior descending coronary artery. In both **A** and **B** the infarcted myocardium is indicated by the broken diagonal lines. The concentric isochronic lines indicate activation times according to the time scale shown below. The activation sequence in **A** was recorded during ventricular tachycardia producing the qS electrocardiographic pattern. The earliest site of epicardial activation was inferior-posterior. The activation sequence in **B** was recorded 30 min. after **A** in the same animal during a ventricular tachycardia with a monophaseic R-wave morphology. The earliest area of epicardial breakthrough in this case was anterior and superior along the margin of the infarcted myocardium. (Reproduced by permission of the American Heart Assoc. from Horowitz et al., 1976.)

in this case was correspondingly late, however, this is not shown in this figure. In Fig. 1B, the electrocardiographic tracing presents a primarily qR pattern and, in this case, the spontaneous rhythm had an early epicardial breakthrough on the left ventricle but in a superior and anterior position along the infarct margin. Again, epicardial activation spread from this point to activate the left and, at a later time, the right ventricle.

Fig. 2 shows analog records taken from another study in which the animal was exhibiting a ventricular tachycardia of the rS variety and had an epicardial activation map indicating an inferior-posterior origin of ventricular activation. In this figure, electrograms were recorded from the bundle of His, the proximal portions of the left bundle branch, a Purkinje fiber within the infarcted zone of the free wall of the left ventricle, and a Purkinje fiber within the border area of the infarct on the left ventricle. In addition, the reference electrogram used for the mapping procedure is also indicated. These records present characteristics which were typical for all of the rhythms following LAD ligation. The Purkinje spike, within the mid-regions of the infarcted myocardium, preceded all other activity and was the earliest activity which we could find in the heart during this rhythm. The sequence of activation in the ventricular conducting system was, therefore, retrograde from its origin in the Purkinje system within the infarct to the bundle branch and then to the His. Further verification that we had located the earliest site of activation within the subendocardial Purkinje system underlying the infarct was accomplished by pacing through the recording electrode which measured this early activation. When this was done, the activation sequence of the conducting system, as well as the surface electrocardiogram and epicardial activation sequence, remained unchanged during overdrive pacing as compared to the spontaneous rhythm. We interpreted this information as confirmatory that we had, in fact, located the area of earliest activation during the ventricular rhythm.

Fig. 3 presents data from another experiment in which the ventricular rhythm had an inferior-posterior origin. This figure compares the relationship of the early epicardial activation to the activation in the conducting system. In Fig. 3A, the anterior and posterior surfaces of the heart are schematized. The cross-hatched area indicates the infarcted myocardium and the dark crescent designates the early area of breakthrough for the spontaneous rhythm which is analyzed in Fig. 3B. Superimposed over a tracing of the lead II electrocardiogram are the relative activation times of left and right ventricular epicardial sites. In addition, Purkinje spikes obtained from the subendocardium, and bundle branch, His and muscle activity from within the ventricular septum are indicated below the electrocardiographic recording on the common-time axis. Time zero of this axis is the occurrence of the earliest

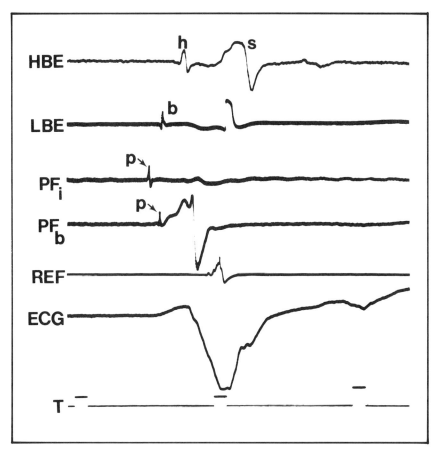

2 Depolarization of the ventricular specialized conducting system during spontaneous ventricular tachycardia, 24 hours following left anterior descending coronary artery occlusion. The records are bipolar recordings from the His bundle (HBE), the left bundle branch (LBE), a Purkinje fiber within the infarct (PF$_i$), a Purkinje fiber in the border zone of the infarct (PF$_b$), non-infarcted myocardium (REF) and a lead II electrocardiogram (ECG). In the HBE record, **h** indicates the retrograde His deflection and **s** indicates the underlying ventricular septal activation. The time signal (T) indicates 100 msec. intervals. The records were obtained during spontaneous ventricular tachycardia originating in the inferior-posterior margin of the infarct. PF$_i$ precedes activation of the proximal conducting system, as well as that of the distal ventricular conducting system and ventricular muscle. (Reproduced by permission of the American Heart Assoc. from Horowitz et al., 1976.)

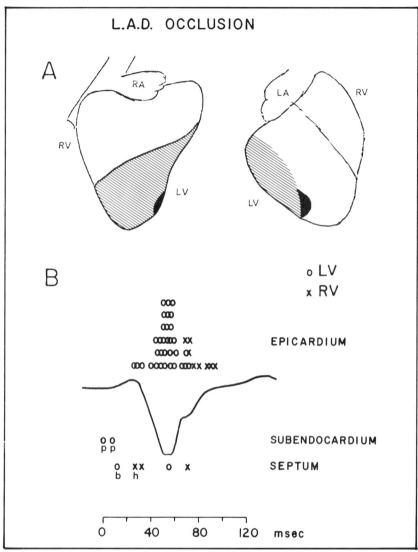

3

A comparison of early epicardial activation and subendocardial Purkinje and septal activation, during a ventricular tachycardia, following left anterior descending coronary artery occlusion. In **A**, the cross-hatched areas indicate the approximate extent of the infarcted myocardium. The dark crescent area designates earliest epicardial activation. In **B**, the electrocardiographic lead II wave form and epicardial, subendocardial and septal activation times are plotted on the common—time axis. The open circles represent left ventricular sites, the x's—right ventricular sites. Epicardial activation times are shown above the ventricular complex, subendocardial and septal activation times are given below the electrocardiographic complex. The **p** below the open circles indicates peripheral Purkinje fiber activations. The **b** below the open circle represents a left bundle activation time and the **h** below the **x** denotes His bundle activation.

recorded Purkinje fiber activity. This was obtained from the sub-endocardium, 1 cm within the infarcted region. This Purkinje fiber activity preceded both left bundle branch and His bundle activity. In addition, Fig. 3B shows that activation of the Purkinje system and the distal bundle branch system occurred before epicardial breakthrough. Also, left ventricular epicardial activation preceded right ventricular epicardial activation. In all 14 of the ectopic ventricular rhythms investigated 24 hr following LAD occlusion, the left ventricular depolarization always occurred earlier than activation of the right ventricle. In animals which exhibited a rhythm originating inferior-posteriorly, right ventricular activation was delayed 20 to 40 msec, whereas in those with the anterior early epicardial breakthrough, right ventricular depolarization began 10 to 20 msec following onset of left ventricular depolarization. The relationship of retrograde His bundle activation to right ventricular epicardial activation, in these studies, suggests that contralateral ventricular activation may have taken place, at least in part, by way of retrograde conduction to the His bundle and antegrade conduction down the right bundle branch to right ventricle. In Fig. 3, retrograde His bundle activation was found to precede earliest right ventricular epicardial activation by 40 msec. In all of the animals which exhibited early posterior-inferior epicardial activation, right ventricular activation followed the His depolarization by 28 to 40 msec. In those animals in which the earliest activation was on the anterior-superior border of the infarct, right ventricular epicardial activation preceded His bundle activation by 2 to 12 msec. This suggests that during the inferior-posterior rhythms, retrograde conduction to the His and antegrade conduction down the right bundle branch may contribute to right ventricular activation.

VENTRICULAR ACTIVATION DURING RHYTHMS INDUCED BY SEPTAL ARTERY OCCLUSION

In those animals which had undergone anterior septal coronary occlusion, the origin of the tachycardia and the ventricular activation were quite different. In contrast to the LAD occlusion, septal occlusion produced rhythms originating in both left and right septal surfaces, causing both left and right early epicardial breakthrough. In all 13 ventricular rhythms, bipolar plunge-electrode recordings localized the earliest areas of activation within the peripheral Purkinje network lying along the ventricular septum. Fig. 4 shows

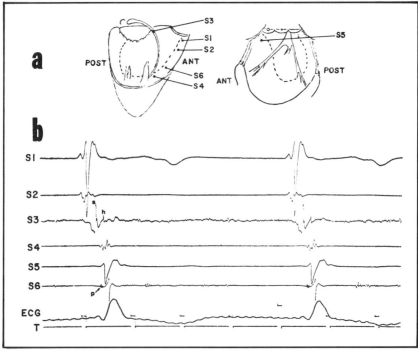

4   Analog records obtained during spontaneous ventricular tachycardia, 24 hours following ligation of the anterior septal coronary artery. In **A** the right and left ventricular septal surfaces are shown schematically. Sites S1 through S5 indicate the approximate areas where the analog records presented in **B** were obtained. In **A**, the dotted lines in the diagrams indicate the approximate borders of the area of infarction within the septum. In **B**, the S3 analog record, **s** indicates ventricular septal activation and **h**—His bundle activation. In the S6 record, **p** denotes a Purkinje fiber spike.

selected analog records obtained from an animal exhibiting a stable ventricular rhythm which originated in the anterior right ventricular septum. The schematics diagrams Fig. 4A show right and left septal surfaces, and locates recording sites of the electrical activity presented in each of the analog records given in Fig. 4B. Our septal recordings indicated that earliest ventricular activity originated within the septum near recording site S2. Recording site S3 was within the penetrating portion of the bundle of His. The analog record shows both the high ventricular septal activation indicated by s and a retrograde His bundle deflection indicated by **h**. These data were typical for all of our studies in that His bundle and bundle branch activity always followed earliest septal activation. Fig. 5 presents data from an experiment, showing the relationship between septal and ventricular conducting system activation and epicardial activation during ventricular tachycardia. In Fig. 5A, the dark crescent indicates the earliest area of epicardial breakthrough which occurred along the anterior margin of the right ventricle near the septum. In this animal, the origin of the activity was within the anterior right septum, approximately underlying this epicardial breakthrough. In all animals, there was a relationship between the area of early septal activation and the ultimate area of epicardial breakthrough on either right or left ventricular surfaces. In Fig. 5B a lead II electrocardiographic complex characteristic for the ventricular rhythm in this animal is exhibited. Both epicardial activation times, and septal myocardial and conduction system activation times are plotted on the common-time axis. Zero time corresponds to the earliest area of activation recorded, which in this case was from the anterior right ventricular septum underlying the early epicardial breakthrough. Notice in Fig. 5B, that this early right ventricular septal activity precedes epicardial breakthrough by 55 msec, and also precedes retrograde His bundle activation by 51 msec. In addition, the data demonstrate that right ventricular epicardial depolarization occurs before left ventricular epicardial depolarization. This activation pattern was most characteristic of the rhythms in our study, and suggests the contribution of retrograde conduction to the His and antegrade conduction down the left bundle branch system to the activation of the left ventricle. In our experiments, the interval between retrograde His bundle activation and activation of the contralateral ventricular epicardium ranged between 15 and 30 msec.

In 5 of the 13 rhythms studied, the left ventricular septum was the site of earliest activation. Fig. 6 presents analog records from one typical study. As before, the schematic diagrams in Fig. 6A indicate the locations of the recording sites for the analog data given in Fig. 6B. Recording and stimulating studies localized the earliest area of ventricular activity to the peripheral Purkinje system indicated by recording site S4. This early Purkinje activity preceded all other recorded activity and took place prior to retrograde His bundle activation by 25 msec. Recording site LV shows the earliest epicardial breakthrough during this rhythm. In contrast to the rhythm in Fig. 5, epicardial breakthrough followed upon early

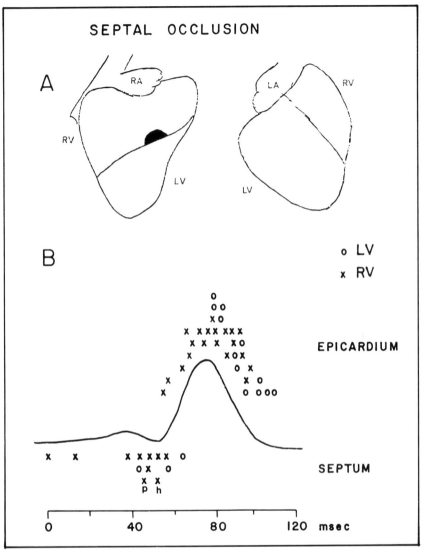

5

The relationship between epicardial activation, septal and ventricular conducting system activation during a ventricular tachycardia, following occlusion of the anterior septal coronary artery. The dark crescent overlying the right ventricle in the schema in **A** indicates earliest epicardial breakthrough during the ectopic rhythm. **B** shows the electrocardiographic configurations as well as the relative times of activation of right and left epicardial and septal sites, plotted on a common-time axis. The open circles are left and the **x**'s—right ventricular activation sites. Epicardial activation is shown above the electrocardiographic complex and septal activation—below. The **p** indicates Purkinje fiber activation; **h** denotes bundle of His activation.

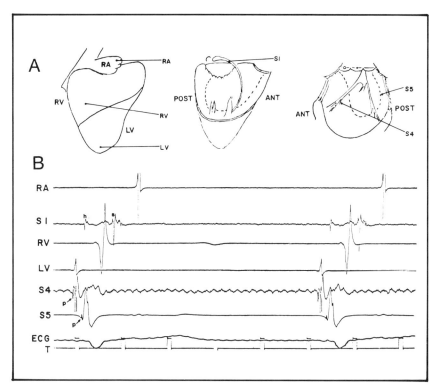

6 Analog records obtained during spontaneous ventricular tachycardia, 24 hours following anterior septal artery occlusion. The schema indicates the approximate recording sites for the analog records displayed below. Records were obtained from the right atrium (RA) and right ventricle (RV), as well as from the earliest left ventricular activation site LV; S1, S4 and S5 indicate septal recording sites. A lead II electrocardiogram (ECG) was recorded simultaneously. The **h** and **s** in the S1 record indicate His bundle and underlying ventricular septal muscle activation. The **p**s designate Purkinje fiber spikes. The timing signal (T) represents 100 msec.

septal activation by 7 msec. This was due to the fact that the epicardial breakthrough was directly overlying the early septal activation site. Fig. 7 correlates the epicardial activation with that in the conducting system and septal myocardium in the same animal. The schema in Fig. 7A, shows early epicardial breakthrough near the left ventricular apex. The data in Fig. 7B indicates the earliest Purkinje fiber activation at time zero, directly underlying this epicardial breakthrough site and contributing to epicardial activa-

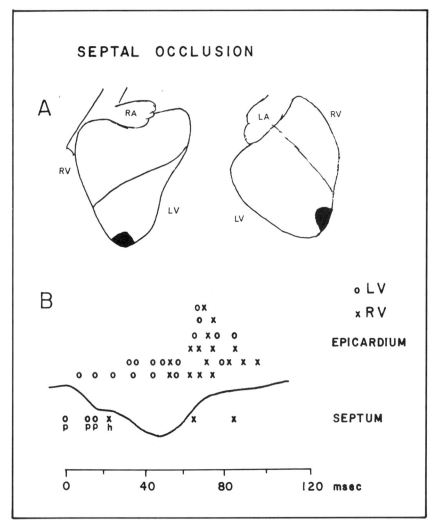

7 Comparison of epicardial and septal activation during spontaneous ventricular tachycardia, following anterior septal artery occlusion. In **A**, the dark crescent indicates earliest epicardial activation occurring in the left ventricle. The following are given in **B**: the electrocardiographic wave form, left and right epicardial and septal activation times plotted on a common-time axis. The open circles are left ventricular sites, the **x**'s—right ventricular sites. Epicardial activation is shown above the electrocardiographic waveform, septal acitvation—below. The **p** indicates Purkinje fiber activation; the **h**—His bundle activation.

tion within 7 msec. It should be noted that epicardial activation, as before, showed an early left ventricular sequence, with the right ventricular epicardial sites following somewhat later. The retrograde His bundle activation is also depicted in this figure. It preceded right ventricular activation by 25 msec, again suggesting that right ventricular activation may, in part, be accomplished by retrograde conduction from the early left septal site to the His and then down the right bundle branch to right ventricular myocardium. In our studies utilizing septal occlusion, the range of time between retrograde His bundle activation and contralateral epicardial activation was from 15 to 30 msec.

DISCUSSION

The analog records of Figs. 2, 4 and 6 demonstrate that the ectopic ventricular rhythms, which occur 24 hr following acute occlusion of either the left anterior descending coronary artery or the anterior septal artery, originate from the peripheral Purkinje system within the region of infarct. In all rhythms, the earliest activity of the total ventricular activation was recorded from the peripheral Purkinje systems. During these rhythms, the bundle branch and His bundle were engaged in a retrograde direction from the ventricle of origin of the rhythm. The peripheral Purkinje system was the site of origin of the ectopic rhythms for the septal infarct as well as the LAD infarct. In the case of the septal occlusion, the His, the right and left bundle branch systems, as well as some of the peripheral Purkinje system, lie within the infarcted region. This implies that the peripheral Purkinje system is more influenced by the process of infarction than is the His or bundle branch system since the ectopic rhythms originate in the peripheral system and not in the His or bundle branches.

The timing of the retrograde His bundle activation, following an ectopic beat originating in one ventricle relative to the early activation of the contralateral ventricle, implies that conduction over the His and bundle branch-Purkinje system may contribute to contralateral ventricular activation. The rhythms originating in either the right or left ventricular septum (Figs. 4, 5, 6 and 7) and those rhythms arising from the inferior-posterior margin of the LAD infarct (Figs. 1A, 2 and 3) all exhibit a retrograde His bundle deflection, preceding the earliest activation of the contralateral ventricle by 15 to 40 msec. Thus there is sufficient time for conduction down the contralateral bundle branch system to contribute at least partially to the activation of the ventricular chamber opposite the site of origin of the ectopic activity. The fact that retrograde His bundle activation follows the initiation of right ventricular epicardial activation, during left-sided rhythms originating in the superior anterior border of the LAD infarct (Fig. 1B), indicates that right ventricular activation in these cases is probably not primarily by way of contralateral bundle branch conduction.

The origins of the ectopic activity in the experiments involving LAD occlusions, as well as anterior septal occlusions, occur at some distance from their earliest epicardial breakthrough. In the case of the LAD occlusions, the activity originated within the infarcted myocardium in the subendocardial Purkinje fibers and then, by way of Purkinje fiber conduction, reached the viable myocardium at the borders of the infarct, producing the earliest area of epicardial activation. In the case of the septal occlusion, while there was a fixed relationship between the location of the septal activation and the ultimate epicardial breakthrough on the surface, the early septal activation usually occurred at some distance from the ultimate epicardial breakthrough. In addition, the time from earliest septal activation to earliest epicardial breakthrough could be as much as 52 msec (Fig. 5). The fact that the origin of the ventricular ectopic activity may lie at some distance from the early epicardial breakthrough, means that the epicardial mapping technique, used with the view of locating an irritable focus for possible surgical resection, might not in itself provide sufficient information for locating the origin of the ectopic ventricular rhythm. Transmural recordings may be necessary to pinpoint exactly the source of the rhythm.

ACKNOWLEDGMENTS

These studies were supported, in part, by Grants 16076-02 and HE-4885-15 from the National Heart and Lung Institute, N.I.H., and by Grant 75-733 from the American Heart Association.

A report of the data from the septal artery occlusion experiments was presented at the 33rd meeting of the American Federation for Clinical Research (Michelson et al., 1976). The data from the left anterior descending coronary artery occlusion experiments have also been previously published (Horowitz, et al., 1976).

The author is an Established Investigator of the American Heart Association.

REFERENCES

El-Sherif, N., Scherlag, B. J., and Lazzara, R.: Conduction disorders in the proximal His-Purkinje system following acute myocardial ischemia. *Circulation* 49:837-857 (1974).

Friedman, P. F., Fenoglio, J. J., and Wit, A. L.: Time course of reversal of electrophysiological and ultrastructural abnormalities in subendocardial Purkinje fibers surviving extensive myocardial infarction in dogs. *Circ. Res.* 36:127 (1975).

Friedman, P. L., Steward, J. R., Fenoglio, J. J., and Wit, A. L.: Survival of subendocardial Purkinje fibers after extensive myocardial infarction in dogs, *Circ. Res.* 33:597 (1973).

Harris, A. S.: Delayed development of ventricular ectopic rhythms following experimental coronary occlusion. *Circulation* 1:1318 (1950).

Horowitz, L. N., Spear, J. F., and Moore, E. N.: Subendocardial origin of ventricular arrhythmias in 24-hour-old experimental myocardial infarction. *Circulation* 53:56-63 (1976).

Kastor, J. A., Spear, J. F., and Moore, E. N.: Localization of ventricular irritability by epicardial mapping. Origin of digitalis-induced unifocal tachycardia from left ventricular Purkinje tissue. *Circulation* 45:952 (1972).

Lazzara, R., El-Sherif, N., and Scherlag, B. J.: Electrophysiological properties of canine Purkinje cells in one-day-old myocardial infarction. *Circ. Res.* 33:722 (1973).

Lumb, G., Shacklett, B. S., and Dawkins, W. A.: The cardiac conduction tissue and its blood supply in the dog. *Am. J. Pathol.* 35:467 (1959).

Michelson, E. L., Spielman, S. R., Spear, J. F., and Moore, E. N.: The origins of late ventricular rhythms and their activation patterns in experimental septal infarction in dogs. *Clin. Res.* 24:23/A (1976).

Nachlas, M. M., and Shnitka, T. K.: Macroscopic identification of early myocardial infarcts by alterations in dehydrogenase activity. *Am. J. Pathol.* 42:379 (1963).

Scherlag, B. J., El-Sherif, N., Hope, R., and Lazzara, R.: Characterization and localization of ventricular arrhythmias resulting from myocardial ischemia and infarction. *Circ. Res.* 35:372 (1974).

Spear, J. F., and Moore, E. N.: Influence of brief vagal and stellate nerve stimulation on pacemaker activity and conduction within the atrioventricular conduction system of the dog. *Circ. Res.* 32:27 (1973).

3

Pathophysiology of Second-Degree and Paroxysmal Atrioventricular Block in Acute Myocardial Infarction

NABIL EL-SHERIF
BENJAMIN J. SCHERLAG
RALPH LAZZARA

INTRODUCTION

Two types of second-degree atrioventricular (AV) block were originally described by Wenckebach (1899, 1906) and Hay (1906) from an analysis of the a-c interval of the jugular pulse. After the introduction of the electrocardiogram, these were classified by Mobitz (1924) as types I and II. Type I AV block, also known as Mobitz type I or the Wenckebach phenomenon, is defined as intermittent failure of AV conduction, preceded by progressive lengthening of AV conduction times. Type II AV block, also known as Mobitz type II block, is characterized by intermittent failure of AV conduction that occurs "suddenly" and in which the PR intervals remain constant before the dropped beat. The clinical significance of these two types of AV conduction disorders was first recognized by Mobitz who suggested that type II block may be the first step

toward Adams-Stokes attacks and complete permanent AV dissociation (Mobitz, 1924). This observation was later confirmed in
several clinical reports (Kaufman et al., 1961; Langendorf and
Pick, 1968). However, in clinical electrocardiography, it has been
recognized that a stable complete AV dissociation carries a less
serious immediate threat to life as compared to the so-called paroxysmal AV block. The latter may be defined as the sudden occurrence of a repetitive block of the atrial impulse during 1:1 AV
conduction (or occasionally 2:1 AV block), resulting in a transient
total interruption of AV conduction (El-Sherif et al., 1974a). The
onset of the arrhythmia is usually associated with a period of ventricular asystole before the return of conduction or the escape of a
subsidiary pacemaker. This period of ventricular asystole represents the crucial pathological manifestation since it often leads to
syncope or, possibly sudden death. Although the incidence of the
latter occurring is not precisely known, it is generally thought that
the propensity to develop paroxysmal AV block is the single most
important clinical consequence of AV conduction disorders.

With the introduction of intensive care and electrocardiographic monitoring for acute myocardial infarction, there was a
renewed interest in the distinction between type I and type II AV
blocks. Several anatomical (Blondeau et al., 1961; Sutton and
Davies, 1968) and clinical (Langendorf and Pick, 1968; Chamberlain and Leinbach, 1970; Rotman et al., 1973; Waugh et al., 1973)
studies have shown that the two types of second-degree AV block
are associated with different anatomical localizations of the infarction and carry a different electrophysiological and clinical significance. Type I AV block is seen when diaphragmatic infarction is
associated with reversible ischemia of the AV node, and it commonly runs a benign course. In contrast, type II AV block is observed in anterior infarction and is associated with necrosis of the
bundle branches and a more grave prognosis. Studies conducted a
few years ago, which utilized His bundle electrocardiography in
patients with acute myocardial infarction (Rosen et al., 1970;
Touboul et al., 1972), have generally confirmed the specific localization of the two types of second-degree AV block. More recently,
however, and mainly through investigations of experimental myocardial infarction, doubt was cast on the distinction between Mobitz
type II and the Wenckebach type of conduction, which were shown
to represent different degrees of the same disorder rather than being two distinct electrophysiological processes (El-Sherif et al.,
1975a). This chapter reviews our recent studies on the evolution of

second-degree AV block in acute myocardial infarction and its relationship to paroxysmal AV block. An attempt is made here to correlate clinical, experimental and basic electrophysiological observations.

PATHOPHYSIOLOGY OF SECOND DEGREE AND PAROXYSMAL AV BLOCK IN THE ISCHEMIC HIS-PURKINJE SYSTEM

Experimental Observations

A recently described experimental model for the study of AV conduction disorders, after ligation of the anterior septal artery in the dog (Scherlag et al., 1974), offered a unique opportunity to analyze the evolution of second-degree AV block (El-Sherif et al., 1974a, 1974b, 1975a). Ligation of the artery produces acute ischemic injury of the proximal His-Purkinje system. Evidence has been accumulated, during both *in vivo* and *in vitro* studies, utilizing the same experimental model, to suggest, for the first time, that Mobitz type II and the Wenckebach type of second-degree AV block represent different degrees of the same disorder rather than two distinct electrophysiological processes. The *in vivo* observations have shown that some increment of conduction delay almost always precedes the blocked impulse. The increment may be as small as 1 or 2 msec at an earlier stage in the experiment and may gradually increase later to 180-200 msec. Although an increment of 1 or 2 msec is usually within the measurement error of most *in vivo* recordings, it is possible that, at a more rapid recording speed, an increment of a fraction of a millisecond could be detected. Notably, *in vitro* observations, which are usually made at more rapid recording sweeps, have consistently shown some increment in conduction time prior to the blocked impulse (El-Sherif et al., 1975a). Also, *in vitro*, the process of recovery during superfusion provided an opportunity to observe the correlate of the *in vivo* pattern of evolution of second-degree AV block, but in the reverse order. Thus, early after excision, a higher degree of increment in conduction delay can be found, e.g., 50-100 msec in the course of second-degree block. With recovery during superfusion, the increment prior to block gradually decreases to only a few milliseconds.

Fig. 1 is taken from one of our *in vivo* studies and offers typical example of the gradual evolution of second-degree AV block in the His bundle, following ligation of the anterior septal artery

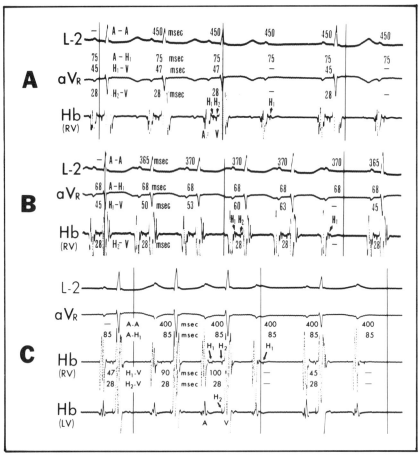

1 Electrode cathether recordings of the His-bundle electrogram from the right ventricle (Hb-R) showing evolution of second-degree intra-His-bundle block, following ligation of the anterior septal artery in the dog. Panels A, B and C were obtained 90, 105 and 150 min, respectively, after ligation. Note gradual increase of the increment in intra-His bundle conduction time (H_1-H_2 interval) prior to the block, from 2 msec in panel A to 15 msec in panel B and 55 msec in panel C. See text for further details. Times lines in this and subsequent records are set at 1 sec intervals.

in the dog. In experiments showing an intra-His bundle lesion, the His-bundle potential usually splits into two deflections (H_1 and H_2), and an increase in the HV interval of 10-20 msec is observed before intermittent block of the impulse develops either spontaneously or in response to atrial pacing (El-Sherif et al., 1974a, 1975a).

Panels A to C, in Fig. 1, show the characteristic pattern for the evolution of second-degree intra-His bundle block. Panel A was recorded 90 min after ligation of the anterior septal artery and shows the sudden occurrence of an intra-His bundle block, with a barely perceptible 2-msec increment in the H_1-H_2 interval in the last conducted beat prior to the block, compared to the first conducted beat subsequent to the block. This arrangement corresponds to the so-called Mobitz type II block. Panel B was obtained 15 min later and shows that, during atrial pacing at a rate of 162/min, a gradual increment of H_1-H_2 intervals of 18 msec occurred prior to failure of AV conduction. This increment in AV conduction delay, clearly indicated in the His-bundle recording at 100 mm/sec paper speed, may be difficult to detect with the standard ECG leads at conventional paper speed of 25 mm/sec. Panel C, which was obtained 2½ hr after ligation, shows the development of a clear Wenckebach periodicity in the ECG leads and an increment of 57 msec in the H_1-H_2 intervals prior to block of the atrial impulse. This example typifies some of the evidence which strongly suggests that the so-called Mobitz type II block and the Wenckebach type of conduction are not two distinct electrophysiological processes but rather represent different degrees of the same phenomenon.

During the study of the evolution of a second-degree AV block in the His-Purkinje system, a clear temporal association was observed between the occurrence of early stages of second-degree AV block, with no perceptible or a few msec increment of conduction delay, and the induction or spontaneous onset of paroxysmal AV block (El-Sherif et al., 1974a, 1974d). Parosyxmal AV block that occurrs abruptly during sinus rhythm or which is induced by rapid atrial pacing were both considered to be tachycardia-dependent, since slowing the heart rate in both instances allowed immediate resumption of 1:1 conduction. Fig. 2 gives an example of tachycardia-dependent paroxysmal intra-His bundle block. The tracings in Panel A were obtained 2 hr after ligation of the anterior septal artery and show a spontaneous second-degree intra-His bundle block, with no perceptible increment of conduction delay prior to the block (the equivalent of so-called Mobitz type II block). Panel B shows distal His-bundle pacing from the catheter electrode in the aortic root. Panel C was obtained 5 min later. The first two beats represent 1:1 AV conduction at a rate of 153/min. Atrial pacing started at the third P wave (PI), with a gradual increase of the pacing rate. A 2:1 intra-His bundle block developed and was followed by complete intra-His bundle block at a critical shortening of the atrial cycle length to 290 msec (rate 207/min).

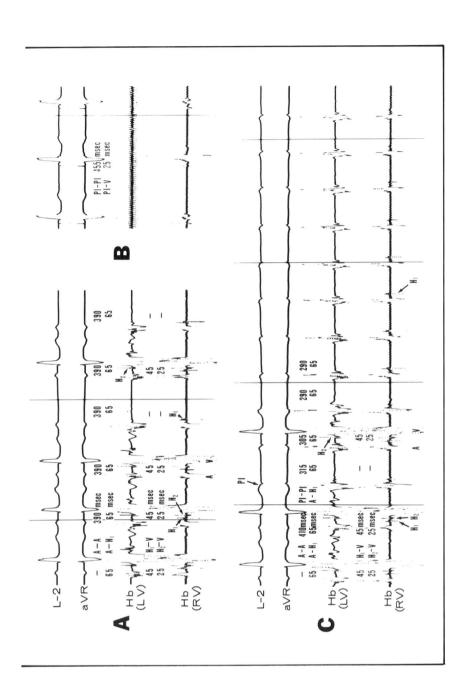

Clinical Observations

Recently, we were able to correlate some clinical findings with the above experimental observations on the evolution of second-degree AV block in the ischemic His-Purkinje system. We studied the evolution of second-degree AV block in the His-Purkinje system in 4 patients with acute myocardial infarction. The patients' clinical and electrocardiographic data are given in Table 1 and results of the electrophysiological studies are summarized in Table 2. His-bundle recordings were obtained during the insertion of a temporary ventricular pacemaker within the first 24 hr of the onset of symptoms of acute myocardial infarction. A second His-bundle recording was made during the removal of the temporary pacemaker 7-14 days after the first recording. In all patients, temporary pacing was instituted because of the presence of second-degree AV block.

Patients 1-3 showed a characteristic pattern of evolution of second-degree block in the His-Purkinje system. The first His-bundle electrogram obtained early in the course of infarction revealed second-degree AV block, with minimal increment of conduction delay (3-10 msec) prior to the blocked beat (the equivalent of Mobitz type II block). The second His-bundle recording, made 7-14 days later, showed the development of a significant increment in conduction delay (35-210 msec) prior to block (the equivalent of Wenckebach type of conduction).

Previous electrocardiograms of patient 1 indicated right bundle-branch block, left anterior hemiblock and anteroseptal myocardial infarction. Electrocardiograms taken on last admission showed evidence of a recent latero-posterior infarction (pathologic Q waves in V_6, leads I and aVL, and prominent R waves in V_1 and V_2), (upper panel in Fig. 3). Twelve hours after admission (18 hr after onset of chest pain), the rhythm strip showed a Mobitz type II second-degree AV block (see rhythm strip in Fig. 3). A

---

2 Electrode catheter recordings of the His-bundle electrogram from the left and right sides of the heart (Hb-L and Hb-R, respectively) obtained from a canine experiment, following ligation of the anterior septal artery. The records illustrate the temporal association of second-degree block, with no perceptible increment in conduction delay (panel A) and tachycardia-dependent paroxysmal intra-His-bundle block (panel C). Panel B shows distal His-bundle pacing. See text for further details.

Table 1. Clinical and electrocardiographic data in 4 patients with acute myocardial infarction and second-degree AV block in the His-Purkinje System

Patient	Age & Sex	Site of Infarction in ECG	IV Conduction Disorder	Initial AV Conduction Disorder	Management	Follow-up ECG
1	72, male	Old anteroseptal MI, recent latero-posterior MI	Old RBBB & LAH	Mobitz type II AV block	Temporary, followed by a permanent pace-maker	RBBB, LAH and 2:1 AV conduction 6 months later
2	68, male	Recent antero-septal MI	Acute RBBB & LAH	Mobitz type II AV block	Temporary, followed by a permanent pace-maker	1:1 AV conduction 6 months later
3	57, male	Recent antero-septal MI	Acute RBBB & LAH	Mobitz type II AV block	Temporary, followed by a permanent pace-maker	RBBB, LAH and 1:1 AV conduction 9 months later
4	67, male	Recent anterior MI	Acute RBBB	Wenckebach type 2° AV block	Temporary, followed by a permanent pace-maker	1:1 AV conduction 10 months later

IV = intraventricular; LAH = left anterior hemiblock;
MI = myocardial infarction; RBBB = right bundle-branch block

Table 2. Electrophysiological data in 4 patients with acute myocardial infarction and second-degree AV block in the His Purkinje System

Patient	First His-Bundle Study		Second His-Bundle Study	
	Time of Study (Hr after Onset of Chest Pain)	Findings	Time of Study (Day in Hospital)	Findings
1	18 hr	HV interval = 60 msec, 2° block in HPS with 5-10 msec ICD	14th day	2° block in HPS with 125-210 msec ICD
2	12 hr	HV interval = 65 msec, 2° in HPS with 2-5 msec ICD	7th day	2° block in HPS with 35-50 msec ICD
3	18 hr	HV interval = 70 msec, 2° block in HPS with 3-10 msec ICD	9th day	2° block in HPS with 40-55 msec ICP
4	24 hr	HV interval = 70 msec, 2° block in HPS with 40-60 msec ICD	10th day	1:1 AV conduction during NSR at 80-95/min, 3:2 block in HPS with 5-10 msec ICD on atrial pacing at 104/min; 4:1 & 6:1 block in HPS on atrial pacing at 133/min

HPS = His-Purkinje system
ICD = increment in conduction delay

His-bundle electrogram obtained during the insertion of a temporary ventricular pacemaker is shown in the lower panel of Fig. 3. The record revealed a prolonged His-Purkinje conduction time (HV interval of 60 msec). The block was localized distal to the His-bundle recording site and there was a 5-10 msec increment in HV intervals prior to the blocked impulse. Rhythm strips obtained for the next 3 days showed either 1:1 AV conduction, 2:1 AV block, or a Mobitz type II block. AV conduction appeared to be tachycardia dependent and varied in relation to spontaneous changes in the sinus rate. On the 4th hospital day, the patient experienced a

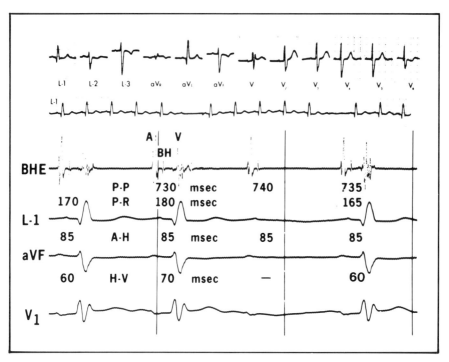

3 Patient 1. Upper panel illustrates the 12-lead ECG obtained on admission, showing right bundle-branch block, left anterior hemiblock, and latero-posterior infarction. The rhythm strip indicates a Mobitz type II AV block. Lower panel illustrates the bundle of His electrogram (BHE) obtained during insertion of a temporary ventricular pacemaker. The record reveals a 2° AV block in the His-Purkinje system, with a 10-msec increment in HV interval prior to the blocked beat.

prolonged chest pain and the electrocardiogram showed extensive ST-T depression in the chest leads (compare lead V_4 in Figs. 3 and 4). A second rise in the cardiac enzymes suggested the occurrence of a fresh subendocardial infarction. The rhythm strips obtained a few hours after the onset of chest pain showed second-degree AV block of the Wenckebach type. The upper rhythm strip in Fig. 4 (lead aVL) indicates periods of 3:2 AV block, with significant increment in the PR interval prior to the block. The lower rhythm strip (lead V_4) illustrates long cycles of second-degree AV block. The relatively constant PR intervals in several beats preceding the blocked impulse should be noted. The PR interval of the beat im-

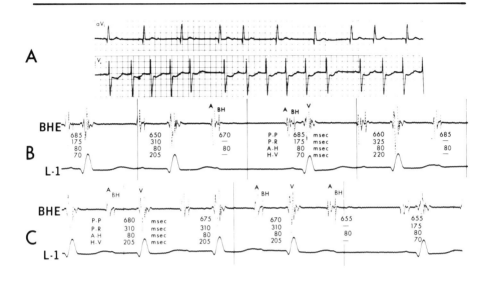

4

Patient 1. Recordings obtained 14 days after the acute ischemic episode. The upper rhythm strip shows 2:1 and 3:2 Wenckebach conduction while the lower one illustrates long Wenckebach cycles with prolonged and almost constant PR intervals prior to the blocked beat and marked shortening of the PR following the block. Records B and C illustrate the bundle of His electrograms (BHE) that correspond to the two rhythm strips. Record B shows a 3:2 Wenckebach conduction in the His-Purkinje system with 135-150 msec increment of HV intervals prior to block. Record C illustrates the last 3 beats of a long Wenckebach cycle, with constant HV intervals prior to block. Note marked shortening of HV of the first conducted beat. This pattern represents one variant of atypical Wenckebach periodicity.

mediately following the block shows significant shortening and the next PR interval—a significant increment. This arrangement represents a variant type of Wenckebach conduction. The AV conduction disorder which was commonly tachycardia dependent persisted in rhythm strips obtained over the next 10 days. Panels B and C in Fig. 4 and panel A in Fig. 5 demonstrates His-bundle recordings made during the removal of the temporary pacemaker on the 14th hospital day. Panels B and C, in Fig. 4 illustrate His-bundle electrograms that corresponded to the two rhythm strips in panel A. Panel B shows periods of 3:2 Wenckebach conduction in the His-

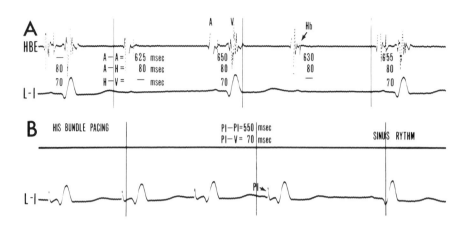

5   Patient 1. Recordings obtained during the same study as shown in Fig. 4. Record A illustrates the bundle of His electrogram (BHE) showing 2:1 block in the His-Purkinje system at a sinus rate of 92-95/min. Record B demonstrates 1:1 His bundle pacing at a faster rate of 109/min. This suggests that the conduction block is localized in the His bundle. See text for more details. PI = paced impulse.

Purkinje system, with an increment of 135-150 msec in the HV interval prior to block. Panel C illustrates the last three beats of a long Wenckebach cycle. Note the markedly prolonged and constant HV intervals preceding the block and the significant shortening of the HV interval in the beat immediately following it. The block is associated with a minimal (15-msec) decrease in the atrial cycle. Panel A in Fig. 5 shows that, during spontaneous acceleration of the sinus rate, 2:1 AV conduction consistently developed, thus revealing the tachycardia-dependent nature of the AV conduction disorder. Panel B in Fig. 5 illustrates His-bundle pacing, via the electrode catheter, obtained during the same setting. It is interesting to observe that 1:1 His-bundle pacing could be achieved at cycle lengths significantly shorter than those during 2:1 AV conduction in Panel A. The paced beats showed a spike-to-V interval (PI-V) of 70 msec, equal to the HV interval during 2:1 AV conduction. This strongly suggests that conduction delay and block are probably localized in the His bundle, and that pacing of the distal His bundle could drive the His-Purkinje system at much higher rates (Touboul et al., 1972, Narula, 1973).

Patients 2 and 3 showed an evolution of second-degree AV block in the His-Purkinje system, that followed the same pattern as described for patient 1, but differed both in the time course and degree of changes. Both patients were admitted with evidence of acute antero-septal infarction, and developed right bundle· branch block and left anterior hemiblock 5 and 9 hr after admission, respectively. Second-degree AV block of the Mobitz II type followed the bundle-branch block pattern by 1-3 hr (12 and 18 hr after the onset of chest pain in patients 2 and 3, respectively). A His-bundle recording, made during the insertion of a temporary ventricular pacemaker, localized the block in the His-Purkinje system and indicated a 3-10 msec increment in the HV interval prior to block. Rhythm strips obtained during the next few days showed second-degree AV block, with some increment of the PR interval prior to block, suggestive of a Wenckebach type of conduction. A repeat His-bundle study, performed on the 7th hospital day in patient 2 and on the 9th—in patient 3, confirmed the presence of a Wenckebach type of conduction in the His-Purkinje system, with an increment of the HV interval of 35-55 msec prior to block.

Patient 4 illustrated the reverse order of the findings obtained in the other three patients. The patient was admitted to the Coronary Care Unit 22 hr after the onset of chest pain. The electrocardiogram on admission revealed an acute anterior-wall myocardial infarction, right bundle-branch block and a normal frontal-plane axis (upper panel, Fig. 6). The rhythm strip showed a Wenckebach type second-degree AV block (see rhythm strip in Fig. 6). The lower panel in Fig. 6 illustrates the His-bundle electrogram made during the insertion of a temporary ventricular pacemaker. The record reveals a Wenckebach type second-degree AV block in the His-Purkinje system, with an increment in the HV interval of 50 msec prior to block. The patient's rhythm strips obtained after the 2nd hospital day showed 1:1 AV conduction. Figs. 7 and 8 illustrate the second His-bundle recordings made on the 8th hospital day, while the temporary pacemaker was removed. The patient showed 1:1 AV conduction during sinus rhythm, at a rate of 80-95/min. On atrial pacing at a rate of 104/min, 3:2 AV conduction developed (Fig. 7). Analysis of the HV intervals revealed a minimal increment of 5-10 msec prior to block distal to the His bundle recording site. Thus the patient's records showed a change

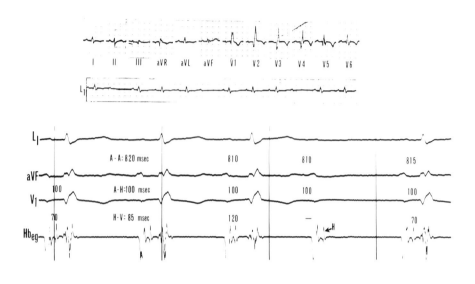

I   II   III   aVR   aVL   aVF   V1   V2   V3   V4   V5   V6

L_I

L_I

A - A: 820 msec   810   810   815

aVF

V_1 100   A-H:100 msec   100   100   100

70   H-V: 85 msec   120   —   70

Hb eg

A   V

6   Patient 4. Upper panel illustrates the 12-lead ECG obtained on admission, showing acute anterior myocardial infarction, right bundle-branch block and normal frontal-plane axis. The rhythm strip demonstrates a Wenckebach type second-degree AV block. The His-bundle electrográm (Hb e.g.), obtained during the insertion of a temporary ventricular pacemaker, reveals that the Wenckebach-type of conduction is occurring in the His-Purkinje system. The 4:3 Wenckebach cycle represents one variant of atypical Wenckebach periodicity. See text for details.

from a second-degree AV block in the His-Purkinje system, with significant increment in conduction delay early after the infarction, to a second-degree AV block, with minimal increment of conduction delay later in the course of the infarction. However, the patient was admitted relatively late after the onset of chest pain and, when first seen, was already showing second-degree AV block, with significant increment in conduction delay prior to block. In this patient, it is possible that the earlier stages of second-degree AV block showed a minimal increment in conduction delay prior to failure of impulse propagation.

Fig. 8 demonstrates that further increase in the atrial pacing rate resulted in a high degree of block in the His-Purkinje system.

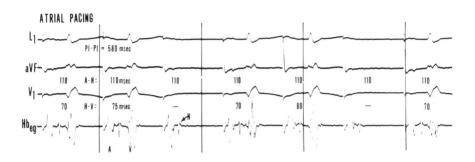

ATRIAL PACING

7

Patient 4. His-bundle electrogram (Hb e.g.) obtained 8 days after admission. 1:1 AV conduction was present during normal sinus rhythm. Atrial pacing at a rate of 104/min resulted in 3:2 AV block in the His-Purkinje system, with a minimal increment (5-10 msec) of HV intervals prior to block.

At an atrial pacing rate of 132/min, alternating 4:1 and 6:1 AV conduction developed. Termination of atrial pacing would result in immediate resumption of 1:1 AV conduction (Fig. 8, record A). This revealed a tachycardia-dependent repetitive block in the His-Purkinje system. Atrial pacing at still higher rates resulted in an interplay between AV nodal and His-Purkinje blocks. Fig. 8, record B shows that, at an atrial pacing rate of 177/min, alternating 3:1 and 4:1 AV conduction developed. This was explained by alternating 3:2 and 4:3 AV nodal Wenckebach block on top of the tachycardia-dependent block in the His-Purkinje system. AV nodal block consistently resulted in a longer HH interval and successful His-Purkinje conduction.

PATHOPHYSIOLOGY OF SECOND-DEGREE AND PAROXYSMAL AV BLOCK IN THE ISCHEMIC AV NODE

Early clinical (Lewis, 1925; Katz and Pick, 1956) and experimental observations (Hoffman and Cranefield, 1960; Watanabe and Dreifus, 1967), as well as relatively recent studies utilizing His-bundle electrocardiography in man (Narula et al., 1971, Narula, 1973), have clearly shown that both the normal and diseased AV

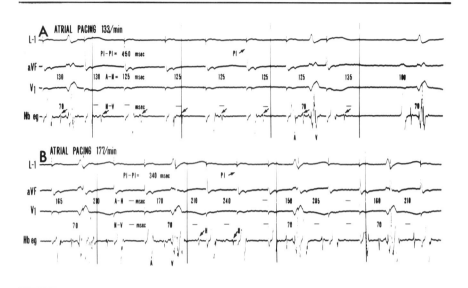

8

Patient 4. His bundle electrograms (Hb e.g.) obtained during the
same study shown in Fig. 7. Record A shows that atrial pacing at
a rate of 133/min resulted in repetitive block in the His-Purkinje
system (6:1 AV ratio). Termination of atrial pacing was followed by
immediate resumption of 1:1 AV conduction. Record B shows atrial
pacing at a faster rate of 177/min, with alternating 3:1 and 4:1
AV conduction. This is explained by interplay of AV nodal
Wenckebach conduction and block in the His-Purkinje system. See
text for more details. PI = paced impulse.

nodes respond to increase in atrial driving frequency by a Wenckebach type second-degree AV block. In the normal AV node, a fast
atrial rate is required to elicit second-degree AV block of the
Wenckebach type, while an AV node with depressed conduction
may show block at relatively long cycles. Few experimental and
clinical reports (Rosen et al., 1971; Spear and Moore, 1971; Yeh
et al., 1972) have suggested that the AV node may occasionally
show a Mobitz type II second-degree AV block. Critical analysis of
some of these records reveals that they actually represent a variant
type of Wenckebach conduction, in which the last conducted beats
of a Wenckebach cycle—prior to the blocked impulse—show no
perceptible or a few millisecond increment in conduction delay,
while the first conducted beat, subsequent to block, indicates a sig-

nificant shortening of AV nodal conduction time. Other published records (Rosen et al., 1971; Spear and Moore, 1971), however, showed a slight (less than 20-msec) increment in conduction delay, as calculated in the beat immediately preceding and the one immediately following the blocked impulse. This arrangement can simulate very closely a Mobitz type II block in the standard ECG, at a relatively slow paper speed. In these cases, there was generally a marked prolongation of AV nodal conduction time before and after block developed. No ready explanation was offered for this peculiar behavior which is distinctly different from the usual response of the normal or diseased AV node. Some authors suggested spontaneous variation in the vagal tone (Narula, 1973) or slight sinus arrhythmia in the presence of marked depression of conduction in the AV node (Spear and Moore, 1971). This may account for the sudden occurrence of block without prior prolongation of the PR interval, but will not explain why AV nodal conduction time fails to significantly shorten following the block, as is normally the case during typical or atypical Wenckebach type of conduction. No electrophysiological or clinical significance was specifically attached to this unusual behavior of the AV node other than that it might be mistaken for a more serious His-Purkinje disease, which is better known to be associated with the so-called Mobitz type II block.

We have recently observed AV nodal second-degree block, with minimal increment in conduction delay, in two different experimental models of acute ischemic injury of the AV node in dogs (El-Sherif et al., 1974c, 1975b). In one experimental model, combined ligation of the AV nodal and anterior-septal arteries produced acute ischemic injury of the AV node and the proximal His-Purkinje system (El-Sherif et al., 1974c). Because of the dual blood supply of the canine AV node, ligation of either artery alone has little functional effect on it. In the second experimental model, ischemia of the AV node was induced by inflow occlusion of major venous return (El-Sherif et al., 1975b). The earliest change in the ischemia of the AV node was an increase in the AV nodal conduction time (first-degree AV nodal block). This was followed by intermittent failure of conduction (second-degree block). In 60% of the experiments, there was a large increment in conduction delay prior to the blocked beat (a Wenckebach type of conduction). In the remaining experiments, second-degree AV nodal block occurred with a minimal increment in conduction delay prior to the block. In these dogs only, increasing the heart rate by atrial pacing re-

sulted in paroxysmal AV nodal block. In dogs showing the Wenckebach type second-degree AV nodal block, rapid atrial pacing usually
produced a higher degree AV block (2:1, 4:1 ratio) rather than a
paroxysmal AV block. Figs. 9 and 10 illustrate one of the inflow-
occlusion experiments. Fig. 9, panel A, shows the control recording
during sinus rhythm. Panel B depicts the response of the normal
AV node to rapid atrial pacing (PI). Note the development of a
second-degree AV nodal block of the Wenckebach type at an atrial
cycle length of 185 msec, with 100-msec increment in AV nodal
conduction time (AH interval) prior to block. Panel C was obtained
5 min after inflow occlusion and shows the occurrence of AV nodal
Wenckebach conduction at a relatively slower atrial pacing rate,
compared to control. The overall AV nodal conduction time is also
longer although the degree of increment of conduction delay prior
to block is not much different from control. This behavior represents a typical AV nodal response to ischemia or hypoxia. Panel D
was obtained 10 min after inflow occlusion and shows a second-
degree AV nodal block during sinus rhythm at a slower atrial rate,
compared to panel C. The overall AV nodal conduction time is significantly prolonged, however; in contrast to the conduction pattern
in panel C, panel D shows only minimal increment in conduction
delay (15 msec) prior to the block, closely simulating the so-called
Mobitz type II block. Records in Fig. 10 were obtained 2 min after
the record in Fig. 9, panel D. The first part of the top panel in Fig.
10 shows a 2:1 AV nodal block. Rapid atrial pacing (PI) produced
a tachycardia-dependent paroxysmal AV block. Termination of
atrial pacing, in the last part of the bottom panel, resulted in
prompt resumption of AV nodal conduction. It should be noted that,
during paroxysmal AV nodal block, AV nodal automaticity was
suppressed and a slow idioventricular escape focus was observed.
This and similar experimental findings did not only document the
occurrence of second-degree AV nodal block, with minimal increment in conduction delay (so-called Mobitz type II block), but also
clearly showed its temporary association with tachycardia-dependent paroxysmal AV nodal block.

CELLULAR ELECTROPHYSIOLOGY OF SECOND-DEGREE AND PAROXYSMAL AV BLOCK IN ACUTE MYOCARDIAL INFARCTION

The characteristics of conduction in a certain pathway are determined by the sum of responses of myriads of individual cells,

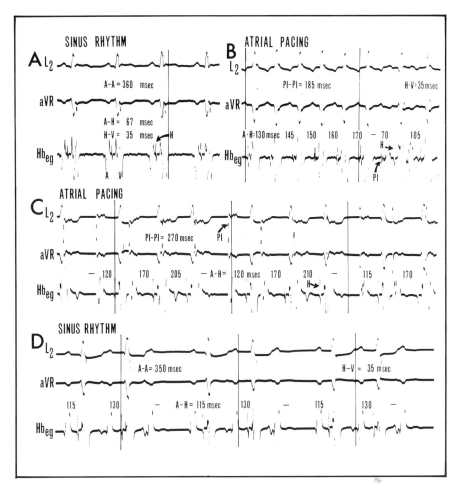

9 Electrode catheter recordings from a canine experiment illustrating the effect of occlusion of major venous return on AV nodal conduction. Panels A and B represent control recordings during normal sinus rhythm and rapid atrial pacing, respectively. Panel C was obtained 5 min following occlusion and shows the occurrence of AV nodal Wenckebach conduction at a relatively slower atrial pacing rate, compared to the control tracing in panel B. Also overall AV nodal conduction times are longer. Panel D was obtained 10 min after occlusion and shows second-degree AV nodal block during sinus rhythm, with prolonged AV nodal conduction time but a minimal increment in conduction delay (15 msec) prior to block, simulating the so-called Mobitz type II block.

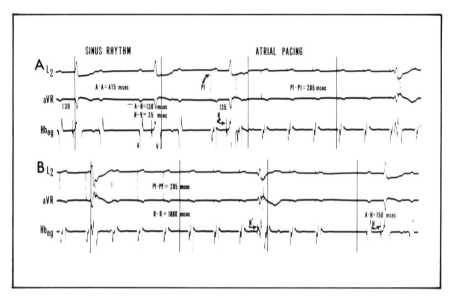

10 Electrode catheter recording from the same canine experiment as shown in Fig. 9, obtained 2 min following the recording in Fig. 9, panel D. The record illustrates a tachycardia-dependent paroxysmal AV nodal block induced by rapid atrial pacing (PI). Note the escape of a slow idioventricular focus. See text for further details. H' represents a retrograde His-bundle potential.

which may exhibit varying degrees of abnormal behavior. Thus, trying to conceptualize a characteristic pattern of conduction from analysis of action potentials of one or a few impaled cells may be sometimes extremely difficult. In a recent study (El-Sherif et al., 1975a), however, the remarkable similarity of action-potential changes and electrical properties of cells in the AV node, where conduction is normally slow, and in the depressed His-Purkinje system has been emphasized. Conduction in the His-Purkinje system can be depressed by a variety of pathophysiological interventions, including acute ischemic injury (El-Sherif et al., 1975a; Lazzara et al., 1975b) or increased extracellular potassium concentration (Cranefield et al., 1971). Depressed cells with slow-conduction characteristics have a low resting potential, slow depolarization phase, reduced membrane responsiveness and a time-dependent refractoriness that frequently outlasts the duration of the action potential. (Cranefield et al., 1971; El-Sherif et al., 1975a; Lazzara et al., 1975b). This last characteristic is of vital significance in understanding a tachycardia-dependent block, which can occur at cycle lengths that far exceed the recorded action-potential duration. The refractoriness contingent on time probably also underlies the tachycardia-dependent intermittent complete failure of transmission (paroxysmal block) (El-Sherif et al., 1975a). This phenomenon represents repetitive and consistent failure on the part of a group of depressed cells to exhibit a regenerative response, capable of stimulating a distal pathway, when they are challenged to conduct at critically short cycle lengths. The exact intracellular ionic derangement that underlies this characteristic conduction failure has not yet been successfully unravelled.

Similar changes in the duration and configuration of action potentials have been observed in both the AV node (Hoffman, 1961; Mendez and Moe, 1966) and the depressed His-Purkinje system (Cranefield, 1971; El-Sherif et al., 1975a; Lazzara et al., 1975b), depending on the state of transmission and the temporal relation of impaled cells to areas of slow propagation and block. Hump-like inflections on the repolarization limb and slow initial steps on the depolarization limb have been ascribed to electronic spread to cells upstream and downstream, respectively, to areas of slow propagation. Aborted action potentials or local responses are usually seen at the site of block. These changes were considered by several authors (Watanabe and Dreifus, 1963, and 1967; Spear and Moore, 1973) as evidence of non-homogeneous, asynchronous and dissociated spread of the activation wave front, resulting in decremental conduction. The interaction by electronic spread of a slowly conducting depolarizing wave with upstream cells, giving rise to a hump-like prolongation of their action potentials, has been used to explain the Wenckebach type of second-degree block, which is characterized by gradual increment of conduction delay prior to failure of conduction (Schaffer, 1971).

Our recently reported *in vitro* findings (El-Sherif et al., 1975a; Lazzara et al., 1975b) indicate that an increment in conduction delay consistently precedes the blocked impulse in the ischemic His-Purkinje preparation. Specifically, we have shown that the same *in vitro* experiment may reveal a greater increment in conduction delay prior to block (equivalent to Wenckebach conduction), which on recovery during superfusion can gradually decrease to a few milliseconds, simulating the so-called Mobitz II block (see Fig. 11). This, in addition to our *in vivo* observations utilizing the same experimental model, strongly suggests that the two types of second-

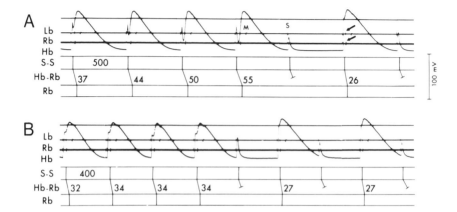

11 Recordings from the proximal His-Purkinje system in an ischemic preparation, showing change from a Wenckebach type of conduction (record A) to a Mobitz type II block (record B) on recovery during superfusion. The preparation was stimulated from a proximal His-bundle position (S) with an intracellular recording electrode in the penetrating portion of the His bundle (Hb), and extracellular bipolar electrodes from the proximal right (Rb) and left (Lb) bundles (marked by arrows). Note that in record B a constant Hb-Rb conduction time precedes the blocked beat but, after the block, there is a 7-msec shortening of the Hb-Rb conduction time, together with a noticeable increase in the amplitude of the Hb action potential.

degree block represent different degrees of the same pathophysiological process. However, the exact mechanism that underlies the evolution from second-degree block with minimal increment in conduction delay to one that shows a higher degree of increment is still conjectural. Some of the factors involved may include a greater extent of deterioration of membrane responsiveness, or a larger population of cells with an abnormal response. Thus, second-degree AV block, with a minimal increment in conduction delay, may represent a lesser derangement of membrane responsiveness, or involvement of a relatively small but strategically positioned area of depressed cells, or both. In this regard, it should be emphasized that slow conduction should not be equated with conduction failure. Slow conduction is probably more linked to the size of the cell population showing degressed responses, whereas very slow conduction may be explained by a summation of a series of slow or even discontinuous propagation waves (Cranefield et al., 1971). On the other hand, intermittent failure of conduction can occur when there is a relatively lesser degree of slow conduction. As a matter of fact, it has been amply documented, in both *in vivo* and *in vitro* experiments, that in the presence of second-degree block with minimal rather than marked increment in conduction delay repetitive complete conduction failure is more likely to occur (El-Sherif 1974a, 1975a).

Recently, several lines of evidence have been reported to suggest that the cardiac action potential might be composed of a fast and a slow component (Carmeliet and Vereecke, 1969; Beeler and Reuter, 1970; Cranefield et al., 1972). The fast component, which gives rise to the initial spike in normal cardiac muscle, is linked to the rapid sodium channel (Weidman, 1955). The slow component seems to be related to the slow inward channel which may be used by either a sodium or calcium ion. It has been suggested that both the action potential and conduction characteristcs of the AV node might represent properties of the slow response (Paes de Carvalho et al., 1969). The slow response has also been described in several experimental preparations, including Purkinje strands exposed to increased potassium ion, or increased potassium ion plus epinephrine (Cranefield et al., 1971, 1972). Some time ago, we suggested that conduction characteristics in the ischemic His-Purkinje system may represent properties of the slow response (El-Sherif et al., 1975a). However, more recently, we have demonstrated that verapamil and D-600, both of them known to block the inward calcium current while markedly delaying conduction in the AV node, have no effect on conduction in the ischemic His-Purkinje system (unpublished observations). On the other hand, lidocaine was shown to have a significant depressant effect on depolarized ischemic muscle and His-Purkinje cells probably related to the drug's action on a slow sodium current (Lazzara et al., 1975a). By contrast, lidocaine has usually little effect on AV nodal cells. Thus it seems that, although conduction in the AV node and depressed His-Purkinje system may have similar electrophysiological characteristics, the ionic basis of the conduction abnormality and the slow response at both sites may be different.

ELECTROPHYSIOLOGICAL COMMON DENOMINATOR
OF PAROXYSMAL AV BLOCK

Since early clinical observations by Mobitz (1924), second-degree AV block, with no perceptible or a minimal increment of conduction delay prior to block (Mobitz type II block), was associated with paroxysmal AV block and Adams-Stokes syndrome. It was suggested (Langendorf and Pick, 1968) and later confirmed, using His-bundle electrocardiography (Narula et al., 1971; Narula, 1973), that this type of block is commonly localized in the His-Purkinje system. We have recently demonstrated, in a study correlating experimental and clinical findings (El-Sherif et al., 1974d), that paroxysmal AV block following acute myocardial infarction is due to a tachycardia-dependent repetitive decremental conduction in the ischemic His-Purkinje system, commonly localized in the His bundle. Paroxysmal AV block was temporally associated with the occurrence of second-degree AV block, with minimal increment in conduction delay. On the other hand, although both clinical reports (Langendorf and Pick, 1956; Langendorf et al., 1965) and electrophysiological studies, utilizing the microelectrode technique (Moe et al., 1964), have demonstrated repetitive concealed conduction in the AV node, paroxysmal AV block in the AV node is a less known entity in spite of occasional reports of its presence (Rosen et al., 1973). In a series of experimental observations, we have recently documented the occurrence of tachycardia-dependent paroxysmal AV block in the ischemic AV node (El-Sherif et al., 1975b). Furthermore, this type of block was temporally related to the development of a characteristic type of second-degree AV block, with a typical marked prolongation of AV nodal conduction time but a minimal increment in conduction delay prior to the blocked beat, thus simulating Mobitz II block (Figs. 9 and 10). An analysis correlating our observations in both the ischemic His-Purkinje system (El-Sherif et al., 1974d) and the AV node (El-Sherif et al., 1975b) reveals that tachycardia-dependent paroxysmal AV block is temporally related to the development of second-degree AV block, with minimal increment in conduction delay. The propensity for developing a tachycardia-dependent paroxysmal AV block was absent when second-degree AV block with greater increment in conduction delay occurred at both sites. This finding strongly suggests that a characteristic pathophysiological disorder rather than the site of lesion seems to be the common denominator of tachycardia-dependent paroxysmal AV block.

Tachycardia-dependent paroxysmal AV block does not necessarily encompass all cases of paroxysmal AV block. Several examples of bradycardia-dependent paroxysmal AV block have been described and the phenomenon was attributed to enhanced diastolic depolarization in the His-Purkinje system (Rosenbaum et al.,

1973). However, as recently pointed out (Langendorf, 1973), this phenomenon cannot be responsible for the majority of cases of paroxysmal AV block, which are closely associated with type II AV block. Furthermore, our recent observations have shown that bradycardia-dependent block may be connected with depressed rather than enhanced diastolic depolarization (El-Sherif et al., 1974e; 1976a, 1976b).

A UNIFIED HYPOTHESIS OF SECOND-DEGREE AV BLOCK AND ITS CLINICAL IMPLICATIONS

Our recent experimental and clinical findings have demonstrated that an increment in conduction delay almost always precedes the blocked impulse in second-degree AV block. This increment may be as small as 1 or 2 msec but can also be in the order of several hundred msec. An increment of only a few msec can only be detected at rapid recording speeds. This observation was also emphasized in a recent study where 99% of intracellular records of second-degree block showed various degrees of increment in conduction delay when tracings were obtained at more rapid sweep speeds (Anderson and Bailey, 1973). Thus, the term "Mobitz II block" does not represent an electrophysiological entity but probably an imaginary line of departure from the characteristic response of the normal to the depressed His-Purkinje system (El-Sherif et al., 1975a).

On the basis of the latest experimental and clinical findings, it is suggested that second-degree AV block should be classified according to the degree of increment in conduction time, as calculated in the beat immediately preceding the blocked impulse and the one immediately following it (El-Sherif et al., 1975a). This classification does not primarily consider the behavior of PR intervals preceding the blocked impulse nor the duration of the QRS complex in conventional leads (Dreifus et al., 1971). The diagram in Fig. 12 gives an illustration of second-degree AV block, based on the suggested electrophysiological mechanism. Panel A presents the pattern of second-degree AV block in the normal AV node. This can always be induced at relatively short cycle lengths and is characterized by a large increment in conduction delay prior to block, while AV nodal conduction time of the beat following the block is within normal limits. Diagram B depicts second-degree AV block in the depressed AV node. It differs from tachycardia-induced

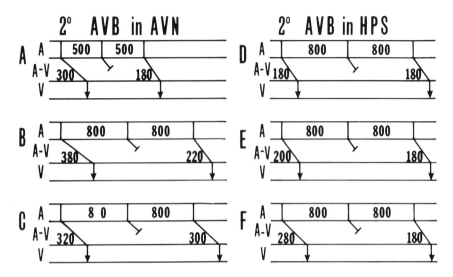

12 Diagrammatic illustration of second-degree AV block, based on the unifield hypothesis. See text for details. The diagram depicts only the beat immediately preceding and the one immediately following the blocked impulse. A, AV and V represent activation of the atrial, AV junction and ventricles, respectively. All values are in milliseconds.

block in the normal AV node in that it occurs at relatively long cycle lengths, and is commonly associated with a greater degree of increment in conduction delay and a prolonged AV nodal conduction time in the beat following the block. This is usually reflected as a prolonged PR interval in the electrocardiogram. Diagram C illustrates a characteristic pattern of second-degree AV block in the depressed AV node. This pattern is associated with marked AV nodal conduction time but a minimal increment in conduction delay. The ECG shows that the PR interval of the beat following the block is markedly prolonged, compared to normal PR. Diagram D represents a second-degree AV block in the His-Purkinje system, showing no perceptible increment in conduction delay. Recordings at a more rapid sweep speed will almost always reveal a one- or few-millisecond increment in conduction delay. Diagram E illustrates second-degree AV block in the His-Purkinje system, associated with a slight increment in conduction delay. This degree of increment may be difficult to detect at the conventional ECG paper speed but can be easily discerned at rapid sweep speeds. Diagram F demonstrates a second-degree AV block in the His-Purkinje system, with a large increment in conduction delay that can be easily diagnosed in the standard electrocardiogram.

Comparative analysis of the six patterns of second-degree AV block in Fig. 12 shows that patterns A and B in the AV node, and pattern F in the His-Purkinje system are almost indistinguishable in the standard electrocardiogram, apart from the relatively fast heart rate in A. These patterns correspond to the conventional Wenckebach type of second-degree AV block. Pattern D can be almost exclusively confined to the His-Purkinje system. Pattern C in the AV node and pattern E in the His-Purkinje system may look superficially similar since both show a minimal increment of conduction delay. These two patterns, however, should be clearly differentiated from one another by the markedly prolonged PR interval of the beat following the block in pattern C. Although theoretically, pattern E associated with a constant marked first-degree AV nodal block may closely simulate pattern C, this situation should be rare indeed. It must be emphasized that the diagrammatic analysis in Fig. 12 is only valid in case that the first beat after the block represents genuine AV conduction and not an AV junctional escape beat (El-Sherif et al., 1975a)—a situation which is not very common and not very difficult to exclude either (Barold and Friedberg, 1974; El-Sherif et al., 1975a).

As already stressed in the introduction to this review, one of the main reasons for the continued interest in different "types" or "patterns" of second-degree AV block is early recognition of the close temporal association of certain of these "types" with paroxysmal AV block, Adams-Stokes syndrome and permanent complete AV dissociation. In recent years, it has been emphasized that the so-called Mobitz type II block is exclusively localized in the His-Purkinje system and is intimately associated with paroxysmal AV block, while the Wenckebach type of second-degree AV block is AV nodal in origin and has a more benign prognosis. The several lines of evidence examined here clearly show that these concepts are not totally valid. Both recent clinical and experimental observations have shown that second-degree AV block, with either minimal or marked increment in conduction delay, can occur at the AV node or the His-Purkinje system. At least, the experimental findings have demonstrated that tachycardia-dependent paroxysmal AV block could be associated with second-degree AV block, with minimal increment in conduction delay at either the AV node or His-

Purkinje system (El-Sherif et al., 1975a, 1975b). If these observations are confirmed by further experimental and clinical studies, a significant step forward would be taken in favor of the unified hypothesis of second-degree AV block presented in this review. This would specifically suggest that the immediate serious prognosis of second-degree AV block, with minimal increment in conduction delay, is related to a characteristic pathophysiological disorder rather than to the site of lesion in the AV conduction system. Such a development may also make it easier for the clinician to prognosticate utilizing the standard ECG in which a minimal increment in conduction delay is usually difficult to identify. It is generally agreed that the standard ECG will remain the most commonly available tool for diagnosis and management of AV conduction disorders in clinical practice. This concept may also limit the need for more sophisticated electrophysiological studies to localize the site of second-degree AV block. However, the problem of whether the long-term prognosis of second-degree AV block, with minimal increment in conduction delay, is similar in both the AV node and His-Purkinje system can only be solved by further clinical and experimental investigations. This and similar unanswered questions clearly emphasize the significant gaps in our understanding of the pathophysiology of second-degree and paroxysmal AV block. This is one reason why it would be premature to discourage the use of the conventional classification of second-degree AV block by clinicians until a more complete formulation of the pathophysiology and clinical history of second-degree and paroxysmal AV block is made available, based on the accumulation of considerably more evidence. However, it is only appropriate that both clinicians and electrophysiologists become wary of some of the limitations inherent in the use of the terms "Mobitz II" and "Wenckebach type" blocks.

ACKNOWLEDGMENT

This work was supported in part by Contract No. 72-2972-M from the National Heart, Lung and Blood Institute, N.I.H.

REFERENCES

Anderson, G. J., and Bailey, J. C.: Conduction delay and block within the peripheral Purkinje system. In *Cardiac Arrhythmias*, L. S. Dreifus and W. Likoff, eds. Grune & Stratton, New York (1973), p. 203.

Barold, S. S., and Friedberg, H. D.: Second degree atrioventricular block. A matter of definition. *Am. J. Cardiol.* 33:311 (1974).

Beeler, G. W., Jr., and Reuter, H.: Membrane calcium current in ventricular myocardial fibers. *J. Physiol.* (Lond.) 207:191 (1970).

Blondeau, M., Rizzon, M., and Lenegre, J.: Les troubles de la conduction auriculoventriculaire dans l'infarctus myocardique récent. II. Etude anatomique. *Arch. Mal. Coeur* 54:1104 (1961).

Carmeliet, E., and Vereecke, J.: Adrenaline and the plateau phase of the cardiac action potential: Importance of Ca^{++}, Na^+ and K^+ conductance. *Pflueger Arch.* 313:300 (1969).

Chamberlain, D., and Leinbach, R.: Electrical pacing in heart block complicating acute myocardial infarction. *Br. Heart J.* 32:2 (1970).

Cranefield, P. F., Klein, H. O., and Hoffman, B. F.: Conduction of the cardiac impulse. 1. Delay, block and one-way block in depressed Purkinje fibers. *Circ. Res.* 28:199 (1971).

Cranefield, P. F., Wit, A. L., and Hoffman, B. F.: Conduction of the cardiac impulse. III. Characteristics of very slow conduction. *J. Gen. Physiol.* 59:227 (1972).

Dreifus, L. S., Watanabe, Y., Haiat, R., and Kimbiris, D.: Atrioventricular block. *Am. J. Cardiol.* 28:371 (1971).

El-Sherif, N., Scherlag, B. J., and Lazzara, R.: Conduction disorders in the canine proximal His-Purkinje system following acute myocardial ischemia. I. The pathophysiology of intra-His bundle block. *Circulation* 49:837 (1974a).

El-Sherif, N., Scherlag, B. J., and Lazzara R.: Conduction disorders in the canine proximal His-Purkinje system following acute myocardial ischemia. II. The pathophysiology of bilateral bundle branch block. *Circulation* 49: 848 (1974b).

El-Sherif, N., Scherlag, B. J., and Lazzara, R.: The effect of combined ligation of the anterior septal artery and the AV nodal artery on the canine AV conduction system. *Circulation* (Suppl. III) 50:171 (Abstr.) (1974c).

El-Sherif, N., Scherlag, B. J., and Lazzara, R.: Pathophysiology of second degree atrioventricular block: A unified hypothesis. *Am. J. Cardiol.* 35-412 (1975a).

El-Sherif, N., Scherlag, B. J., and Lazzara, R.: Experimental production of "Mobitz II" and paroxysmal block in the AV node. *Clin. Res.* 23:181A (Abstr.) (1975b).

El-Sherif, N., Scherlag, B. J., and Lazzara, R.: Bradycardia-dependent conduction disorders. (Editorial) *J. Electrocardiol.* 9(1):1 (1976a).

El-Sherif, N., Scherlag, B. J., and Lazzara, R.: Bradycardia-dependent conduction disorders. Clinical and experimental correlation. *Am. J. Cardiol.* 37:13 (1976b).

El-Sherif, N., Scherlag, B. J., Lazzara, R., Hope, R., Williams, D. O., and Samet, P.: The pathophysiology of paroxysmal AV block after acute myocardial ischemia. Experimental and clinical observations. *Circulation* 50: 515 (1974d).

El-Sherif, N., Scherlag, B. J., Lazzara, R., et al.: The pathophysiology of tachycardia- and bradycardia-dependent block in the canine proximal His-Purkinje system following acute myocardial ischemia. *Am. J. Cardiol.* 33: 529 (1974e).

Hay, J.: Bradycardia and cardiac arrhythmia produced by depression of certain of the functions of the heart. *Lancet* 1:139 (1906).

Hoffman, B. F.: Electrical activity of the atrio-ventricular node. In *Specialized Tissue of the Heart*, A. Paes de Carvalho, W. C. deMello and B. F. Hoffman, eds. Elsevier Publishing Co., Amsterdam (1961).

Hoffman, B. F., and Cranefield, P. F.: *Electrophysiology of the Heart*. McGraw-Hill Book Company, Inc., New York (1960), p. 132.

Katz, L. N., and Pick, A.: *Clinical Electrocardiography. Part I. The Arrhythmias*. Lea and Febiger, Philadelphia (1956), p. 526.

Kaufman, J. G., Wachtel, F. W., Rothefield, E., and Bernstein, A.: The association of complete heart block and Adams-Stokes syndrome in two cases of Mobitz type of block. *Circulation* 23:253 (1961).

Langendorf, R.: The role of spontaneous diastolic depolarization in second degree AV block. The mechanism of "paroxysmal" AV block and of a new form of pseudo-supernormal AV conduction (Editorial). *Chest* 63:652 (1973).

Langendorf, R., and Pick, A.: Concealed conduction. Further evaluation of a fundamental aspect of propagation of the cardiac impulse. *Circulation* 13:381 (1956).

Langendorf, R., and Pick, A.: Atrioventricular block type II (Mobitz)—its nature and clinical significance. (Editorial) *Circulation* 38:819 (1968).

Langendorf, R., Pick, A., Edelist, A., and Katz, L. N.: Experimental demonstration of concealed AV conduction in the human heart. *Circulation* 32:386 (1965).

Lazzara, R., El-Sherif, N., Befeler, B., and Scherlag, B. J.: Lidocaine action on depressed cardiac cells. *Circulation* (Suppl. II) 52:85 (Abstr.) (1975a).

Lazzara, R., Scherlag, B. J., and El-Sherif, N.: Cellular electrophysiology of the ischemic His bundle. *Circ. Res.* 36:444 (1975b).

Lewis, T.: *The Mechanisms and Graphic Registration of the Heart Beat*. Shaw and Sons, Ltd., London (1925), p. 177.

Mendez, C., and Moe, G. K.: Some characteristics of transmembrane potentials of AV nodal cells during propagation of premature beats. *Circ. Res.* 19:933 (1966).

Mobitz, W.: Uber die unfallständige Störung der Erregungsüberleitung zwischen Vorhof and Krammer des menschlichen Herzens. *Z. Ges. Exp. Med.* 41:180 (1924).

Moe, G. K., Abildskov, J. A., and Mendez, C.: An experimental study of concealed conduction. *Amer. Heart J.* 67:338 (1964).

Narula, O. S.: Conduction disorders in the AV transmission system. In *Cardiac Arrhythmias*, L. S. Dreifus and W. Likoff, eds. Grune & Stratton, New York (1973), p. 259.

Narula, O. S., Scherlag, B. J., Samet, P., and Javier, R. P.: Atrioventricular block: Localization and classification by His bundle recordings. *Am. J. Med.* 50:146 (1971).

Paes de Carvalho, A., Hoffman, B. F., and dePaula Carvalho, M.: Two components of the cardiac action potential. I. Voltage-time course and the effect of acetylcholine on atrial and nodal cells of the rabbit heart. *J. Gen. Physiol.* 54:607 (1969).

Rosen, K. M., Loeb, H. S., Chuquimia, R., Sinno, M. Z., Rahimtoola, S. H., and Gunnar, R. M.: Site of heart block in acute myocardial infarction. *Circulation* 42:925 (1970).

Rosen, K. M., Loeb, H. S., Gunnar, R. M., and Rahimtoola, S. H.: Mobitz type II block without bundle branch block. *Circulation* 44:1111 (1971).

Rosen, K. M., Loeb, H. S., and Rahimtoola, S. H.: Mobitz type II block with narrow QRS complex and Stokes-Adams attacks. *Arch. Intern. Med.* 132: 595 (1973).

Rosenbaum, M. B., Elizari, M. V., Levi, R. J., and Nau, G. J.: Paroxysmal atrioventricular block related to hypopolarization and spontaneous diastolic depolarization. *Chest* 63:678 (1973).

Rotman, M., Wagner, G. S., and Waugh, R. A.: Significance of high degree atrioventricular block in acute posterior myocardial infarction. *Circulation* 47:257 (1973).

Schaffer, A. J.: Mechanism of the Wenckebach type of atrioventricular block. (Annotations) *Am. Heart J.* 79:138 (1971).

Scherlag, B. J., El-Sherif, N., and Lazzara, R.: Experimental model for study of Mobitz type II and paroxysmal atrioventricular block. *Am. J. Cardiol.* 34:309 (1974).

Spear, J. J., and Moore, E. N.: Electrophysiological studies on Mobitz type II second degree heart block. *Circulation* 44:1087 (1971).

Spear, J. F., and Moore, E. N.: Intranodal conduction. In *Cardiac Arrhythmias*, L. S. Dreifus and W. Likoff, eds. Grune and Stratton, New York (1973), p. 298.

Sutton, R., and Davies, M.: The conduction system in acute myocardial infarction complicated by heart block. *Circulation* 38:987 (1968).

Touboul, P. ,Clement, C., Porte, J., Magrina, J., and Delahaye, P.: Etude électrophysiologique des troubles de conduction auriculoventriculaire dans l'infarctus myocardique récent. *Arch. Mal. Coeur* 65:1287 (1972).

Watanabe, Y., and Dreifus, L. S.: Inhomogeneous conduction in the AV node: A model for re-entry. *Am. Heart J.* 70:505 (1963).

Watanabe, Y., and Dreifus, L. S.: Second degree atrioventricular block. *Cardiovasc. Res.* 1:150 (1967).

Waugh, R. A., Wagner, G. S., Haney, T. L., Rosati, R. A., and Morris, J. J., Jr.: Immediate and remote prognostic significance of fascicular block during acute myocardial infarction. *Circulation* 47:765 (1973).

Weidman, S.: The effect of cardiac membrane potential on the rapid availability of the sodium carrier system. *J. Physiol.* (Lond.) 127:213 (1955).

Wenckebach, K. F.: Zur Analyse des unregelmässigen Pulses. *Z. Klin. Med.* 37:475 (1899).

Wenckebach, K. F.: Beiträge zur Kenntniss der menschlichen Herztätigkeit. *Arch. Anat. Physiol. (Physiol. Abteil.)* 297 (1906).

Yeh, B. K., Tao, P., and deGuzman, N.: Mobitz type II AV block as a manifestation of digitalis toxicity. *J. Electrocardiol.* 5:74 (1972).

4

Mechanism of Action of Antiarrhythmic Agents

LEONARD S. DREIFUS
SATOSHI OGAWA
MARY JANE OSMICK
YOSHIO WATANABE

INTRODUCTION

While many important studies have been carried out in cardiac pharmacology during the past decade, a rational basis for the selection and electropharmacological action of antidysrhythmic agents is still lacking, the situation being hopelessly confused. Vaughan Williams (1970) first attempted to categorize known antidysrhythmic agents according to their individual electrophysiological and pharmacological actions. The problems of classification became compounded by the lack of a reliable animal model, the use of a wide variety of methods for inducing dysrhythmia, such as coronary ligation, ischemia, aconitine, chloroform, epinephrine, digitalis excess, electrical stimulation, etc. Furthermore, it is generally acknowledged that these interventions have more than one class of action. Admittedly, we still have an incomplete understanding of the mechanisms engendering various cardiac arrhythmias, despite the recent contributions by investigators using ultramicroelectrode and His-bundle techniques. Too often the clinician, surprised by the actions of a specific agent, may be unable to predict whether the drug will be beneficial or precipitate more hazardous problems. This is particularly true when one antiarrhythmic agent is used in the wake of another, since the interactions of various antiarrhythmic drugs still remain unclear (Dreifus et al., 1974b). Recent reviews have brought into sharp focus both the electrophysiology and pharmacology of antiarrhythmic agents (Dreifus et al., 1974b; Rosen and Hoffman, 1973; Rosen et al., 1975b; Wit et al., 1974a; Gettes, 1971; Watanabe et al., 1963). It is the purpose of this discussion to relate some of the currently available antiarrhythmic drugs to their possible modes of action on impulse formation and conduction. Previously documented data will be summarized and newer information presented to define the present state of our knowledge, in the hope that this will serve as a basis for future investigation.

For purposes of classification, Hoffman and Bigger (1971) have summarized the possible membrane effects of antiarrhythmic agents and have divided these compounds into several groups. As shown in Table 1, Group I includes the quinidine-like drugs, such as quinidine, propranolol, and procainamide. To the original list, we can add antihistamines, a new ester of ajmaline (17-monochloroacetyl ajmaline hydrochloride-MCAA), aprindine, disopyramide phosphate and potassium. These agents are classified together because they appear to decrease automaticity and responsiveness, and prolong the refractory period.

A second group of antiarrhythmic drugs includes diphenylhydantoin (DPH), lidocaine and, under certain conditions, the catecholamines. Lidocaine and DPH decrease automaticity, and increase responsiveness and the refractory period. However, this last group is far more heterogeneous with respect to membrane effects, and several investigators have observed sharp differences in their action, particularly when the drug and potassium concentrations have a wide range. (Watanabe et al., 1963, 1969, 1972; Singh, 1971b; Davis and Temte, 1969; Shigenobu et al., 1966; Gettes, 1971; Dreifus et al., 1969; Jensen and Katzung, 1970; Bigger and Mandel, 1970; Dreifus and Watanabe, 1970; Bigger et al., 1968a 1968b; Sano et al., 1968; Strauss et al., 1968; Weidman, 1956; Helfant et al., 1967; Singh, 1971a, 1971c; Rosati et al., 1967; Wit et al., 1970a; Obayashi et al., 1975; Pamintuan et al., 1970).

Bretylium tosylate, a beta-blocking agent with potent antiarrhythmic action, does not belong in the first two groups and could possibly be included a third. (Bigger et al., 1968b; de Azevedo et al., 1974; Bacaner, 1968; Singh and Vaughan Williams, 1970; Sanna and Arcidiatoho, 1973). Several other agents, such as sotalol (MJ-1999), the beta blockers of the ethanolamine class and the anti-

Table 1. Classification of antiarrhythmic agents

I	II	III	IV
QUINIDINE	LIDOCAINE	BRETYLIUM	VERAPAMIL
PROCAINAMIDE	DPH**	AMIODARONE	D-600
PROPRANOLOL		SOTALOL	LANTHIUM
17-MCAA*		NIFENALOL	MANGANESE
APRINDINE			
DISOPYRAMIDE			
PHOSPHATE			
ANTIHISTAMINES			
POTASSIUM			

*17-MCAA = monochloroacetyl ajmaline hydrochloride
**DPH = diphenylhydantoin

anginal drug, amiodarone, have a Group III effect (Vaughan Williams, 1970) by virtue of their ability to prolong the duration of the action potential.

Such agents as verapamil and manganese (Posner et al., 1975; Imanishi and Surawicz, 1975; Schamroth et al., 1972; King et al., 1974; Rosen et al., 1974b) appear to have a very selective action on the slow response mediated through the calcium/sodium (Ca^{++}/Na^{+}) channels. These agents, which appear to slow intranodal conduction and also offer potent antiarrhythmic action, will be discussed as a possible fourth subset of drugs (Table 1).

While it is generally acknowledged that antiarrhythmic agents cannot be classified in a precise manner, the tentative format shown in Table 1 will be used as an approach to this overview. Several antiarrhythmic drug interactions will be discussed when it is considered of clinical or electrophysiological importance. Finally, it should be emphasized that hypopotassemia may completely nullify the depressive or antiarrhythmic effects of the drugs in question, while hyperpotassemia or concomitant administration of potassium salts may enhance the development of serious intoxication (Watanabe et al., 1963; Singh, 1971b; Pamintuan et al., 1970).

METHODS

All ultramicroelectrode experiments described by the authors were carried out on isolated perfused rabbit hearts, employing the techniques of isolation and perfusion previously reported (Watanabe and Dreifus, 1968). A modified Chenoweth's solution was used, with the following composition in millimoles per liter: NaCl — 119.8; KCL — 4.5; $CaCl_2$ — 2.4; $MgCl_2$ — 2.1; $NaHCO_3$ — 25.0, and dextrose — 10.0. The perfusate was saturated with 95% oxygen plus 5% CO_2. Ventricular electrograms were recorded by two small surface electrodes attached to the right ventricular apex and left ventricular base. A bipolar stimulating electrode was placed near the sinus node and the heart was electrically driven at a constant rate of 10-15 beats per minute higher than the intrinsic rate. Glass microelectrodes filled with 3M KCl with tip resistances of 10-25 megohms were used to record transmembrane potentials from either the atrioventricular (AV) junctional or ventricular fibers. The potentials were amplified by a neutralized input-capacity amplifier and Tektronix amplifiers. A Grass camera was used to photograph tracings from a Tektronix oscilloscope.

Catheter electrode studies to test the refractory periods of the atria, AV node, and His-Purkinje system were carried out in intact dogs. The animals, weighing from 18-22 kg, were anesthetized with sodium pentobarbital and maintained on a respirator for the period of the experiment. A tripolar His-bundle recording catheter was positioned across the tricuspid valve to record His potentials. The sinus node was crushed and a close bipolar teflon-coated stimulating electrode was placed in the high right atrium, near the sinus node, to directly stimulate the atrium and introduce premature atrial stimuli. A multichannel oscilloscope recorder was used at paper speeds of 100 and 200 mm per second. Atrial stimulation was performed with a programmable stimulator (M. Bloom, Philadelphia), using stimuli of 1.5 msec duration, at approximately twice diastolic threshold. Refractory periods were determined by means of the extra-stimulus technique. Beginning late in the cardiac cycle, a premature atrial stimulus (S_2) was introduced after every 8th driven beat (S_1) in all animals. The prematurity of the S_2 was decreased in 10 to 20-msec steps until the atrial refractory period was encountered, so that the entire atrial cycle was scanned. Lidocaine 5mg/kg, procainamide 5mg/kg, deslanoside C 0.05 mg/kg, propranolol 0.1 mg/kg, and aprindine 10 mg/kg were administered after control refractory periods for the AV transmission system were obtained. Measurements of the intracardiac conduction intervals and refractory periods were accomplished according to standard techniques (Wit et al., 1970b).

A_1 and H_1 are the atrial and His electrograms resulting from either spontaneous sinus beats or driven atrial beats, S_1.

A_2 and H_2 represent the atrial and His electrograms obtained upon premature atrial stimulus, S_2.

The refractory periods for the AV conduction system were defined as follows: Atrial effective refractory period (atrial ERP) = longest $S_1 - S_2$ interval not resulting in atrial capture by S_2. Atrial functional refractory period (atrial FRP) = shortest $A_1 - A_2$ interval achievable. AV nodal effective refractory period (AV nodal ERP) = longest $A_1 - A_2$ interval in which A_2 does not conduct to the His bundle. AV nodal functional refractory period (AV nodal FRP) = shortest $H_1 - H_2$ interval achievable by atrial stimulation. All determinations could not be made in all animals, particularly in respect to the effective refractory period of the AV node.

DIGITALIS

Cellular Physiology

While it has been generally accepted that digitalis inhibits the active transport of sodium and potassium across the cell (Hoffman and Bigger, 1971; McCans et al., 1973; Surawicz, 1963), it appears that the potassium ion is more important than the sodium one. (Hoffman and Bigger, 1971; Watanabe, 1970; Vassalle et al., 1962). In fact, relative intracellular vs. extracellular potassium concentration may be crucial in the genesis or termination of cardiac arrhythmias (Hoffman and Bigger, 1971; Watanabe, 1970; Kunin et al., 1962). Several recent reviews are available describing the precise electrophysiological action of digitalis (Rosen et al., 1975b; Hoffman, 1972; Dreifus and Watanabe, 1972). A number of extensive studies on the action of digitalis glycosides on transmembrane potentials of ventricular fibers are in general agreement that digitalis shortens the action-potential duration (Surawicz, 1963; Vassalle et al., 1962; Cannon and Sjostranol, 1953; Woodbury and Hecht, 1952; Stutz et al., 1954; Dudel and Trautwein, 1958; Watanabe, 1965). On the other hand, its effects on membrane action and resting potentials, and the rate of depolarization have been less consistent (Woodbury and Hecht, 1952; Stutz et al., 1954; Dudel and Trautwein, 1958; Watanabe, 1965). Digitalis in excessive doses may affect automaticity. The increase in phase 4 depolarization may result in threshold potential being reached and in automatic rhythm (Rosen et al., 1975b). A transient sequence of oscillations from membrane potential and subsequent electrical quiescence can occur

(Rosen et al., 1975b; 1973a, 1973b; Hashimoto and Moe, 1973; Ferrier et al., 1973; Davis, 1973; Hogan et al., 1973). When this takes place in specialized conducting cells, it is referred to as a low-amplitude potential (Rosen et al., 1973a), a transient depolarization (Ferrier et al., 1973), or enhanced diastolic depolarization (Davis, 1973). Rosen et al. (1975b) have shown that, following excessive ouabain administration, phase 4 depolarization can be produced. Furthermore, discontinuation of the stimulus can be succeeded by a stable spontaneous rhythm at a slower rate than the drive stimulus. Discontinuation of the stimulus results in a subthreshold depolarization, followed by repolarization, and no further electrical activity is seen.

Other investigations have shown oscillatory phenomena due to digitalis administration (Davis, 1973). Aronson and Cranefield (1974) demonstrated oscillations or after-potentials in slow cardiac fibers. Depolarization occurs to the extent that the normal mechanism for phase 4 depolarization and the fast inward sodium current are inactivated, and only the slow response and its accompanying automaticity remain. These observations follow completion of the action-potential repolarization in cells that now have low resting and maximal diastolic potentials (Aronson and Cranefield, 1974). Cranefield has identified these observations as delayed after-depolarization. Rosen et al. (1975b) suggest that this not only is an appropriate description of the oscillatory events that occur during phase 4, but distinguishes them from those oscillations which may be seen prior to full repolarization and, hence, are designated as "early after-depolarization." It has now been shown that, under certain conditions, digitalis-induced delayed after-depolarizations can reach threshold potential and initiate spontaneous action potentials (Ferrier et al., 1973; Davis, 1973; Hogan et al., 1973). Rosen et al. (1975b) further described that when an appropriate coupling interval or rate of sinus stimulus is attained, after depolarization will reach threshold and initiate a variable number of spontaneous action potentials. These authors further suggested that two distinct types of automatic activity may occur as the result of digitalis toxicity. Either the automatic activity is seen in the ventricular escape beat or the delayed after-potentials reach thresholds which result in a variable number of propagated action potentials (Wit et al., 1974b). These abnormal automatic responses are much less prone to develop when the potassium concentration is between 4 and 5.5 mM (Wit et al., 1974b). It should be pointed out that manganese and verapamil decreased the magnitude of digitalis-induced delayed after-depolarization (Ferrier and Moe, 1973; Rosen et al., 1974a).

King et al. (1974) showed suppression of ouabain-induced ventricular ectopy with verapamil and reversal with calcium. Rosen et al. (1974a) found that verapamil counteracted the effects of digitalis on the slope of phase 4 depolarization. Hence, it can be concluded that an inward current carried by calcium could be responsible, at least in some part, for the changes in diastolic membrane potential induced by digitalis. Finally, it has been shown that the interactions between digitalis-induced delayed after-depolarizations and premature action potentials can result in concealment of conduction within the His-Purkinje system, and produce complex disturbances of rhythm, including re-entry (Rosen et al., 1975b).

Effect of Digitalis on AV Transmission

Recently, Goodman et al. (1975) demonstrated that the electrophysiological effects of digitalis on atrioventricular conduction, in man, are most marked in the AV node and appear dependent on cardiac innervation. Both the AV nodal functional and effective refractory periods were prolonged by digitalis and were unrelated to changes in cycle length (Goodman et al., 1975). However, no significant alterations were seen in patients with denervated hearts. Prolongation of the effective refractory period in the AV junction is caused partly by vagal activation and partly by a direct effect on the nodal fibers themselves (Vassalle et al., 1962; Watanabe, 1965; Mendez and Mendez, 1953; Watanabe and Dreifus, 1966, 1970, 1972a). Characteristically, digitalis engenders a low amplitude and phase 0 upstroke velocity (V max) of the action potentials from the N region of the AV node (Watanabe and Dreifus, 1966). The rate of rise of phase 0 (V max) in nodal His (NH) fibers also appears to be decreased. Hence, a greater decrement and failure of propagation may result within the AV node (Watanabe and Dreifus, 1970). Furthermore, part of the increase in the so-called effective refractory period of the AV transmission system results from concealment of rapid atrial impulses into the AV junction; this occurs especially in the presence of atrial fibrillation and to a lesser extent —of atrial flutter. Hence, in the presence of repetitive concealment, partial penetration into and conceivable re-entry within the AV junction could inhibit subsequent AV transmission (Watanabe and Dreifus, 1965, 1972a).

The interrelation of digitalis with potassium and propranolol appear most important in the management of patients with supra-ventricular arrhythmias.

Interrelation of Digitalis and Potassium

It seems that the primary effects of cardiac glycosides and potassium are exerted on different portions of the AV conducting system (Watanabe and Dreifus, 1966, 1967). Lanatoside C almost selectively depresses conduction across the AV node, with little or no delay in the intra-atrial and His-Purkinje transmission (Watanabe and Dreifus, 1966, 1970).

In contrast, high potassium concentration will slow intra-atrial (Sano et al., 1967) and subnodal conduction, and provide protective action for intranodal conduction (Watanabe and Dreifus, 1967). Hence, elevation of potassium may counteract the depressant effect of cardiac glycosides on intranodal transmission, but could cause further delay above and below the AV node (Fig. 1).

If intranodal conduction is severely depressed by toxic doses of cardiac glycosides, the beneficial action of an elevated potassium concentration may be insufficient to restore 1:1 conduction across the crucial N region of the AV node. Significant prolongation of intra-atrial conduction by cardiac glycosides is seen only in the presence of a high potassium level. The delay is attributed to potassium alone (Dreifus et al., 1974b; Watanabe and Dreifus, 1967).

Since cardiac glycosides increase diastolic depolarization in His-Purkinje fibers (Wit et al., 1974b; Vasalle et al., 1962) and, since the resultant loss of membrane potential could cause a decreased rate of phase 0 depolarization (V max) and slower conduction velocity (Singer et al., 1967), suppression of automaticity by a high concentration of potassium may sometimes improve His-Purkinje conduction. However, it has been pointed out that, in the presence of a severe conduction disturbance in the more proximal portion of the AV tranmission system (e.g., the AV node), such suppression of His-Purkinje automaticity may result in abolition of subsidiary pacemakers and ventricular standstill. For this reason, great caution must be exercised in the administration of potassium in patients with AV block and possible excess of digitalis.

Interrelation of Digitalis and Propranolol

The combined use of digitalis and propranolol probably represents one of the most significant advances in the control of supra-

CONDUCTION IN THE AV TRANSMISSION SYSTEM

	SLOWS	ENHANCES
ATRIAL	QUINIDINE	LOW K^+
	PROCAINEAMIDE	
	PROPRANOLOL	
	MCAA	
	APRINDINE	
	TETRODOTOXIN	
AV NODE	DIGITALIS	ISOPOTERENOL
	VERAPAMIL	QUINIDINE
	PROPRANOLOL	HIGH K^+
	BRETYLIUM	DPH
	APRINDINE	
	LOW K^+	
	LOW Na^+	
	AMIODARONE	
PURKINJE	QUINIDINE	LOW K^+
	PROCAINEAMIDE	
	MCAA	
	DISOPYRAMIDE	
	HIGH K^+	
	TETRODOTOXIN	
	APRINDINE	

1 Effect of electrolytes and antiarrhythmic agents on AV transmission.

ventricular arrhythmias (Dreifus et al., 1974b; Pamintuan et al., 1970). The complementary action of these agents slows the ventricular rate in the presence of atrial flutter and fibrillation. Propranolol has been shown to depress both intra-atrial and His-Purkinje conduction, with little effect on intranodal conduction in rabbit hearts (Pamintuan et al., 1970; Dreifus and Josipovic, 1968) (Figs. 1,2).

Further studies in the dog demonstrated an increase in the functional and effective refractory periods by digitalis alone, with an additional increase when digitalis and propranolol were combined (Fig. 3). Although the AH interval and the refractory periods were prolonged by digitalis and further extended by the addition of

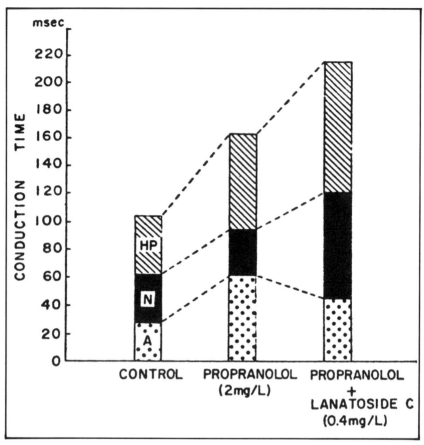

2 Site of AV conduction delay in the presence of propranolol and lanatoside C in isolated rabbit heart. Intra-atrial conduction (A); intranodal conduction (N); His-Purkinje conduction (HP). Propranolol (2.0 mg/l) increases the A and HP conduction time, with only a small increment in intranodal conduction. After administration of lanatoside C (0.4 mg/l), the intranodal time is prolonged (Fig. 3).

propranolol, measurement of these parameters is not sufficient to precisely characterize conduction across the AV node (Watanabe and Dreifus, 1967). This may, in part, explain the confusion concerning the actions of antiarrhythmic agents and electrolytes on AV conduction.

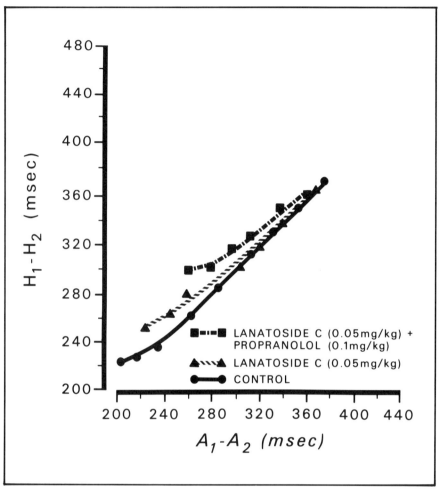

3

Effect of lanatoside C (0.05 mg/kg) and propranolol (0.1 mg/kg) on the AV nodal refractory periods. A_1-A_2 = the interval between the last driven atrial beat and the premature atrial stimulus; H_1-H_2 = the interval between the last driven His-bundle deflection, and the His-bundle deflection resulting from the premature stimulus. The AV nodal effective and functional refractory periods are increased after lanatoside C and further prolonged after the addition of propranolol.

GROUP I

Quinidine

Cellular physiology

Agents which decrease automaticity and responsiveness, and prolong the refractory period are included in the so-called Group I drugs (Hoffman and Bigger, 1971). However, there are notable exceptions among the substances in Table 1. These differences will be discussed subsequently.

Weidmann (1955), Johnson (1956; Johnson and McKinnon, 1957), Hecht (1957), Gettes et al. (1962), and Watanabe and co-workers (Watanabe, 1965; Watanabe et al., 1962; Dreifus et al., 1962) have demonstrated a decrease in the maximal rate of depolarization (V max) in the presence of quinidine and quinidine-like agents. Furthermore, suppression of the spontaneous pacemaker activity of the Purkinje fibers by these drugs was also reported by Hoffman (1958) and Weidmann (1955). Other investigators emphasized the importance of the delay in repolarization following the administration of quinidine (Hoffman, 1958; West and Amory, 1960). Although the action-potential duration was increased by quinidine recovery of excitability lagged further behind the completion of repolarization (Watanabe et al., 1963; Rosen and Hoffman, 1973). Restoration toward normal of the action-potential amplitude, resting potential and phase 0 depolarization (V max) occurred in the presence of a lowered potassium concentration (Watanabe et al., 1963) (Fig. 4).

Effect of quinidine and potassium on atrioventricular conduction

Quinidine, in the presence of normal potassium, markedly prolonged AV conduction time, with a further increase by high potassium (Johnson, 1956). Quinidine or a high potassium concentration prolongs the AV interval by slowing intra-atrial, His-Purkinje, and intraventricular conduction (Watanabe and Dreifus, 1967). Lowering the potassium level in the presence of quinidine shortens the AV interval of enhancing His-Purkinje conduction. Josephson et al. (1974) found that quinidine routinely prolonged His-Purkinje and intraventricular-conduction time in man. In addition, the refractory periods of the atria and His-Purkinje system were extended while the effective refractory period of the AV node was consistently

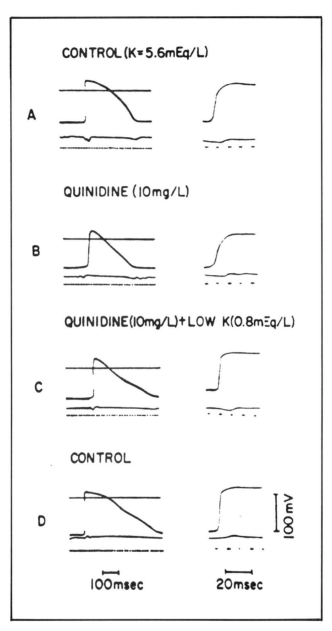

4 Effect of lowering of the potassium concentration on phase-0 depolarization (Vmax). Control (A) quinidine reduced V max (B), lowering of potassium (K = 0.8 mEq/l) restored phase 0 depolarization towards normal (C). Control (D) (Fig. 1).

Table 2. Electrophysiological effects of quinidine and propranolol
combination on ventricular fibers

	CONTROL	CONTROL + QUINIDINE (5 mg/l)	QUINIDINE (mg/l) PROPRANOLOL (0.5 mg/l)
APA	79.9 ± 4.9	77.2 ± 2.2	74.6 ± 6.8
MRP	60.5 ± 3.4	57.5 ± 3.7	59.6 ± 5.6
OS	19.4 ± 4.9	19.7 ± 3.4	15.0 ± 2.2 ‡‡
APD	126.0 ± 19.0	149.0 ± 13.7**	165.4 ± 12.8 ‡
MRD	81.7 ± 17.6	44.5 ± 12.0*	36.2 ± 13.3*

* P < 0.001   Abbreviations: APA = action-potential amplitude in millivolts
** P < 0.01   MRP = membrane-resting potential in millivolts
‡ P < 0.02   OS = overshoot in millivolts
‡‡P < 0.05   APD = action-potential duration in milliseconds
                                    MRD = maximal rate of Phase 0 depolarization in volts/sec

shortened. These and other investigators thought that procainamide had effects similar to quinidine but different from diphenylhydantoin, lidocaine and propranolol (Josephson et al., 1972; Damato and Lau, 1970; Gallagher et al., 1972, 1973; James and Nadeau, 1964; Caracta et al., 1973). The above findings were consistent
with those obtained in rabbit hearts by Watanabe and Dreifus
(1967). These studies suggest that quinidine has anticholinergic
properties which can be of clinical significance. Josephson et al.
(1974) noted an apparent shortening of the effective refractory
period of the His-Purkinje system in one patient. However, when
low potassium effects predominated, the AV interval could remain
relatively unchanged before second-degree block would occur. In
short, different portions of the AV conduction system can be selectively influenced by quinidine and potassium (Watanabe and Dreifus, 1967). In the presence of low potassium and quinidine, AV
conduction depends on the net results of their antagonism within
individual fibers.

Effect of quinidine and propranolol on atrioventricular conduction

While propranolol has similar membrane effects to quinidine
in that it decreases automaticity, slows the rate of depolarization,

Table 3. Effect of propranolol on AV conduction time
(in msec)

	CONTROL	PROPRANOLOL (2 mg/l)	P % Change Value
Intra-atrial	32.0 ± 4.09	73.8 ± 12.91	+130.6**<0.05
Intranodal	41.7 ± 6.79	51.8 ± 6.76	+ 24.2 <0.1
His-Purkinje	37.5 ± 3.07	72.2 ± 5.04	+ 92.5* <0.01
Total AV conduction	110.8 ± 10.15	192.7 ± 15.20	+ 73.9* <0.01

* P < 0.01
** P < 0.05

and reduces responsiveness, it has little or no effect on the action-potential duration (Hoffman and Bigger, 1971). However, the shortening of the action-potential duration is probably less marked than that of the refractory period. Further studies of the interaction of propranolol and quinidine show that V max was decreased by quinidine and this change was further enhanced by the addition of propranolol (Table 2). The effect of propranolol alone on AV conduction is shown in Table 3. Propranolol significantly increased intra-atrial and His-Purkinje conduction time, without significantly prolonging that of intranodal conduction (Pamintuan et al., 1970). However, the addition of propranolol to quinidine further depressed intra-atrial, intranodal, and His-Purkinje conduction (Table 4).

Clinical use has shown that the combination of quinidine and propranolol is extremely effective in the management of cardiac arrhythmias. This may be explained by their additive action on cellular electrophysiology and AV conduction (Pamintuan et al., 1970; Stern, 1966; 1967, 1971).

Disopyramide Phosphate

A new antiarrhythmic agent, disopyramide phosphate (Norpace®) has been successfully used for the treatment of various cardiac arrhythmias, including atrial fibrillation and ventricular tachycardia (Dreifus et al., 1973; Vismara et al., 1974; Ryan et al., 1974; Dreifus, 1975). The drug appears to be effective in the presence of paroxysmal atrial and nodal tachycardia. The membrane effects of disopyramide phosphate include an increase in the action-potential duration and refractory period, with a decrease in the rate

Table 4. Electrophysiological effects of quinidine and propranolol
combination on AV conduction
(in msec)

	CONTROL	CONTROL + QUINIDINE (5 mg/l)	QUINIDINE (5 mg/l) + PROPRANOLOL (0.5 mg/l)
Intra-atrial	18.8 ± 4.4	38.4 ± 13.5‡	54.0 ± 19.2‡
Intranodal	42.4 ± 19.4	69.6 ± 12.1**	109.2 ± 25.7**
His-Purkinje	31.4 ± 9.2	52.2 ± 19.7‡	90.8 ± 51.2**
Total AV conduction	92.6 ± 16.3	160.2 ± 17.8*	254.0 ± 59.9*

  * P < 0.01
 ** P < 0.02
 ‡ P < 0.05

of phase 0 depolarization (V max) (Dreifus et al., 1973; Dreifus, 1975) (Fig. 5). Similarly to quinidine and other antiarrhythmic agents (Watanabe et al., 1962, 1963, 1965; Dreifus et al., 1962), lowering the potassium concentration tended to reverse the membrane effects of Norpace (Fig. 5) (Table 5). Disopyramide phosphate appears to increase intra-atrial, intranodal, and His-Purkinje conduction time (Dreifus et al., 1973; Dreifus, 1975) (Fig. 6) (Table 6). The slowing of conduction within the N fibers of the AV node may contribute to the marked effectiveness of this drug in terminating reciprocating atrial tachycardias.

17-Monochloroacetyl Ajmaline Hydrochloride (MCAA)

The alkaloids of rauwolfia serpentia have been employed for some time in the treatment of cardiac arrhythmias of supraventricular and ventricular origin (Slama et al., 1963; Kleinsorge and Gaida, 1962). The effects of ajmaline, the principal alkaloid used, have a brief duration. Beccari (1963) studied the antiarrhythmic action of some ajmaline derivatives and concluded that the esterification of 2-hydroxyls of ajmaline caused a potentiation of the antiarrhythmic action. However, when these compounds are introduced into the organism, the action of the precursor is enzymatically regenerated. From an electrophysiological standpoint, there is a sig-

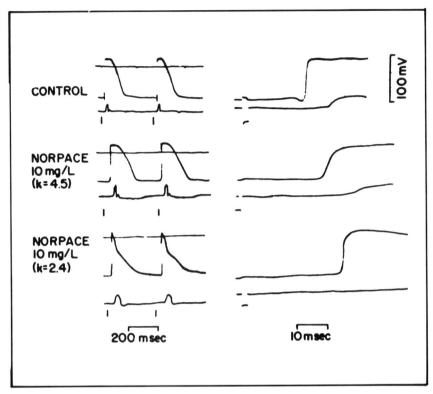

5

Effect of disopyramide phosphate (Norpace®) on rabbit ventricular fibers. Norpace showed phase 0 depolarization and prolonged the action-potential duration (middle curve). Lowering potassium from 4.5 to 2.4 mEq restored phase 0 depolarization towards normal (lower curve).

Table 5. Electrophysiological effects of disopyramide on ventricular fibers

	APA	MRP	OS	APD	MRD
Control	91.4 ± 14.9	69.1 ± 15.6	23.8 ± 10.2	125.3 ± 16.8	149.3 ± 57.7
Disopyramide 10 mg/l (K=4.5)	91.5 ± 17.0	69.6 ± 16.1	$20.9 \pm 6.1*$	$164.5 \pm 24.0*$	$46.0 \pm 18.1*$
Disopyramide 10 mg/l (K=2.7)	$100.4 \pm 14.6*$	$85.5 \pm 8.3*$	15.0 ± 8.3	$168.5 \pm 50.3*$	$140.5 \pm 46.0*$

* $P < 0.02$
Abbreviations: see Table 2

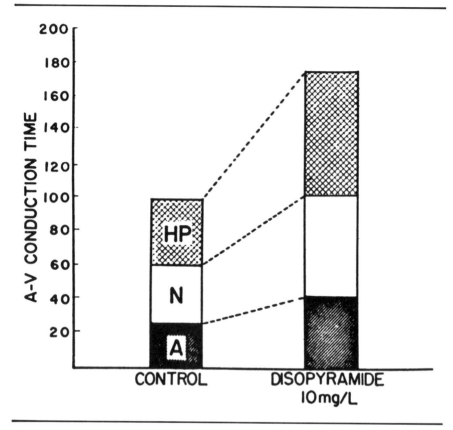

6 Effect of disopyramide phosphate (Norpace®) on AV conduction. Conduction time is prolonged in all three regions of the AV transmission system. The greatest increases occurred within the AV node and His-Purkinje system.

nificant decrease in the action-potential amplitude, overshoot, and maximal rate of depolarization (V max), as well as an increase in the action-potential duration (de Azevedo et al., 1975). These findings are similar to those obtained with quinidine as far as ventricular fibers are concerned, although studies on Purkinje fibers exposed to epinephrine were not performed. Nevertheless, it can be speculated on the basis of these data, that MCAA probably has antiarrhythmic effects similar to those of quinidine (Table 7).

Intra-atrial, nodal, and total AV conduction times are prolonged by this drug (Fig. 7). Thus, in contrast to what happens with

Table 6. Electrophysiological effects of disopyramide phosphate
on AV conduction time
(in msec)

	CONTROL	DISOPYRAMIDE PHOSPHATE (10 mg/l) K+ (4.5 mEq/l)	DISOPYRAMIDE PHOSPHATE (10 mg/l) Low K+ (2.7 mEq/l)
Intra-atrial	24.8 ± 3.3	45.3 ± 10.1**	26.2 ± 6.8
Intranodal	32.0 ± 10.2	56.0 ± 9.0**	66.1 ± 37.5
Intra-His-Purkinje	39.2 ± 6.5	74.5 ± 12.6*	46.7 ± 11.2*
Total AV conduction	96.0 ± 8.2	175.8 ± 18.9*	139.0 ± 43.8

* P < 0.001
** P < 0.01

quinidine, the slowing of conduction—especially in the atria and AV node—could offer important advantages in the treatment of supraventricular tachycardias, atrial fibrillation, flutter, and tachycardias associated with the Wolff-Parkinson-White syndrome. MCAA may offer potent antiarrhythmic effects and deserves more extensive clinical evaluation.

Aprindine

Aprindine is an antiarrhythmic agent with local anesthetic properties similar to those of lidocaine (Reid and Varghese, 1974). It appears effective both orally and parenterally according to Van Durme et al. (1974). The latter also found aprindine to be superior to procainamide and quinidine in a crossover experiment in patients with stable ventricular dysrhythmias, following healed myocardial infarction. The effectiveness of this agent seems related to its plasma level. Zipes et al. (1975) reported a high incidence of ventricular fibrillation in dogs with acute left anterior descending-artery ligation upon rapid infusion of aprindine. Initiation of ventricular fibrillation was related to a critical myocardium, rapid heart rate and ischemia. When aprindine is administered intravenously in a high concentration, it binds preferentially and immediately to the myocardium, the serum level of the drug representing only 1-2% of the total dose. It was further observed that, when the myocardial aprindine level fell rapidly, ventricular fibrillation could no

Table 7. Electrophysiological effects of MCAA on ventricular fibers

	CONTROL	CONTROL + MCAA (3 mg/l)
APA	84.1 ± 6.0	75.2 ± 5.8*
MRP	61.0 ± 5.8	59.1 ± 6.7
OS	23.1 ± 5.9	16.1 ± 2.9**
APD	119.8 ± 12.6	135.6 ± 25.1**
MRD	63.4 ± 30.8	40.7 ± 19.7*

MCAA = 17-monochloroacetyl ajmaline hydrochloride
* P < 0.01
** P < 0.05

Abbreviations: see Table 2

longer be produced (Zipes et al., 1975). Hence, rapid infusion rates plus ischemia plus high myocardial aprindine concentrations produced asynchronous ventricular excitation, leading to ventricular fibrillation.

The membrane effects of aprindine were studied by Greenspan et al. (1974) in normal non-automatic Purkinje fibers. Aprindine depressed the rate of rise of phase 0, with concomitant reduction in action-potential amplitude, duration and—at times—membrane potential. After prolonged superfusion, conduction became altered, with varying degrees of block, and exhibited the clinical counterpart of the Wenckebach structure. In Purkinje fibers rendered automatic by stretch, hypoxia, digitalis or catecholamines, the slope of phase 4 depolarization was reduced and, eventually, abolished by aprindine. Conduction depression and block at high doses also occurred in muscle fibers with this agent, but the latter tissue was less sensitive than Purkinje fibers. Greenspan and coworkers (1974) suggested that the alteration in conduction, associated with abolition of automaticity, would abolish tachycardia. All investigators found that the action of aprindine persisted at low doses and after long periods of time.

Aprindine significantly prolongs the effective refractory period of the atrium, AV junction and ventricular myocardium. The conduction times of the atria, AV, and HV were also increased, according to Reid and Varghese (1974); these authors found a return of the functional refractory periods to control values while the relative refractory periods remained above those of controls after 2 hr.

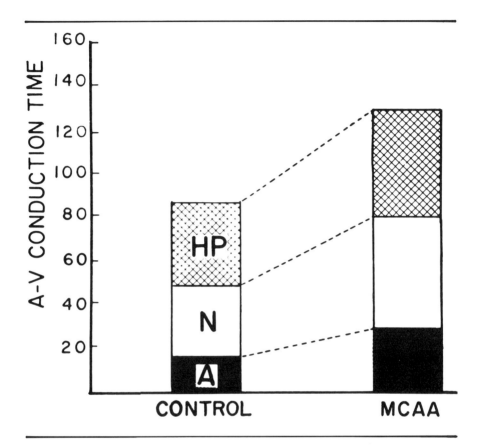

7

Effect of MCAA on AV transmission. The intra-atrial and intranodal conduction times were significantly prolonged, while the intra-His-Purkinje conduction time was increased to a lesser degree than the intranodal conduction delay. The total AV conduction time was markedly extended (Fig. 3). MCAA = 17-monochloroacetyl ajmaline hydrochloride.

Our recent study of atrial conduction revealed that aprindine was a potent depressant, especially of the conduction through atrial muscle to the appendages. This was evidenced by prolongation of conduction time and refractory period after administration of the drug. In contrast, inter-atrial conduction was relatively insensitive to aprindine and, consequently, a Wenckeback block was observed within the atrial appendages in the presence of 1:1 conduction through the inter-atrial paths to the left atrium.

GROUP II

Lidocaine

Cellular Electrophysiology

The electrophysiological and pharmacological effects of lidocaine have been extensively reviewed by Rosen et al. (1975a). For this reason, we shall discuss here only the interrelation of lidocaine, a Group II agent, with procainamide and propranolol, drugs often used clinically in combination.

It appears that lidocaine will produce a concentration-dependent decrease in V max and depression of membrane responsiveness (Rosen et al., 1975a). This depression of conduction by the drug could theoretically convert areas of unidirectional conductional block into bidirectional block, thereby abolishing re-entry. This may be of particular importance since lidocaine exerts a differential effect on healthy and diseased tissues (Rosen et al., 1975a). Maximum diastolic-potential amplitude and V max are reduced or further depressed by therapeutic concentrations of lidocaine.

The action-potential duration and effective refractory period of Purkinje fibers are decreased by lidocaine (Bigger and Mandel, 1970). The degree of alteration is related to the location of the particular Purkinje fiber, since the most significant effects of lidocaine are seen at a site close to the insertion of the free-running strands into the ventricular myocardium (Wittig et al., 1973; Myerburg et al., 1970). Furthermore, the drug causes the greatest changes in action-potential duration and refractoriness in normal Purkinje fibers in which these parameters have initially the highest value (Wittig et al., 1973).

Lidocaine suppresses spontaneous diastolic depolarization and automatic impulse formation, at membrane potentials between -90 and -60 mV, due to a time- and voltage-dependent decrease in an outward K^+ current (iK_2) (Wit et al., 1974a). This occurs at lidocaine concentrations that do not influence sinus-node automaticity.

The action-potential amplitude and V max are reduced by lidocaine, but to a lesser degree than by procainamide, according to Singh and Hauswirth (1974); these authors attributed the effects of lidocaine on V max to a decrease in membrane conductance for Na^+.

Recent studies in our laboratory, carried out on rabbit ventricular fibers, confirm the reduction in V max; however, no sig-

Table 8. Electrophysiological effects of lidocaine and procainamide
combination on ventricular fibers

	CONTROL	CONTROL + LIDOCAINE (10 mg/l)	LIDOCAINE (10 mg/l) + PROCAINAMIDE (5 mg/l)
APA	100.2 ± 12.1	102.5 ± 14.4	99.6 ± 10.4
MRP	72.5 ± 11.1	76.0 ± 11.8	86.0 ± 10.2
OS	28.0 ± 8.9	26.5 ± 6.6	27.7 ± 5.8
APD	127.9 ± 35.8	144.8 ± 17.3	132.3 ± 22.1
MRD	103.1 ± 16.8	44.6 ± 14.2*	41.7 ± 7.5

* $P < 0.01$
Abbreviations: see Table 2

nificant change was observed in the action-potential amplitude and duration, or the membrane resting potential (Dreifus et al., 1974a) (Table 8). Addition of procainamide to lidocaine engendered a smaller drop in V max. (Table 8). When the drugs were administered in reverse fashion, the effect on phase-0 depolarization (V max) was additive (Table 9) (Fig. 8). There was no further increase in the action-potential duration when lidocaine was added to procaine amide (Table 9). Han et al. (1974) found that both procainamide and lidocaine were effective in decreasing automaticity since they significantly increased post extra-systolic escape intervals of idioventricular beats. Although procainamde failed to abolish the re-entrant beats, induced by early premature beats, lidocaine eliminated these beats in a considerable number of the dogs studied. These results suggest that lidocaine is more effective than procainamide in preventing ventricular re-entrant activity induced by early premature beats. Thus, the interrelation of procainamide and lidocaine could be useful in the management of resistant cardiac arrhythmias. Kabela (1973) noted a lesser sensitivity of atrial fibers to lidocaine than to procainamide, and attributed this to a smaller efflux of potassium from atrial—as opposed to ventricular-muscle and Purkinje fibers. This may explain the inconsistent effect of lidocaine on atrial arrhythmias.

From earlier studies on the interrelation between antiarrhythmic agents and potassium, it became apparent that the divergence of effects seen with lidocaine resulted from a wide variation of

Table 9. Electrophysiological effects of procainamide and lidocaine combination on ventricular fibers

	CONTROL	CONTROL + PROCAINAMIDE (5 mg/l)	PROCAINAMIDE (5 mg/l) + LIDOCAINE (10 mg/l)
APA	79.7 ± 5.3	78.6 ± 5.1	75.7 ± 6.7
MRP	58.8 ± 5.4	58.9 ± 5.7	59.7 ± 7.4
OS	20.9 ± 7.6	19.7 ± 6.3	16.0 ± 4.4
APD	126.0 ± 42.7	132.3 ± 42.0**	137.3 ± 44.4
MRD	115.0 ± 23.3	54.0 ± 11.7*	44.8 ± 20.2*

* $P < 0.01$
** $P < 0.05$
Abbreviations: see Table 2

potassium levels in the animal models (Watanabe et al., 1962, 1963; Watanabe, 1970; Watanabe and Dreifus, 1967; Dreifus et al., 1962, 1973). Studies by Singh and Vaughan Williams (1971) indicated that at a 5.6 mM potassium concentration, lidocaine reduced the maximum rate of depolarization of phase 0. This potassium level compared favorably to those found in the blood of successfully treated patients. However, at lower potassium levels of 3.0 mM, lidocaine did not necessarily change the electrophysiological parameters. Our recent studies (Dreifus et al., 1974a) showed a marked reduction in the maximum rate of depolarization (V max) in the presence of a potassium concentration of 4.5 mM.

Effect of lidocaine and procaine amide on atrioventricular conduction

The above discussion indicated that the effect of lidocaine on AV conduction must necessarily be related to the potassium level (Rosen et al., 1970). Previous electrophysiological studies, employing His-bundle recordings, have demonstrated no significant depression of intra-atrial, AV nodal, or intraventricular conduction (Bekheit et al., 1973). However, investigations using ultramicroelectrode techniques demonstrated a significant increase in intra-atrial and intranodal conduction time, with a net prolongation in the total AV interval, following lidocaine administration in rabbit hearts (Drei-

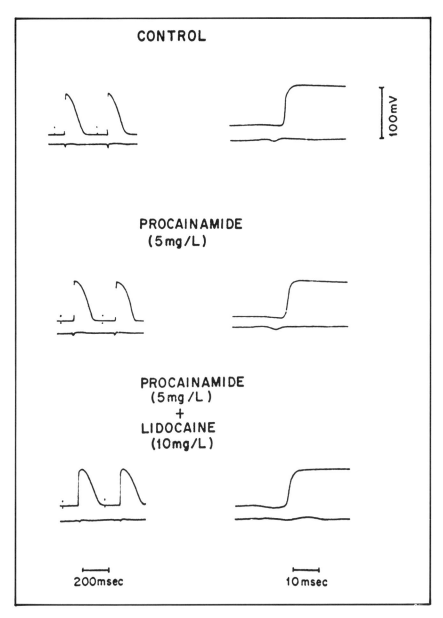

8

Effect of lidocaine on ventricular fibers. Procainamide increased action-potential duration and phase 0. Addition of lidocaine to procainamide caused a further decrease in the maximum rate of depolarization of phase 0.

Table 10. Electrophysiological effects of lidocaine and procainamide combination on AV conduction

		CONTROL + LIDOCAINE (10 mg/l)	LIDOCAINE (10 mg/l) PROCAINAMIDE (5 mg/l)
Intra-atrial	20.9 ± 8.3	35.1 ± 3.8*	30.3 ± 11.8
Intranodal	39.0 ± 10.2	53.1 ± 9.3*	54.9 ± 9.7
His-Purkinje	27.4 ± 8.6	24.2 ± 6.2	42.6 ± 10.6*
Total AV conduction	83.3 ± 11.6	112.4 ± 19.6*	127.8 ± 10.0*

* $P < 0.01$

fus et al., 1974a) (Table 10). When procainamide was added, no further increase was seen in intra-atrial or intranodal conduction time but the usual extension in His-Purkinje conduction time was observed. Both the effective and functional refractory periods of the AV junction were prolonged upon lidocaine administration (3mg/kg) and were further increased after the addition of procainamide (3mg/kg) (Fig. 9).

Although lidocaine and procainamide show several dissimilar electrophysiological actions, there appear to be significant additive effects when these agents are administered together. It is not unusual for lidocaine and procainamide to be used in combination in the presence of resistant cardiac arrhythmias and, from the electrophysiological studies presented, it would seem that some beneficial effects could be expected.

Diphenylhydantoin

Although diphenylhydantoin (DPH) has been in clinical use for more than 25 years, its precise role in the treatment of heart disease is still unsettled (Dreifus and Watanabe, 1970). Several clinical reports as early as 1939 suggested that this drug may exhibit antiarrhythmic effects on the heart (Williams, 1939). Although DPH still appears to have only limited value in the therapy of cardiac arrhythmias, its unique electrophysiological properties render it extremely useful as a pharmacological tool.

DPH seems to depress automaticity, and enhance conduction and responsiveness, thus, differing from Group I agents in several

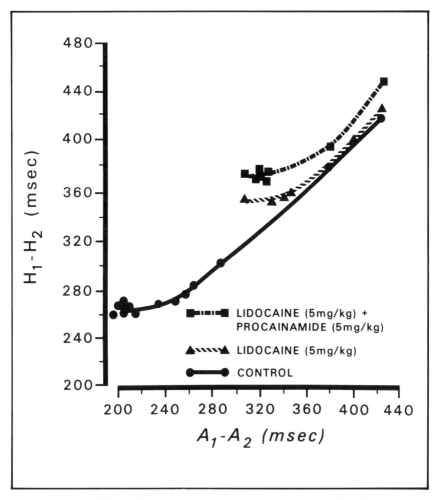

9

Effect of lidocaine and procainamide on the functional and
effective refractory periods of the AV node. Addition of lidocaine
(3 mg/kg) increased the effective and functional refractory periods.
A further prolongation of the refractory periods was seen following
the addition of procainamide (3 mg/kg).

respects (Pamintuan et al., 1970; Cohen, 1975; Bigger et al., 1968;
Helfant et al., 1967; Scherlag et al., 1968). However, Strauss et al.
(1968), using higher concentrations of DPH (10^5 M), showed a decrease in the slope of phase 4 depolarization in sinoatrial and
venous automatic tissue. Sano et al. (1968) demonstrated a reduc-

tion in phase 0 over a wide range of concentrations and an increase in the action-potential duration with higher DPH levels. It appears that any particular action of the drug is essentially related to its concentration. Further studies, using ultramicroelectrode techniques with higher levels of 10mg/liter, showed an increase in intra-atrial as well as His-Purkinje conduction time (Dreifus and Watanabe, 1970). However, Scherlag et al. (1968) noted a decrease in the His-ventricular activation time measured by intracardiac catheters. It is reasonable to suspect that in arrhythmias which are mainly a result of re-entry due to depressed conduction, DPH in low concentrations may be effective in terminating the disturbance by improving the conduction (Pamintuan et al., 1970). Like lidocaine, DPH diminishes the action-potential duration. However, the effective refractory period is reduced to a lesser degree and, therefore, the ratio of abbreviation of the effective refractory period to action-potential duration remains less than 1. Since the rate of action-potential propagation depends on V max, DPH will increase conduction at voltages where membrane responsiveness is altered (Bigger, 1972).

Studies by Sasyniuk and Dresel (1968) suggest that DPH prolonged the AV interval. Again, it should be stressed that, in most studies, DPH enhanced AV conduction. Inter-species variation, drug level and the underlying potassium concentration will affect the action of DPH on AV transmission time. Our group has occasionally observed slowing of the ventricular rate, in the presence of atrial flutter or fibrillation, as well as high-grade AV heart block. Thus, extreme care must be taken when using this agent in the presence of underlying AV conduction disorders.

GROUP III

Bretylium Tosylate

Cellular electrophysiology

It is difficult to place bretylium tosylate in either of the two previous groups of antiarrhythmic drugs because the primary effects of this agent do not appear to decrease automaticity and responsiveness, or prolong the refractory period. In fact, automaticity has actually been increased by bretylium, and spontaneous firing in quiescent fibers in preparations of papillary muscle and Purkinje fibers has been observed (Wit et al., 1970a; Bigger and Jaffe, 1971). This response is usually transient and is abolished by pre-

Table 11. Effects of quinidine and bretylium on the ventricular
fibers of rabbit heart

	APA	MRP	APD	MRD
Control	90.0 ± 9.1	64.8 ± 10.3	118.0 ± 22.0	57.5 ± 14.6
Quinidine alone	93.0 ± 11.3	69.4 ± 13.1	147.0 ± 25.6*	36.0 ± 8.9*
Quinidine and bretylium	92.8 ± 13.3	67.1 ± 9.6	135.0 ± 25.2[+]	42.1 ± 12.1

* P < 0.01
[+] P < 0.05
Abbreviations: see Table 2

treatment with reserpine. Wit et al. (1970a) noted occasional hyperpolarization induced by bretylium, especially when the membrane resting potential was reduced or the tissue was considered hypoxic. They explained such findings by possible release of catecholamines from the sympathetic nerve endings. It is conceivable that this mechanism played a role in the hyperpolarization and increased conduction velocity observed in our previous experiments (Watanabe et al., 1969). It is unlikely, however, that the same mechanism prevailed in our recent study of isolated hearts (Dreifus et al., 1974a) perfused through the coronary system, since myocardial oxygenation in this setting should be better than in a tissue-bath experiment, and recirculation of released catecholamines should not play a major role (Watanabe et al., 1969). Absence of this mechanism may explain why the addition of bretylium to quinidine did not change the membrane resting potential or the action-potential amplitude and overshoot (de Azevedo et al., 1974) (Table 11).

All the effects of bretylium cannot be attributed to catecholamine release, since this agent shortened the action-potential duration, both alone in the tissue-bath experiments and in the perfused heart in the presence of quinidine. Furthermore, if catecholamine release were solely responsible for the electrophysiological action of bretylium, one would not expect significant depression of intranodal conduction by this agent, whether used alone or after perfusion with quinidine. Cervoni et al. (1971) showed that bretylium increased the fibrillation threshold in both reserpine-pretreated and chronically sympathectomized dog hearts, and concluded that the antiarrhythmic effects of this drug are due to a direct action on the myocardium rather than to its adrenergic blocking action or its ability to release norepinephrine. In their study, the positive inotropic effect of bretylium was apparently not dependent on catecholamine release since it was demonstrated after sympathectomy and in reserpinized dogs. In our experiments, using normal potassium concentration (K = 4.5 mM), the membrane resting potential, action-potential amplitude and maximal rate of depolarization were increased, while the action-potential duration and effective refractory periods were decreased (Pamintuan et al., 1970; de Azevedo et al., 1974; Watanabe et al., 1969). These findings were in contrast to those obtained by Bigger and Jaffe (1971), and could be related to the 4.5 mM potassium concentration of the perfusate in our experiments (de Azevedo et al., 1974), as opposed to the 2.7 mM concentration employed by other investigators (Bigger and Jaffe, 1971).

The important electrophysiological mechanisms of bretylium may be connected directly with its capacity for chemical defibrillation (de Azevedo et al., 1974). Fig. 10 shows that bretylium produced a more normal looking action potential following a premature depolarization. As a result, after bretylium administration, the earliest premature response arises at a more negative level of membrane potential, and conducts at a more rapid velocity than the earliest premature depolarization evoked after washout of the drug. Improved propagation of premature systoles may not entirely abolish ectopic beating but may, instead, engender more efficient conduction and, consequently, provide less of a chance for microreentry and ventricular fibrillation.

Quinidine alone produced an increase in the action-potential duration and a decrease in V max. Following the addition of bretylium, there was a significant shortening of the action-potential duration, with no change in action-potential amplitude, membrane resting potential and V max. Hence, the addition of bretylium to quinidine decreased the action-potential duration and, in general, appeared to have the opposite effect than quinidine (Table 11).

Effect of bretylium tosylate on atrioventricular conduction

Bretylium alone selectively increased intranodal conduction time (Fig. 11). Furthermore, when quinidine and bretylium were combined, the latter exerted an antagonistic effect on the increased intra-atrial and His-Purkinje conduction time (Table 12). Hence,

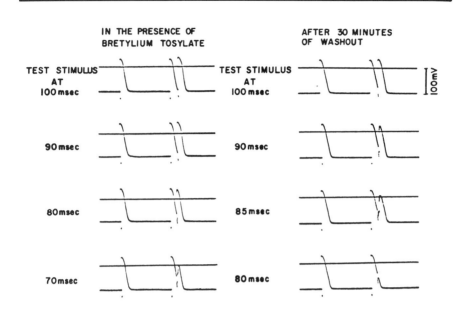

10 Effect of bretylium tosylate on the action potential of a premature stimulus. Left column: bretylium (20 mg/L). Right column: after washout of bretylium. Premature systole 90 msec following the last driven beat produced a smaller action-potential amplitude with a slowly rising phase 0, as compared to the action potential in the presence of bretylium. At 85 msec, there is a further deterioration of the action-potential configuration after washout, while a rather normal-appearing action potential is seen in the presence of bretylium. At 80 msec, there is a failure of activation of the fiber while an abortive action potential is seen after the premature stimulus is delivered 70 msec following the last driven beat.

bretylium depresses intranodal conduction similarly to low potassium, digitalis and propranolol, with little or no effect on intra-atrial or His-Purkinje conduction. However, the combined effect of quinidine and bretylium tended to prolong the total AV interval (Table 12).

Although bretylium may never gain widespread popular use as a primary antiarrhythmic drug because of its hypotensive effects, it deserves further study in order to identify its antiarrhyth-

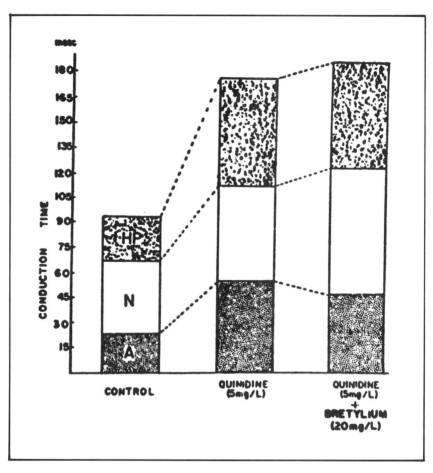

11 Effect of bretylium tosylate on AV conduction. Bretylium markedly increased intranodal conduction, with no effect on intra-atrial or His-Purkinje conduction time.

mic and antifibrillatory actions. Its effects which are in contrast to those of Group I or Group II agents indicate that this drug is a very interesting pharmacological tool. It is obvious, however, that bretylium should not be used together with either Group I or Group II agents, since such a combination may completely nullify the anti-arrhythmic effects of either drug alone (de Azevedo et al., 1974).

Table 12. Combined effects of quinidine and bretylium on AV conduction time (means ± standard errors)

	CONTROL (msec)	QUINIDINE (msec)	QUINIDINE + BRETYLIUM (msec)
Atrial	25.6 ± 11.6	75.0 ± 6.6	63.6 ± 56.6
Nodal	43.8 ± 13.4	69.0 ± 37.5	100.2 ± 52.2**
His-Purkinje	30.2 ± 12.3	70.6 ± 24.7*	69.4 ± 28.8
AV interval	99.6 ± 36.0	214.6 ± 102.8**	233.2 ± 105.4

* $P < 0.01$
** $P < 0.05$

GROUP IV

Verapamil

As opposed to the other possible classifications of antiarrhythmic agents, verapamil appears to have a rather selective action on fibers dependent on a slow inward current. Wit and Cranefield (1974) demonstrated that this drug decreased the action-potential amplitude in the upper and mid-AV nodes so that maximum depolarization was below 0, without reducing maximum diastolic potential. However, action potentials in the lower AV node were not affected. Verapamil prolonged the time-dependent recovery of excitability and the effective refractory period of AV nodal fibers. Premature impules would be blocked in the AV node, preventing the conduction delay necessary for AV nodal re-entry and tachycardia. Verapamil had no effect on the ventricular diastolic threshold or amplitude of atrial or His-bundle action potentials. King et al. (1974) showed that verapamil blocked the slow ionic current carried by calcium and/or sodium, but not the rapid current carried by sodium alone. The drug suppressed ouabain-induced ventricular ectopy and this suppression was reversed by calcium administration. Rosen et al. (1974b) demonstrated that verapamil, at concentrations of 2×10^{-6} M, decreased action-potential amplitude, membrane resting potential, maximum rate rise of phase 0 and membrane responsiveness. Changes in the effective refractory period were compatible with those in action-potential duration. Conduction velocity was slowed only by the higher concentrations of verapamil. The drug also suppressed automaticity and calcium-induced low-amplitude potentials. These effects on the action potential and low-amplitude potentials were partially reversible by increasing calcium concentration (Rosen et al., 1974b). Its effects on the action-potential plateau were consistent with blockade of an inward calcium current and suggest that verapamil may suppress arrhythmias produced by calcium-induced slow potentials. Lower concentrations of verapamil did not alter phase 4 depolarization or conduction but did suppress low-amplitude potentials. These authors suggest that verapamil acts by a mechanism different from those of other antiarrhythmic agents (Rosen et al., 1974b).

Imanishi et al. (1975) also found that verapamil-induced suppression was partially restored by increasing extracellular calcium concentration. These investigators compared the effects of lidocaine with verapamil and found that slow channel-dependent rhythmic automatic depolarizations in depolarized ventricular myocardium could be suppressed by moderately high doses of verapamil, but not by very high doses of lidocaine. The unique action of verapamil appears to be quite different from those of the other antiarrhythmic agents discussed so far, suggesting a possible fourth group of these drugs. The clinical effects of verapamil, particularly in suppressing supraventricular arrhythmias, and slowing the ventricular rate in the presence of atrial fibrillation and atrial flutter, as first reported by Schamroth et al. (1972), appear to have received an electrophysiological confirmation.

It is known from human (Heng et al., 1975) and animal studies (Ogawa and Dreifus, 1976) that a single dose of verapamil elicits an acute depressive effect on the AV node, with the prolongation of the AH interval and effective refractory period. These values appear to return to control levels within one hour. In contrast, verapamil could produce more potent and prolonged effects in the presence of sympathetic denervation with propranolol and, therefore, potentiation of verapamil by propranolol must be considered when these agents are combined.

Recent extensive reviews (Dreifus et al., 1974b; Watanabe, 1970; Watanabe and Dreifus, 1972b) on the interaction of magnesium, potassium, and sodium and tetrodotoxin are available and will not be discussed in this overview.

REFERENCES

Aronson, R. S., and Cranefield, P. F.: The effect of resting potential on the electrical activity of canine cardiac Purkinje fibers exposed to Na-free solution or to ouabain. *Pfluegers Arch.*, 347:101 (1974).

Bacaner, M. B.: Quantitative comparison of bretylium with other anti-fibrillatory drugs. *Am. J. Cardiol*, 21:504 (1968).

Beccari, E.: Latenziamento dell'ajmalina. *Farmaco* 18:65 (1963).

Bekheit, S. Murtagh, J. G., Morton, P., and Fletcher, E.: Effect of lidocaine on conduction system of human heart. *Br. Heart J.* 35:305 (1973).

Bigger, J. T., Jr.: Arrhythmias and antiarrhythmic drugs. *Ad. Intern. Med.* 18:251 (1972).

Bigger, J. T., J., Bassett, A. L., and Hoffman, B. F.: Electrophysiological effects of diphenylhydantoin on canine Purkinje fibers. *Circ. Res.* 22:221 (1968a).

Bigger, J. T., Jr., and Jaffe, C. C.: The effect of bretylium tosylate on the electrophysiologic properties of ventricular muscle and Purkinje fibers. *Am. J. Cardiol.* 27:82 (1971).

Bigger, J. T., Jr., and Mandel, W. J.: Effect of lidocaine on the electrophysiological properties of ventricular muscle and Purkinje fibers. *J. Clin Invest.* 49:63 (1974).

Bigger, J. T., Jr., and Mandel, W. J.: Effect of lidocaine on the transmembrane potentials of ventricular muscle and Purkinje fibers. *J. Clin Invest.* 49:63 (1970).

Bigger, J. T., Jr., Schmidt, D. H., and Kutt, H.: Relationship between the plasma level of diphenylhydantoin sodium and its cardiac antiarrhythmic effects. *Circulation* 38:363 (1968b).

Cannon, F., and Sjostrand, T.: The occurrence of a positive after-potential in the ECG in different physiological and pathological conditions. *Acta Med. Scand.* 146:191 (1953).

Caracta, A. R., Damato, A. N., Josephson, M. E., Gallagher, J. J., Ricciutti, M., and Lau, S. H.: Electrophysiology of diphenylhydantoin. *Circulation* 47:1234 (1973).

Cervoni, P., Ellis, C. H., and Mazwell, R. A.: The antiarrhythmic action of bretylium in normal reserpine-pretreated and chronically denervated dog hearts. *Arch. Int. Pharmacodyn.* 190:91 (1971).

Cohen, L.: Diphenylhydantoin sodium (dilantin). In *Drugs in Cardiology*, Part 1, E. Donoso, ed. Stratton Intercontinental Medical Book Corp., New York (1975), p. 49.

Damato, A. N., and Lau, S. H.: The clinical value of the electrogram of the conducting system. *Prog. Cardiovasc. Dis.* 13:119 (1970).

Davis, L. D.: Effect of changes in cycle length on diastolic depolarization produced by ouabain in canine Purkinje fibers. *Circ. Res.* 32:206 (1973).

Davis, L. S., and Temte, J. V.: Electrophysiological actions of lidocaine on canine ventricular muscle and Purkinje fibers. *Circ. Res.* 24:639 (1969).

de Azevedo, I. M., Dreifus, L. S., and Watanabe, Y.: Electrophysiologic effects of a new ester of ajmaline 17-mono chloroacetyl ajmaline hydrochloride

(MCAA). *Eur. J. Cardiol.* 2/3:321 (1975).

de Azevedo, I. M., Watanabe, Y., and Dreifus, L. S.: Electrophysiologic antagonism of quinidine and bretylium tosylate. *Am. J. Cardiol.* 33:633 (1974).

Dreifus, L. S.: Electrophysiology of Norpace. *Angiology* 26:111 (1975).

Dreifus, L. S., de Azevedo, I. M., and Dreifus, H. N. and Watanabe, Y.: Interaction of procainamide and lidocaine, *Circulation* 50 (Suppl III) 170 (Abstr.) (1974a).

Dreifus, L. S., de Azevedo, I. M., and Watanabe, Y.: Electrolyte and drug interaction. *Am. Heart J.* 88:95 (1974b).

Dreifus, L. S., Filip, Z., Sexton, L., and Watanabe, Y.: Electrophysiological and clinical effects of a new antiarrhythmic agent: disopyramide. *Am. J. Cardiol.* 31:129 (Abstr.) (1973).

Dreifus, L. S., and Josipovic, V.: Effects of propranolol on A-V transmission. *Fed. Proc.* 27:226 (Abstr.) (1968).

Dreifus, L. S., and Watanabe, Y.: Current status of diphenylhydantoin, *Am. Heart J.* 80:709 (1970).

Dreifus, L. S., and Watanabe, Y.: Clinical correlates of the the electrophysiologic action of digitalis on the heart. *Drug Treatment* 2:179 (1972).

Dreifus, L. S., Watanabe, Y.: Cardanas, N., and Volastro, P.: Newer antiarrhythmic drugs. *Cardiovasc. Clin.* 1:3 (1969).

Dreifus, L. S., Watanabe, Y., Sirlin, N., and Katz, M.: Potassium and the action of quinidine. *J. Lab. Clin. Med.* 60:870 (1962).

Dudel, J., and Trautwein, W.: Elektrophysiologische Messungen zur Strophanthinwirkung am Herzmuskel. *Arch. Exp. Pathol.* 232:393 (1958).

Ferrier, G. R., and Moe, G. K.: Effect of calcium on acetylstrophanthidin-induced transient depolarizations in canine cardiac tissues. *Circ. Res.* 33:508 (1973).

Ferrier, G. R., Saunders, J. H., and Mendez, C.: A cellular mechanism for the generation of ventricular arrhythmias by acetylstrophanthidin. *Circ. Res.* 32:600 (1973).

Fisch, C., Steinmetz, E. F., Fasola, A. F., and Martz, B. L.: Effect of potassium and "toxic" doses of digitalis on the myocardium. *Circ. Res.* 7:424 (1959).

Gallagher, J. J., Damato, A. N., Caracta, A. R., Varghese, P. J., Josephson, M. E., and Lau, S. H.: Gap in A-V conduction in man: Types I and II. *Am. Heart J.* 85:78 (1973).

Gallagher, J. J., Damato, A. N., Varghese, P. J., and Lau, S. H.: Localization of an area of maximum refractoriness or "gate" in the ventricular specialized conduction system in man. *Am. Heart J.* 84:310 (1972).

Gettes, L. S.: The electrophysiologic effects of antiarrhythmic drugs. *Am J. Cardiol.* 28:526 (1971).

Gettes, L. S., Surawicz, B., and Shiue, J. C.: Magnitude of ventricular transmembrane action and resting potential during development of intraventricular conduction disturbances in rabbit heart: Effects of high and low K+ and quinidine. *Fed. Proc.* 21:134 (1962).

Goodman, D. J., Rossen, R. M., Cannon, D. S., Rider, A. K. and Harrison, D. C.: Effect of digoxin on atrioventricular conduction: Studies in patients with and without autonomic innervation. *Circulation* 51:251 (1975).

Greenspan, K., Steinberg, M., Holland D., and Freeman, A. R.: Electrophysiologic alterations in cardiac dysrhythmias: Antiarrhythmic effects of aprindine. *Am. J. Cardiol* 33:140 (Abstr.) (1974).

Han, J., Goel, B. G., Yonn, M. S., and Rodegs, R.: Effect of procainamide and lidocaine on ventricular automaticity and re-entry during acute coronary occlusion. *Am. J. Cardiol.* 34:171 (1974).

Hashimoto, K., and Moe, G. K.: Transient depolarizations induced by acetyl-strophanthidin in specialized tissue of dog atrium and ventricle. *Circ. Res.* 32:618 (1973).

Hecht, H. H.: Normal and abnormal transmembrane potentials of the spontaneously beating heart. *Ann. N. Y. Acad. Sci.* 65:700 (1957).

Helfant, R. H., Sherlag, B. J., and Damato, A. N.: The electrophysiological properties of diphenylhydantoin sodium as compared to procainamide in the normal and digitalis-intoxicated heart. *Circulation* 36:108 (1967).

Heng, M. K., Singh, B. N., Roche, A. H. G., Norris, R. M., and Mercer, C. L.: Effects of intravenous verapamil on cardiac arrhythmias and on the electrocardiogram. *Am. Heart J.* 90:487 (1975).

Hoffman, B. F.: The action of quinidine and procainamide on single fibers of dog ventricle and specialized conducting system. An. Acad. Brasil. Cience. 29:365 (1958).

Hoffman, B. F.: Effects of digitalis on electrical activity of cardiac membranes. In *Basic and Clinical Pharmacology of Digitalis*, B. H. Marks and A. M. Weissler, eds. Charles C. Thomas, Springfield, Ill. (1972), pp. 118-127.

Hoffman, B. F., and Bigger, J. T., Jr.: Antiarrhythmic drugs. In *Drills Pharmacology in Medicine*, 4th ed., J. R. DiPalma, ed. McGraw Hill Book Company, Inc., New York (1971), pp. 824-852.

Hogan, P. M., Wittenberg, S. M., and Klocke, F. J.: Relationship of stimulation frequency to automaticity in the canine Purkinje fiber during ouabain administration. *Cir. Res.* 32:377 (1973).

Imanishi, S., and Surawicz, B.: Effects of lidocaine and verapamil on slow channel-dependent automatic depolarizations in depolarized guinea pig ventricular myocardium. *Am. J. Cardiol.* 35:145 (Abstr.) 1975.

James, T., and Nadeau, R. A.: The mechanism of action of quinidine on the sinus node studies by direct perfusion through its artery. *Am. Heart J.* 67:804 (1964).

Jensen, R. A., and Katzung, B. G.: Electrophysiological actions of diphenylhydantoin on rabbit atria. *Circ. Res.* 26:17 (1970).

Johnson, E. A.: The effects of quinidine, procainamide and pyrilamine on the membrane resting and action potential of guinea pig ventricular muscle fibers. *J. Pharmacol. Exp. Ther.* 117:237 (1956).

Johnson, E. A., and McKinnon, M. G.: The differential effect of quinidine and pyrilamine on the myocardial action potential at various rates of stimulation. *J. Pharmacol. Exp. Ther.* 120:460 (1957).

Josephson, M. E., Caracta, A. R., Ricciutti, M. A., Lau, S. H., and Damato, A. N.: Correlation of electrophysiological properties of procainamide with plasma levels in man. *Circulation* 46:681 (Abstr.) (1972).

Josephson, M. E., Seides, S. F., Battsford, W. P., Weisfogel, G. M., Akhtar, M., Caracta, A. R., Lau, S. H., and Damato, A. N.: The electrophysiological effects of intramuscular quinidine on the atrioventricular conducting system in man. *Am. Heart J.* 87:55 (1974).

Kabela, E.: The effects of lidocaine on potassium efflux from various tissues of the heart. *J. Pharmacol. Exp. Ther.* 184:611 (1973).

King, R. M., Zipes, D. P., de B. Nicoll, and Linderman, J.: Suppression of ouabain-induced ventricular ectopy with verapamil and reversal with calcium. *Am. J. Cardiol.* 33:148 (Abstr.) 1974.

Kleinsorge, H., and Gaida, P.: Behavior of the serum level after intravenous injections of ajmaline. *Klin. Wochenschr.* 40:149 (1962).

Kunin, A. S., Surawicz, B., and Sims, E. A.: Decrease in serum potassium concentrations and appearance of cardiac arrhythmias during infusion of potassium with glucose in potassium-depleted patients. *N. Engl. J. Med.* 266:228 (1962).

McCans, J. L., Brennan, F. J., Chiong, M. A., and Parker, J. O.: Effects of ouabain and diphenylhydantoin on myocardial potassium balance in man. *Am. J. Cardiol.* 31:320 (1973).

Mendez, C., and Mendez, R.: The action of cardiac glycosides on the refractory period of heart tissues. *J. Pharmacol. Exp. Ther.* 107:24 (1953).

Myerburg, P. J., Stewart, J. W., and Hoffman, B. F.: Electrophysiological properties of the canine peripheral AV conducting system. *Circ. Res.* 20: 361 (1970).

Obayashi, K., Hayakawa, H., and Mandel, W. J.: Interrelationships between external potassium concentration and lidocaine: Effects on canine Purkinje fibers. *Am. Heart J.* 80:221 (1975).

Ogawa, S., and Dreifus, L. S.: Interaction of digitalis and verapamil on AV conduction. *Fed. Proc.* 35:235 (Abstr.) (1976).

Pamintuan, J. C., Dreifus, L. S., and Watanabe, Y.: Comparative mechanisms of antiarrhythmic agents. *Am. J. Cardiol.* 26:512 (1970).

Posner, P., Lambert, C., and Miller, B. L.: Effect of verapamil on ^{42}K transport in canine cardiac Purkinje fibers. *Am. J. Cardiol.* 35:163 (Abstr.) (1975).

Reid, P. R., and Varghese, J. P.: Electropharmacology of aprindine HCL. *Circulation* 50 (Suppl. III): 200 (Abstr.) (1974).

Rosati, R. A., Alexander, J. A., Schaal, S. F., and Wallace, A. G.: Influence of diphenylhydantoin on electrophysiological properties of the canine heart. *Circ. Res.* 21:757 (1967).

Rosen, M. R., Gelband, H., and Hoffman, B. F.: Correlation between effects of ouabain on the canine electrocardiogram and transmembrane potentials of isolated Purkinje fibers. *Circulation* 47:65 (1973a).

Rosen, M. R., Gelband, H., Merker, C., and Hoffman, B. F.: Mechanisms of digitalis toxicity: Effects of ouabain on phase 4 of canine Purkinje fiber transmembrane potentials. *Circulation* 47:681 (1973b).

Rosen, M. R., and Hoffman, B. F.: Mechanisms of action of antiarrhythmic drugs. *Cir. Res.* 32:1 (1973).

Rosen, M. R., Hoffman, B. F., and Wit, A. L.: Electrophysiology and pharmacology of cardiac arrhythmias. V. Cardiac antiarrhythmic effects of lidocaine. *Am. Heart J.* 89:526 (1975a).

Rosen, M. R., Ilvento, J., Gelband, H., and Merker, C.: Effects of verapamil on electrophysiologic properties of canine cardiac Purkinje fibers. *J. Pharmacol. Exp. Ther.* 189:414 (1974a).

Rosen, M. R., Ilvento, J. P., and Merker, C.: The electrophysiological basis for the suppression of cardiac arrhythmias by verapamil. *Am. J. Cardiol.* 33: 166 (Abstr.) (1974b).

Rosen, K. M., Lau, S. H., Weiss, M. B., and Damato, A. N.: The effect of lidocaine on atrioventricular and intraventricular conduction in man. *Am. J. Cardiol.* 25:1 (1970).

Rosen, M. R., Wit, A. L., and Hoffman, B. F.: Electrophysiology and pharmacology of cardiac arrhythmias IV. Cardiac antiarrhythmic and toxic effects of digitalis. *Am. Heart J.* 89:391 (1975b).

Ryan, M. J., Tmete, J., and Lown, B.: Evaluation of a new antiarrhythmic agent, disopyramide phosphate. *Circulation* 49, 50: (Suppl. I): 1-79 (Abstr.) (1974).

Sanna, G., and Arcidiacono, R.: Chemical ventricular defibrillation of the human heart. *Am. J. Cardiol.* 32:982 (1973).

Sano, T., Iida, W., and Yamagishi, S.: Changes in the spread of excitation from the sinus node induced by alterations in extracellular potassium. In *Electrophysiology and Ultrastructure of the Heart*, T. Sano, V. Mizuhira and K. Matsuda, eds. Grune & Stratton, Inc. New York (1967), p. 127.

Sano, T., Suzuki, F., Sato, S., and Iida, Y.: Mode of action of new antiarrhythmic agents. *Jap. Heart J.* 9:161 (1968).

Sasyniuk, B., and Dresel, P.: The effect of diphenylhydantoin on conduction in isolated blood perfused hearts. *J. Pharmacol. Exp. Ther.* 161:191 (1968).

Schamroth, L., Krikler, D. M., and Garrett, C.: Immediate effects of intravenous verapamil in cardiac arrhythmias. *Br. Med. J.* 224:73 (1972).

Scherlag, B., Helfant, R. H., and Damato, A. N.: The contrasting effects of diphenylhydantoin and procainamide on A-V conduction in the digitalis-intoxicated and the normal heart. *Am. Heart J.* 75:200 (1968).

Shigenobu, K., Kamiyama, A., Takagi, K., et al.: Membrane effects of pronethalol on the mammalian heart muscle fiber. *Jap. Heart J.* 7:494 (1966).

Singer, D. H., Lazzara, R., and Hoffman, B. F.: Interrelationship between automaticity and conduction in Purkinje fibers. *Circ. Res.* 21:537 (1967).

Singh, B. N.: A study of the pharmacological actions of certain drugs and hormones with particular reference to cardiac muscle. Ph.D. Thesis, Oxford University, Oxford (1971a).

Singh, B. N.: Comparative mechanisms of antiarrhythmic agents. *Am. J. Cardiol.* 28:240 (1971b).

Singh, B. N.: Explanation for the discrepancy in reported cardiac electrophysiological actions of diphenylhydantoin and lignocaine, *Br. J. Pharmacol.* 41:385P (1971c).

Singh, B. N., and Hauswirth, O.: Comparative mechanisms of action of antiarrhythmic drugs. *Am. Heart J.* 87:367 (1974).

Singh, B. N., and Vaughan Williams, E. M.: The effect of amiodarone, a new antianginal drug on cardiac muscle. *Br. J. Pharmacol.* 39:657 (1970).

Singh, B. N., and Vaughn Williams, E. M.: Effect of altering potassium concentration on the action of lidocaine and diphenylhydantoin on rabbit atrial and ventricular muscle. *Circ. Res.* 29:286 (1971).

Slama, R., Foucault, J. P., and Bouvrain, Y.: Le traitement d'urgence des troubles du rythme cardiaque par l'ajmaline intraveineuse. *Presse Méd.* 71:2250 (1963).

Stern, S.: Synergistic action of propranolol with quinidine. *Am. Heart J.* 72:569 (1966).

Stern, S.: Conversion of chronic atrial fibrillation to sinus rhythm with combined propranolol. *Am. Heart J.* 74:170 (1967).

Stern, S.: Treatment and prevention of cardiac arrhythmias with propranolol and quinidine. *Br. Heart J.* 33:522 (1971).

Strauss, H. C., Bigger, J. T., Jr., Bassett, A. L., and Hoffman, B. F. Actions of diphenylhydantoin on the electrical properties of isolated rabbit and canine atria. *Circ. Res.* 23:463 (1968).

Stutz, H., Feigelson, E., Emerson, J., and Bing, R. J.: The effect of digitalis (cedilanid) on the mechanical and electrical activity of extracted and non-extracted heart muscle preparations. *Circ. Res.* 2:555 (1954).

Surawicz, B.: Electrolytes and the electrocardiogram. *Am. J. Cardiol.* 12:656 (1963).

Van Durme, J. P., Bogaert, M. G., and Rosseel, M. T.: Effectiveness of aprindine, procainamide, and quinidine in chronic ventricular dysrhythmias. *Circulation* 50 (Suppl. III): 248 (Abstr.) (1974).

Vassalle, M., Karis, J., and Hoffman, B. F.: Toxic effects of ouabain on Purkinje fibers and ventricular muscle fibers. *Am. J. Physiol.* 203:433 (1962).

Vaughan Williams, E. M.: Classification of antiarrhythmic drugs. In *Symposium on Cardiac Arrhythmias*, E. Sandoe, E. Flensted-Jensen and K. H. Olsen, eds. A. B. Astra, Sodertalje, Sweden (1970), pp. 449-472.

Vismara, L. A., Mason, D. T., and Amsterdam, R. A.: Disopyramide phosphate: Clinical efficacy of a new oral antiarrhythmic drug. *Clin. Pharmacol. Ther.* 16:330 (1974).

Watanabe, Y.: Antagonism and synergism of potassium and antiarrhythmic agents. In *Electrolytes and Cardiovascular Diseases*, E. Bajusz, ed. S. Karger, Basel (1965), pp. 86-100.

Watanabe, Y.: Effects of electrolytes and antiarrhythmic drugs on atrioventricular conduction. In *Symposium on Cardiac Arrhythmias*, E. Sandoe, E. Flensted-Jensen and K. H. Olesen, eds. A. B. Astra, Sodertalje, Sweden (1970), pp. 535-557.

Watanabe, Y., de Azevedo, I. M., and Dreifus, L. S.: Electrophysiologic antagonism of quinidine and bretylium tosylate. *Circulation* 45, 46 (Suppl. II): 40 (1972).

Watanabe, Y., and Dreifus, L. S.: Inhomogeneous conduction in the AV node: A model for reentry. *Am. Heart J.* 70:505 (5965).

Watanabe, Y., and Dreifus, L. S.: Electrophysiologic effects of digitalis on A-V transmission. *Am. J. Physiol.* 211:1461 (1966).

Watanabe, Y., and Dreifus, L. S.: Interactions of quinidine and potassium on atrioventricular transmission, *Circ. Res.* 20:434 (1967).

Watanabe, Y., and Dreifus, L. S.: Sites of impulse formation within the atrioventricular junction of the rabbit. *Circ. Res.* 22:717 (1968).

Watanabe, Y., and Dreifus, L. S.: Interactions of lanatoside C and potassium on atrioventricular conduction in rabbits. *Circ. Res.* 27:931 (1970).

Watanabe, Y., and Dreifus, L. S.: Levels of concealment in second degree and advanced second degree A-V block. *Am. Heart J.* 84:330 (1972a).

Watanabe, Y., and Dreifus, L. S.: Electrophysiological effects of magnesium and its interactions with potassium. *Cardiovasc. Res.* 6:79 (1972b).

Watanabe, Y., Dreifus, L. S., and Likoff, W.: Electrophysiologic antagonism and synergism of potassium and antiarrhythmic agents. *Am. J. Cardiol.* 12:702 (1963).

Watanabe, Y., Dreifus, L. S., McGarry, T. F., and Likoff, W.: Electrophysiologic antagonism of potassium and antiarrhythmic agents. *Circulation* 26:799 (1962).

Watanabe, Y., Josipovic, V., and Dreifus, L. S.: Electrophysiological mechanisms of bretylium tosylate. *Fed. Proc.* 28:270 (Abstr.) (1969).

Weidmann, S.: Effects of calcium ions and local anesthetics on electrical properties of Purkinje fibers. *J. Physiol.* (Lond.) 129:568 (1955).

Weidmann, S.: Elektrophysiologie der Herzmuskelfaser. Hans Huber Medical Publisher, Bern (1956), p. 42.

West, T. C., and Amory, D. W. Single fiber recording of the effects of quinidine at atrial and pacemaker sites in the isolated right atrium of the rabbit. *J. Pharmacol. Exp. Ther.* 130:183 (1960).

Williams, D.: Treatment of epilepsy with sodium diphenylhydantoinate, *Lancet* 2:678 (1939).

Wit, A. L., and Cranefield, P. F.: Verapamil inhibition of the slow response; A mechanism for its effectiveness against reentrant AV nodal tachycardia. *Circulation* 50 (Suppl. III): 146 (1974).

Wit, A. L., Rosen, M. R., and Hoffman, B. F.: Electrophysiology and pharmacology of cardiac arrhythmias. II. Relationship of normal and abnormal electrical activity of cardiac fibers to the genesis of arrhythmias. A. Automaticity. *Am. Heart J.* 88:515 (1974a).

Wit, A. L., Rosen, M. R., and Hoffman, B. G.: Electrophysiology and pharmacology of cardiac arrhythmias. II. Relationship of normal and abnormal electrical activity of cardiac fibers to the genesis of arrhythmias B. Re-entry. Sections I, II. *Am. Heart J.* 88:64, 798 (1974b).

Wit, A. L., Steiner, C., and Damato, A. N.: Electrophysiologic effects of bretylium tosylate on single fibers of the canine specialized conducting system and ventricle. *J. Pharmacol. Exp. Ther.* 173:344 (1970a).

Wit, A. L., Weiss, M. B., Berkowitz, W. D., Rosen, K. M., Steiner, C., and Damato, A. N.: Patterns of atrioventricular conduction in the human heart. *Circ. Res.* 27:345 (1970b).

Wittig, J., Harrison, L. A., and Wallace, A. G.: Electrophysiological effects of lidocaine on distal Purkinje fibers of canine heart. *Am. Heart J.* 86:69 (1973).

Woodbury, L. A., and Hecht, H. H.: Effects of cardiac glycosides upon electrical activity of single ventricular fibers of the frog heart, and their relation to the digitalis effect of the electrocardiogram. *Circulation* 6:172 (1952).

Zipes, D. P., Nobel, R. J., Carmichael, R. T., Rowell, H., and Fasola, A. F.: Relations between aprindine concentration [APR] heart rate, ischemia, and ventricular fibrillation (VF) in dogs. *Am. J. Cardiol.* 35:179 (Abstr.) (1975).

Pathophysiology and Therapeutics of Myocardial Ischemia

5

Role of the Adrenergic Nervous System in Arrhythmia Produced by Acute Coronary Artery Occlusion

CLAIRE M. LATHERS
GERALD J. KELLIHER
JAY ROBERTS
ANDREW B. BEASLEY

INTRODUCTION

The importance of neural factors in the development of arrhythmias associated with acute coronary occlusion has been discussed by many investigators. In 1963, Costantin made recordings from postganglionic sympathetic nerves in decerebrate cats and noted that the neural discharge associated with the initial drop in blood pressure produced by coronary artery occlusion was decreased in 3 cats and showed no change in 2 additional animals. In the late 1960's and early 1970's, two reports appeared in the literature, describing neural changes in cat preganglionic sympathetic nerves. Malliani et al. (1969) noted that the discharge activity in a majority of nerves increased, although in a few it decreased or showed no change when coronary artery occlusion was produced. In contrast, Gillis (1971) reported that neural discharge increased after coronary artery occlusion and that this increased nerve activity was associated with occlusion-induced arrhythmia. In 1972, Webb et al. observed a high incidence of autonomic disturbance in the acute phase of a coronary attack, in humans, and considered this an important factor in rhythm disturbances occurring in this early period. More recently, Armour et al. (1972) also has stressed that cardiac rhythm disturbances in the cat can be induced by autonomic imbalance.

In addition to the "autonomic imbalance" associated with coronary occlusion-induced arrhythmias, the currently available antiarrhythmic agents have been shown not to be as effective against the fatal rhythm disturbances occurring immediately after myocardial infarction as they are later on when the patient reaches the coronary care unit. For instance, Pantridge and Adgey (1969) reported that lidocaine did not always reverse arrhythmias when the patient was seen within one-half hour of the onset of symptoms. Gamble and Cohn (1972) noted that lidocaine failed to abolish coronary occlusion-induced arrhythmias in 65% of the cats examined. In addition, Lawrence and Kelliher (personal communication) showed that, in cats, intermittent doses of lidocaine did not prevent arrhythmia and death after acute occlusion of the left anterior descending artery. Finally, in 1976, Corr et al. noted that procainamide resulted in a greater incidence of ectopic beats and ventricular fibrillation, in the cat, after acute coronary artery occlusion.

The purpose of this study was twofold. The first series of experiments, conducted in the cat, were designed to determine the role of the postganglionic sympathetic neural innervation to the heart in the production of arrhythmias induced by acute occlusion of the left anterior descending artery. The second phase of this research evaluated the effect of two currently used antiarrhythmic agents, lidocaine and procainamide, on the postganglionic sympathetic neural discharge at the time of acute occlusion-induced arrhythmia.

METHODS

Adult cats of either sex, weighing between 2.5-4.5 kg, were anesthetized with α-chloralose (80 mg/kg, i.v.). The trachea was cannulated and the animals were ventilated with a mixture of O_2 and room air, using a respirator set at a rate of 18 breaths/min. The femoral arteries were then cannulated to monitor mean arterial blood pressure and to collect arterial blood samples at 10 min intervals. Arterial blood pH was maintained between 7.4 and 7.5 by monitoring pO_2 and pCO_2 levels with a blood gas analyzer (Instrumentation Laboratories, Model 113), and adjusting the percentage of O_2 in the inspired air. The femoral vein was cannulated for drug administration, atropine (2 mg/kg) was infused slowly to prevent vagal efferent activity, and gallamine (2 mg/kg) was given periodically to impede spontaneous muscle movement from interfering with the electrical recordings. Body temperature was monitored on a Yellow Springs telethermometer, using a rectal temperature probe, and was maintained at 37-38°C by a hot-water pad (K-Aquamatic).

The chest was opened on the left side between the fourth and fifth ribs. The pericardium was opened, the left anterior descending artery was isolated, and a tie was placed at the origin, ready for the occlusion. The clavicle and first five ribs on the right side were then resected to allow identification of the right stellate ganglion. The right cardiac postganglionic sympathetic nerve fibers were isolated to allow electrical recordings of the nervous activity in the small nerve branches. A pool was formed by tying the cut ends of the ribs, the clavicle, and the skin flaps to a flexaframe support. Oxygenated mineral oil, maintained at 37.5°C by an appropriate thermoregulator, was then added to the pool.

The nerve branches were initially identified as sympathetic nerves by determining their discharge response to an injection of histamine (5 µg/kg, i.v.) as shown in Fig. 1. Nervous activity was elicited by reflex, using a method described by Kelliher and Roberts (1973), in which the drop in blood pressure is produced by histamine. This method identified the recorded nerves as being sympathetic since it has been reported previously that a drop in blood pressure elicits neural discharge via the baroreceptor reflex. Afferent discharge originating from the heart was eliminated by crushing the nerve distal to the recording electrode; the effect of the parasympathetic nervous system on the heart was abolished by the administration of atropine. A nerve-activity ratio (NAR) was computed to relate the changes in nerve discharge with changes in blood pressure, which occurred during the experiment. The nerve-activity ratio was calculated by determining the mean spontaneous discharge (determined by inspection) during a 1 min interval and dividing this by the existing mean arterial blood pressure.

Adrenergic nerve activity was recorded from 1-3 postganglionic cardiac accelerator nerve branches placed on platinum bipolar recording electrodes connected to a Tektronix 122 differential pre-

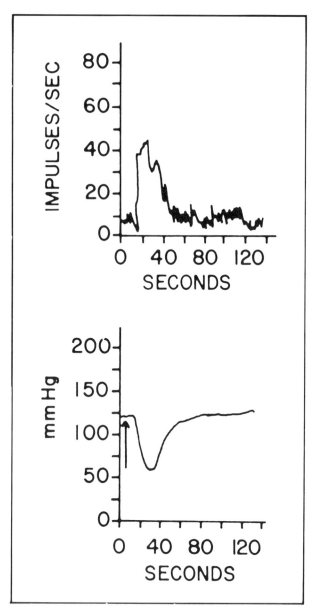

1 Histamine-evoked neural discharge. In the upper graph, postganglionic cardiac accelerator neural discharge in impulses/sec is plotted as a function of time (in sec). In the lower graph, mean arterial blood pressure in mm Hg is presented as a function of time (in sec). The arrow indicates an injection of histamine (5 μg/kg, i.v.). This injection produced a fall in blood pressure that was accompanied by an increase in neural discharge. As the blood pressure began to rise, the nerve activity fell to the pre-injection level.

amplifier. The output of the preamplifier was displayed oscillo-graphically and entered a differential amplitude discriminator. The output of the differential amplitude discriminator was then fed into an integrating circuit which converted mean impulses/sec into DC voltage, and was displayed on a Polygraph (Grass, Model 7), along with mean arterial blood pressure, at a paper speed of 0.25 mm/sec. A sine-wave signal generator, fed into the differential ampli-tude discriminator, provided a calibration signal over the range of 30 to 100 Hz, in 10 Hz increments after each experiment. Since a single efferent unit is not being recorded from, the range of 30 to 100 Hz is inclusive of the experimental values recorded. Lead II ECG was taped, using a suitable tape recorder and, at a later date, was printed on polygraph paper at a speed of 25 mm/sec. The signal from the differential amplitude discriminator was also taped during the experiment.

The stability of the nervous activity as a function of time was determined in a control group ($N = 4$) for 60 min. In the occlusion experiments, 10 min of control spontaneous discharge was always monitored before the artery was occluded.

Statistical analysis was carried out by establishing a 95% confidence interval from the control group for a period of 15 min (Goldstein, 1964). In the experimental group, examined after cor-onary occlusion, nerve-activity ratios determined in the minute be-fore arrhythmia, which were above or below the limits of the con-fidence interval, were considered to be significantly different from control. These values were then placed in either the increased or decreased category of neural activity.

Lidocaine (2 mg/kg, i.v.) or procainamide (5 mg/kg, i.v.) were given as bolus injections alone or within a few seconds after occlusion to determine their effects on both cardiac rhythm and postganglionic cardiac accelerator nerve discharge.

The drugs used in this study were histamine phosphate (Lilly) ; atropine sulfate (K and K Labs) ; a-chloralose (Fisher) ; Flaxedil (Gallamine, Davis and Geck) ; lidocaine hydrochloride (Astra) ; and procainamide hydrochloride (Squibb). The doses used are ex-pressed in terms of the salt.

RESULTS

Control Neural Discharge

Nerve activity from 10 nerves, recorded from 4 cats, was mon-itored as a function of time and the data are summarized in Fig. 2.

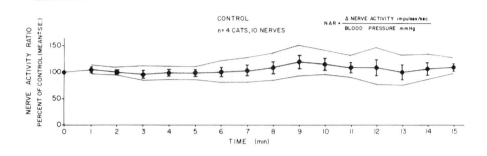

2 Control data in which the nerve-activity ratio [percentage of control (mean ± S.E.)] is given as a function of time (in min). The shaded area represents the 95% confidence limits in this and in Figs. 3, 4, and 5.

The 95% confidence limits were established and are represented by the shaded area in this figure as well as in Figs. 3, 4, and 5. Not shown in this figure is control nerve activity which was monitored for 60 min; however, it was just as stable. The 15 min interval shown in Fig. 2 is the period of time that will be discussed in the following experiments in which the coronary artery was occluded, since arrhythmia and/or ventricular fibrillation always developed during this interval. Note the stability of the preparation throughout the 15 min period.

Neural Activity and Coronary Occlusion-
Induced Arrhythmia

In the next series of experiments, spontaneous discharge was monitored in one postganglionic cardiac accelerator branch before and after the left anterior descending coronary artery was occluded by a tie. The nerve-activity ratio, expressed as a percentage of the control, is plotted as a function of time (in min) in Fig. 3. Data collected from 3 different cats are illustrated. The coronary vessel was occluded at zero time. The triangles represent the increased neural activity obtained in a cat which died in ventricular fibrillation 2 min after the occlusion. The other graphs were obtained from 2 cats that developed arrhythmia but did not die. The nerve-activity ratio (NAR) value increased in one nerve (circles) prior to ar-

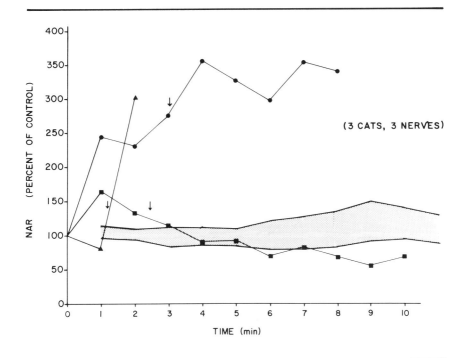

3

Effect of coronary occlusion on spontaneous neural discharge.
Nerve-activity ratio (percentage of control) was calculated after
recording from 3 postganglionic cardiac accelerator nerves in 3
cats. The nerve-activity ratio, percentage of control, is plotted as a
function of time (in min). Occlusion was produced at zero time.
The arrows indicate the time at which arrhythmia developed. The
shaded area represents the 95% confidence limits of the control.

rhythmia. In the third cat, arrhythmia developed 2 min, 28 sec
after the occlusion. The associated neural discharge (squares) was
increased above control; it then began to gradually decrease over
the next 7 min.

Neural activity was also recorded from two or three cardiac
accelerator branches simultaneously in another group of cats before
and after the coronary artery was completely occluded by a tie. The
mean time to arrhythmia for the 8 cats was 0.9 ± 0.4 min. Representative experiments from two animals are shown in Fig. 4. The
coronary vessel was occluded at zero time. In the upper graph, ar-

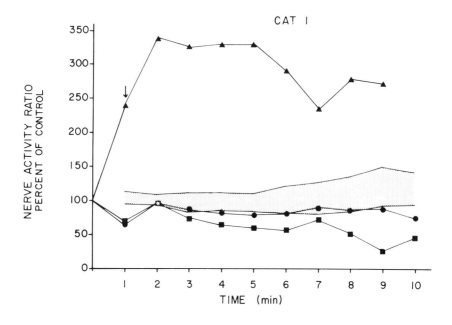

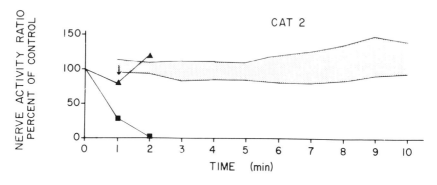

4   Spontaneous discharge, monitored as a function of time, after an acute occlusion of the left anterior descending artery at time 0. The nerve-activity ratio, percentage of control, is shown as a function of time (in min). In the upper graph, the neural discharge was monitored in 3 postganglionic cardiac accelerator branches simultaneously; neural activity was monitored from 2 nerves in a second cat in the lower graph. The arrow indicates the appearance of arrhythmia. The shaded area represents the 95% confidence limits of the control.

Table 1. Effect of coronary artery occlusion on the spontaneous
discharge of postganglionic cardiac accelerator nerves
just prior to arrhythmia

	Percentage of Nerves*
Increase†	47%
Decrease†	40%
No change	13%

*N = 8 cats, 15 nerves.
†Significantly different at the 95% confidence limit.

rhythmia developed 1 min after the occlusion; the nerve activity
associated with arrhythmia increased in one nerve (triangles) and
was depressed in the other two. In the lower graph, arrhythmia
also developed 1 min after occlusion; the associated neural activity
was depressed in both nerves, although in one of them it (squares)
was depressed to a much greater extent. The neural discharge represented by the triangles subsequently increased. Thus a non-
uniform neural discharge was associated with occlusion-induced
arrhythmia, i.e., in some nerves it increased, in others it decreased,
and in some it showed no change. Neural discharge was monitored
in 15 nerves (8 cats) for the minute prior to the development of
the arrhythmia; the data are summarized in Table 1. Mean time
to arrhythmia was approximately 1 min.

Neural Activity and Lack of Arrhythmia after
Coronary Occlusion

When postganglionic cardiac accelerator discharge was monitored in 4 cats that did not develop arrhythmia after the coronary
artery was occluded, the lack of non-uniform neural discharge
within the first 3 min after occlusion was apparent. Representative
data of this relationship are shown for one animal in Fig. 5; the
other three experiments showed a very similar pattern. It should be
emphasized that, if arrhythmia developed, it generally occurred
within the first 3 min.

Examination of three of the hearts obtained from the cats
which did not develop arrhythmia after occlusion of the coronary
artery by latex injection revealed that, in all of the hearts, significant circulation existed which was not occluded by the tie (Fig. 6).

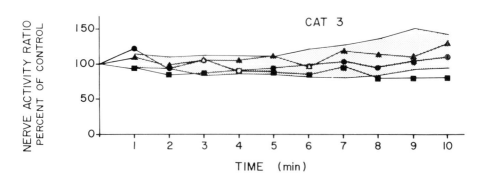

NERVE ACTIVITY RATIO
PERCENT OF CONTROL

150

100

50

0

CAT 3

TIME (min)

1 2 3 4 5 6 7 8 9 10

5   Spontaneous discharge monitored as a function of time after an acute occlusion of the left anterior descending artery at time 0. The axes are the same as in Fig. 4. Arrhythmia did not develop. The shaded area represents the 95% confidence limits.

It should be noted that the tie definitely occluded the left anterior descending artery of the heart shown in the lower portion of the figure. However, the collateral extending from the left circumflex artery appeared to be large enough to deliver a sufficient blood supply to the area of the myocardium, which prevented the development of arrhythmia.

In contrast, in cats that developed arrhythmia, the ties definitely included the left anterior descending artery and its collaterals. This suggests that the production of arrhythmia after coronary occlusion is at least partially related to the extent to which the collaterals have been occluded by the tie.

Standard Deviation of Mean Nerve Activity Ratios (NAR)

The standard deviation indicates how values deviate from the mean, i.e., a small standard deviation shows that most values did not deviate much from the mean, while a large value denotes that many of the results deviated from the mean. Therefore, to determine how the standard deviation of mean NAR values varied in each experimental group, the mean NAR ± the standard deviation was calculated. In Fig. 7, the mean NAR (expressed as a percentage of control, ± the standard deviation) is plotted as a function of

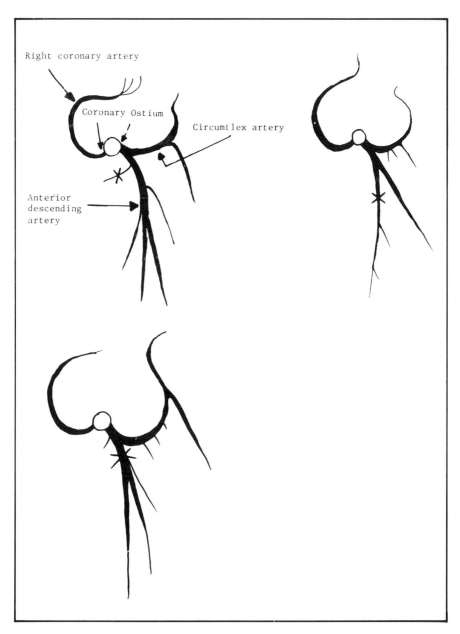

6 Diagrams of coronary vasculature from cats which did not develop arrhythmia after occlusion. Latex was injected at the end of the experiment to delineate the vasculature and drawings were made. The **X**'s represent the site of occlusion.

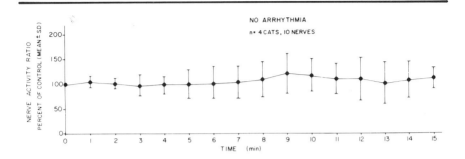

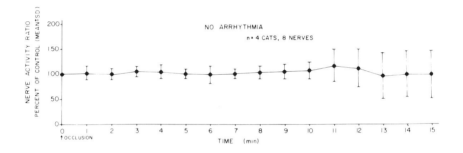

7 Spontaneous discharge monitored as a function of time. The nerve-activity ratio (percentage of control, mean ± standard deviation) is given as a function of time (in min) for both graphs. The data in the upper graph was obtained in the control group of animals; the data in the lower one pertains to the 4 cats which did not develop arrhythmia after coronary occlusion.

time (in min) for two groups of animals. The graph in the upper portion of the figure represents a control, obtained in 4 cats (10 nerves), and illustrates the effect of time on neural discharge. Note the stability of the preparation. A similar pattern was obtained when neural activity was monitored, in 4 cats, where in the 8 nerves tested occlusion failed to produce arrhythmia (lower graph). The standard deviation of the mean NAR for the two groups of animals shown in Fig. 7 is expressed as a function of time (in min) in Fig. 8. The small standard deviation obtained in both the controls (upper graph) and in the group with occlusion but no arrhythmia (lower graph) indicates that the population of nerves examined

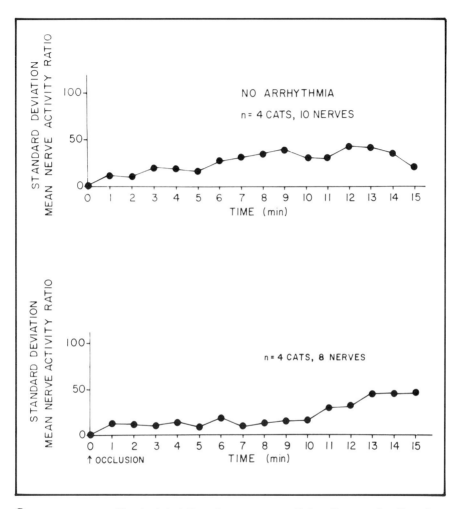

8   Standard deviation of mean nerve-activity ratios as a function of
time (in min) for the two groups of animals described in Fig. 7.

contained a high proportion of values which did not deviate greatly
from the mean.

In contrast are the data shown in the lower graph of Fig. 9.
The standard deviation of the mean nerve activity ratio is plotted
here as a function of time (in min) for 15 nerves monitored in 8
cats. A large standard deviation was associated with the mean time
required for arrhythmia to occur (approximately 1 min). The large

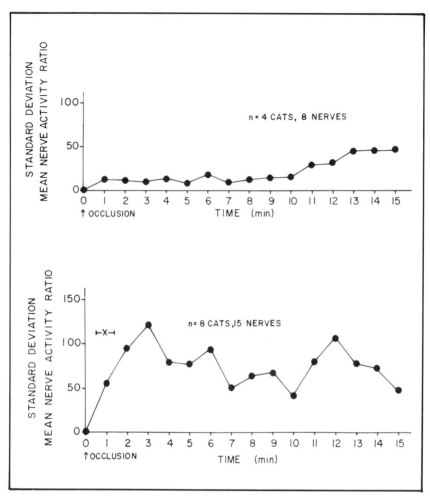

9 Standard deviation of mean nerve-activity ratios as a function of time (in min). Occlusion was performed at time 0 for both groups of animals; arrhythmia (indicated by /-x-/ in this and all subsequent figures) developed only in the 8 animals depicted in the lower graph.

standard deviation indicates that the population of nerves examined contained a high proportion of values that deviated considerably from the mean, i.e., the neural discharge associated with occlusion-induced arrhythmia increased in one group of nerves, decreased in a second, and showed little or no change in a third group. Thus a non-uniform neural discharge was associated with occlusion-induced arrhythmia.

Effect of Lidocaine on Neural Discharge Associated with Occlusion-Induced Arrhythmia

It was considered appropriate to determine whether two drugs commonly used as antiarrhythmic agents, lidocaine and procainamide, would prevent the development of non-uniform neural discharge and the associated occlusion-induced arrhythmia. The upper graph in Fig. 10 depicts the effect of lidocaine (2 mg/kg, i.v. given at 0 time) on postganglionic cardiac accelerator discharge determined in 3 cats in which occlusion of the left anterior descending artery was not performed. Little or no change occurred in the standard deviation, especially in the first minute (the mean time to arrhythmia in the group of cats with occlusion). Conversely, the lower graph, shows a large standard deviation 4 min after coronary occlusion, which was associated with arrhythmia, even though lidocaine (2 mg/kg, i.v.) was injected as a bolus at the time of occlusion (0 min). This dose of lidocaine significantly increased the time to arrhythmia from 0.9 ± 0.4 to 4.2 ± 1.3 min ($p < 0.05$); however, a non-uniform neural discharge was associated with the arrhythmia when it finally occurred. The incidence of death (3 of 8) was the same for the group of cats not receiving lidocaine.

Effect of Procainamide on Neural Discharge Associated with Occlusion-Induced Arrhythmia

The effect of procainamide (5 mg/kg, i.v.), given at zero time, on postganglionic cardiac accelerator discharge was determined in 3 cats in which neural activity was monitored in 8 nerves. Procainamide itself altered neural discharge by either increasing and/or decreasing it. In the case of 3 nerves the results were above the 95% confidence limits, in 1 nerve they were below, and in 4, they were not significantly different in the 3rd min after the injection of procainamide. The time involved is equivalent to the minute preceding the mean time it takes for arrhythmia to occur in cats receiving procainamide at the moment of occlusion. This effect is noted by the large standard deviation seen in the upper graph of Fig. 11. When procainamide was given at the time of the occlusion (lower graph in Fig. 11), no further neural changes took place and arrhythmia developed. However, as with lidocaine, the mean time to arrhythmia was significantly increased from 0.9 ± 0.4 to $4.0 \pm$

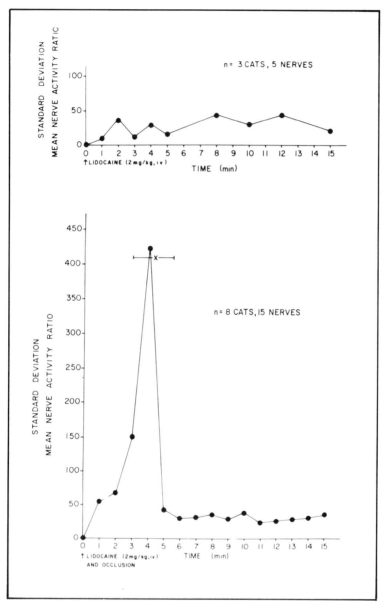

10 Standard deviation of mean nerve-activity ratios presented as a function of time (in min). In the upper graph, a bolus injection of lidocaine (2 mg/kg, i.v.) was injected at time 0. Nerve activity was monitored in 5 nerves of 3 cats. The drug did not induce arrhythmia. In the lower graph, the bolus injection of lidocaine (2 mg/kg, i.v.) was given at the time of occlusion. Mean time to arrhythmia was approximately 4 min.

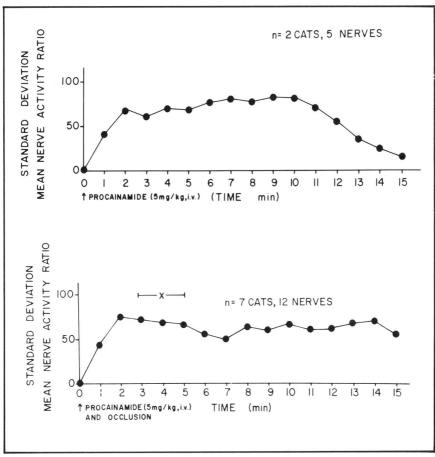

11 Standard deviation of mean nerve-activity ratios plotted as a function of time (in min). In the upper graph, a bolus injection of procainamide (5 mg/kg, i.v.) was injected at time 0. The drug itself did not induce arrhythmia. In the lower graph, the bolus injection of procainamide was given at the time of occlusion. Mean time to arrhythmia was approximately 4 min.

1.1 min (p < 0.05). It is important to note that none of the 7 cats died after occlusion.

Comparison of the Anatomy of the Coronary Collateral Vasculature in Animals Treated with Lidocaine or Procainamide

Examination of two hearts (Fig. 12A) obtained from cats that died in ventricular fibrillation after coronary artery occlusion, even though they received a bolus injection of lidocaine (2 mg/kg, i.v.),

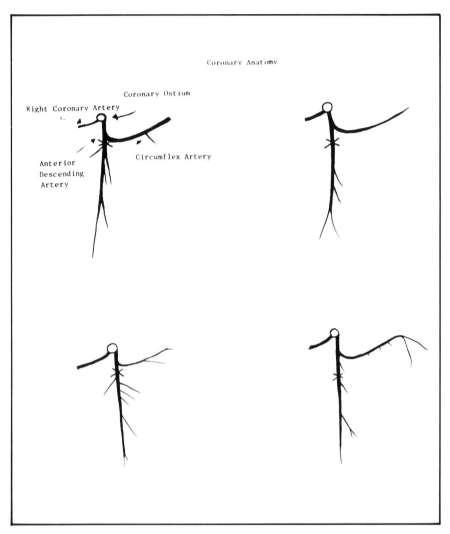

Coronary Anatomy

Coronary Ostium

Right Coronary Artery

Circumflex Artery

Anterior
Descending
Artery

12 Diagrams in the upper portion of the figure are of coronary vasculature from cats which died of ventricular fibrillation after acute coronary occlusion, even though a bolus injection of lidocaine (2 mg/kg, i.v.) was given at the time of the occlusion. Diagrams in the lower part are of coronary vasculature from cats which did not die of ventricular fibrillation after acute occlusion and a bolus injection of procainamide (5 mg/kg, i.v.). Method and labeling as in Fig. 6.

Table 2. Spontaneous discharge of postganglionic cardiac accelerator nerves just prior to arrhythmia produced by coronary occlusion

	Coronary Occlusion* Percentage of Nerves	Lidocaine* (2 mg/kg, i.v.) Coronary Occlusion Percentage of Nerves	Procainamide** (5 mg/kg, i.v.) Coronary Occlusion Percentage of Nerves
Increase†	47%	60%	67%
Decrease†	40%	27%	8%
No change	13%	13%	25%

* N = 8 cats, 15 nerves.

** N = 7 cats, 12 nerves.

† Significantly different at the 95% confidence limits.

revealed that the anatomy, in particular, the small circumflex artery, was very similar to that observed in two hearts (Fig. 12B) obtained from animals that developed occlusion-induced arrhythmias but did not die after procainamide (5 mg/kg, i.v.).

Comparison of Lidocaine and Procainamide on Neural Discharge Associated with Occlusion-Induced Arrhythmia

The effects of lidocaine and procainamide on uniformity of discharge were examined after coronary occlusion and the results are summarized in Table 2. After lidocaine, more nerves responded with an increase and fewer with a decrease in discharge, when compared with the group of animals receiving no drugs. After procainamide, the number of nerves in which increased discharge occurred remained about the same as in the lidocaine group, i.e., 67% vs. 60%, but the number of nerves increased in which discharge was not affected (25%) and fewer nerves responded with a reduced discharge (8%). Thus, the distribution of the occlusion-induced non-uniform neural discharge was altered but not prevented by lidocaine or procainamide.

DISCUSSION

The results of the present study clearly establish that non-uniform neural discharge in postganglionic cardiac accelerator nerves is associated with and may be a mechanism involved in the production of ventricular rhythm disturbances produced by coronary artery occlusion. When recordings were obtained simultaneously from two or three postganglionic branches in the same cat, the onset of occlusion-induced arrhythmias coincided with nonuniform changes in the direction (i.e., increases, decreases, and/or no change) and/or magnitude of spontaneous discharge. Recordings from one postganglionic sympathetic branch in each cat revealed that, prior to occlusion-induced arrhythmia, an increase, a decrease, or no change in spontaneous activity could occur in any one of these animals. These data suggest that neural recordings from one postganglionic cardiac accelerator branch do not reflect the neural discharge in other postganglionic branches in the same cat. The discrepancies in reports of other authors may be partly attributed to the fact that in previous studies, activity had been recorded only in one branch in each animal. This non-uniform neural discharge may be reflected in the heart as non-uniform changes in excitability and conduction. Non-uniform neural discharge and arrhythmia did not develop in animals where the left anterior descending artery was not totally occluded, nor was it found in one cat with total left anterior descending artery occlusion (Fig. 6). This would, therefore, suggest that the extent of occlusion (by tie) of the collaterals is not the sole factor involved in the subsequent arrhythmias and death.

Whether the observed rises in neural discharge are due to increased firing of the original population of nerve fibers or due to the recruitment of additional fibers could not be differentiated in the present experiments. This augmented frequency may be explained by shorter inter spike intervals or by an increased duration of the burst discharge pattern. Thus, in each nerve branch, this pattern may be altered as arrhythmia develops. However, in order to resolve this problem, bursting discharge patterns in control situations must be analyzed in many nerve branches to determine if a definite control pattern does exist.

The non-uniform response of the adrenergic nervous system, which coincides with arrhythmia produced by coronary occlusion, may result from increased afferent discharge to the central nervous system (CNS). The afferent activity may originate within the cardiac muscle as ischemia develops (Malliani et al., 1969). In turn, in the cat, the CNS may increase neural activity via the spinal segments T_1 to mid-T_8 of the thoracolumbar intermediolateral nucleus of the right side (Henry and Calaresa, 1972), producing altered neural discharge in the postganglionic cardiac accelerator nerve branches. It is unlikely that increased afferent activity was responsible for the results of our study since the nerve branches were cut distal to the recording electrode, eliminating any contribution of afferent discharge to the recordings.

The central nervous system may not be the sole mechanism which accounts for the non-uniform neural discharge reported in these studies. Costantin (1963) found increased activity or no change in postganglionic sympathetic nerves after occlusion in decerebrate cats. However, this does not preclude other areas of the CNS from being involved in this response. Thus, one might attribute the non-uniform neural effect, which coincides with occlusion-induced arrhythmia, to the local cardiac reflex described by Malliani et al. (1969), i.e., cardiac afferent activity, initiated by an ischemic response, travels to the stellate ganglia and directly back to the heart via the postganglionic sympathetic nerves.

Finally, it is well known that a drop in blood pressure normally elicits an increased neural discharge in cardiac accelerator nerves. In fact, we make use of this phenomenon to identify and confirm that the nerve we are recording from is sympathetic. Since there is a drop in blood pressure during the first few minutes after coronary occlusion, it is likely that some of the increased neural responses may be explained by this physiological mechanism. The important point is, however, that all nerves show a rise in discharge in response to a lowering in blood pressure, during the control phase of the experiment, but in only 47% is there an increase when the blood pressure drops after coronary occlusion, while in 13% and 40% no change or a decrease, respectively, are found.

Supporting anatomical evidence for the production of arrhythmia by a non-uniform postganglionic cardiac accelerator discharge includes reports that the distribution of the adrenergic nerve fibers in the heart is not uniform (Dahlström et al., 1965); the sinoatrial (SA) and atrioventricular (AV) nodes, and selected areas of the atria and ventricular myocardium receive extensive adrenergic innervation which is lacking in other parts of the myocardium. Dahlström called this type of innervation "patchy." Adrenergic innervation of the Purkinje fibers has also been demonstrated to be sparse or missing altogether in large numbers of these fibers. Excitation of selected nerve filaments induced responses in highly localized regions of the heart (Szentivany et al., 1967; Randall et al., 1968), while stimulation of the left stellate ganglion resulted in little or no change in the conduction velocity of Purkinje tissue (Wallace and Sarnoff, 1964). It should be noted that electrical stimulation of individual cardiac nerves has been shown to produce arrhythmia by Raper and Wale (1969), and Armour et al. (1972).

More recently, Dahlström's concept of "patchy" adrenergic innervation of the myocardium was challenged by Ellison (1974) who found that this type of innervation was evenly distributed in the atria and ventricles, and, therefore, could not be classified as "patchy." Nevertheless, if the neural recordings described in this paper were obtained from branches terminating in different areas of the heart, i.e., atria vs. ventricle, or SA node vs. ventricle, or different areas of a Purkinje fiber, etc., then non-uniform excitability and conduction effects could still be imposed on the various areas of the heart to produce arrhythmia.

In spite of the origin or cause of the occlusion-induced non-uniform neural discharge, it should be noted that we are hypothesizing that the non-uniform neural discharge is manifest in the ventricular structures as non-uniform excitability and conduction, which then produce the ventricular arrhythmias in the manner described by Han and Moe in 1964. Han and co-workers (Han, 1969a, 1969b; Han et al., 1970) recently expanded this hypothesis to indicate that non-uniformity in ventricular structures will lead to occlusion-induced re-entrant arrhythmias. Additional data that provide supporting evidence for non-uniform changes in cardiac muscle, associated with occlusion-induced arrhythmia, was published by Nagy et al. (1975). They recorded monophasic action potentials in four neighboring areas in non-infarcted and in ischemic tissue and found that "inhomogeneity" developed in the repolarization time when the potentials were recorded from the ischemic cardiac muscle.

The dose of lidocaine used (2 mg/kg, i.v.) did not prevent arrhythmia or decrease the incidence of ventricular fibrillation after acute occlusion. This confirms the data of Gamble and Cohn (1972) and Lawrence and Kelliher (personal communication). Recently, Borer et al. (1976) have reported that lidocaine pretreatment reduces significantly the occurrence of ventricular fibrillation after coronary artery ligation in the dog. However, it should be noted that, in their animals, these investigators ligated both the left anterior descending and septal arteries, and that this resulted in fibrillation in 87% of these dogs. Procainamide (5 mg/kg, i.v.) itself altered neural discharge. When given at the time of occlusion, no further neural changes occurred and arrhythmia developed, although no animals died from ventricular fibrillation. The failure of lidocaine and procainamide to abolish acute occlusion-induced arrhythmia may be explained by the fact that, in the doses used, these drugs did not prevent the non-uniform neural discharge associated with the development of arrhythmia.

In the case of lidocaine, a different dose regimen, i.e., pretreatment and/or higher doses, might have prevented the arrhythmia and the associated non-uniform neural discharge. Nevertheless, Lawrence and Kelliher (personal communication) used bolus injections of lidocaine (2, 4, or 6 mg/kg, i.v.), administered in a manner similar to that employed in the present study and noted that arrhythmia and/or death nevertheless followed occlusion. We used lidocaine (4 mg/kg, i.v.) as a bolus injection in two animals, and still noted arrhythmia and the associated non-uniform neural discharge. We are now in the process of determining lidocaine levels produced by the bolus injection of this drug (2 mg/kg, i.v.). We will attempt to obtain higher levels via a bolus and infusion method, to determine if this dose regimen will prevent occlusion-induced arrhythmia and the associated non-uniform neural discharge. Similar analyses will be performed with procainamide.

The time to arrhythmia was significantly increased after lidocaine and procainamide. This suggests that these drugs might be acting on the heart itself. The fact that no animals died in ventricular fibrillation after procainamide but did die after lidocaine, although both groups had very similar coronary vasculatures, suggests that the extent of the occlusion (by tie) of the collaterals is not the sole factor responsible for the subsequent arrhythmias.

Possibly, the size of the infarct was larger in the group receiving lidocaine than in that given procainamide; thus explaining, in part, the absence of ventricular fibrillation in the latter. The design of the present experiment did not allow us to determine infarct size and we were, therefore, not able to evaluate this possibility.

The experimental technique described in this paper involves an acute occlusion of the left anterior descending artery. Perhaps, this technique may provide a model for the pre-hospital phase of myocardial infarction. If this should be the case, then certain antiarrhythmic drugs may prove more effective in the pre-hospital phase while others could be more efficacious against arrhythmias which occur several hours after myocardial infarction, the period of time which often elapses before the patient reaches the hospital intensive care unit (McNeilly and Pemberton, 1968). On the basis of clinical experience, it has been suggested that lidocaine and procainamide are not effective immediately after coronary occlusion (Pantridge and Adgey, 1969). Our results, i.e., that lidocaine and procainamide, given immediately after coronary occlusion failed to prevent arrhythmia and the associated non-uniform neural discharge, may explain these clinical observations.

ACKNOWLEDGMENTS

This project was supported by the Pharmaceutical Manufacturers Association Faculty Development Award, the Merck Grant for Faculty Development, USPHS Grant HL 16283, and a grant from The American Heart Association, Southeastern Pennsylvania Chapter.

The authors would like to express their appreciation to Mr. Arnold Teres for his excellent technical assistance and to Ms. Christina Maya for her help in the preparation of this manuscript.

REFERENCES

Armour, J. A., Hageman, G. R., and Randall, W. C.: Arrhythmias induced by local cardiac nerve stimulation. *Am. J. Physiol.* 223:1068-1075 (1972).

Borer, J. S., Harrison, L. A., Kent, K. M., Levy, R., Goldstein, Robert, E., and Epstein, S. E.: Beneficial effect of lidocaine on ventricular electrical stability and spontaneous ventricular fibrillation during experimental myocardial infarction. *Am. J. Cardiol.* 37:860-863 (1976).

Corr, P. B., Helke, C. J., and Gillis, R. A.: Deleterious cardiac rhythm effect produced by the vagolytic action of procainamide in experimental myocardial infarction. *Am. J. Cardiol.* 37:128 (1976).

Costantin, L.: Extracardiac factors contributing to hypotension during coronary occlusion. *Am. J. Cardiol.* 11:205-217 (1963).

Dahlström, A., Fuxe, K., Mya-Tu, M., and Zetterstrom, B. E. M.: Observations on adrenergic innervation of dog heart. *Am. J. Physiol.* 209:689-692 (1965).

Ellison, J. P.: The adrenergic cardiac nerves of the cat. *Am. J. Anat.* 139: 209-226 (1974).

Gamble, O., and Cohn, K.: Effect of propranolol, procainamide, and lidocaine on ventricular automaticity and re-entry in experimental myocardial infarction. *Circulation* 46:498-506 (1972).

Gillis, R. A.: Role of the nervous system in the arrhythmias produced by coronary occlusion in the cat. *Am. Heart J.* 81:677-684 (1971).

Goldstein, A.: *Biostatistics: An Introductory Text.* New York, Macmillan Company (1964).

Han, J.: Mechanisms of ventricular arrhythmias associated with myocardial infarction. *Am. J. Cardiol.* 24:800-813 (1969a).

Han, J.: Ventricular vulnerability during acute coronary occlusion. *Am. J. Cardiol.* 24:857-864 (1969b).

Han, J., Goel, B., and Hanson, C. S.: Re-entrant beats induced in the ventricle during coronary occlusion. *Am. Heart J.* 80:778-784 (1970).

Han, J., and Moe, G. K.: Nonuniform recovery of excitability in ventricular muscle. *Circ. Res.* 14:44-60 (1964).

Henry, J. L., and Calaresa, F. R.: Distribution of cardioacceleratory sites in intermediolateral nucleus of the cat. *Am. J. Physiol.* 222:700-704 (1972).

Kelliher, G. J., and Roberts, J.: A comparison of the effects of sotalol and of the isomers of practolol on adrenergic nervous activity. *Life Sci.* 13:1231-1243 (1973).

Lawrence, T., and Kelliher, G. J.: *Personal communication.*

Malliani, A., Schwartz, P. J., and Zanchetti, A.: A sympathetic reflex elicited by experimental coronary occlusion. *Am. J. Physiol.* 217:703-709 (1969).

McNeilly, R. H., and Pemberton, J.: Duration of last attack in 998 fatal cases of coronary artery disease and its relation to possible cardiac resuscitation. *Br. Med. J.* 3:139-142 (1968).

Nagy, E., Szekeres, L., and Udvary, E.: Electrophysiological effects of verapamil on the dog heart *in situ* after coronary occlusion. In *Proceedings, 6th International Congress of Pharmacology,* Helsinki, Finland. July 20-25 (1975), p. 376.

Pantridge, J. F., and Adgey, A. A. J.: Prehospital coronary care unit. *Am. J. Cardiol.* 24:666-673 (1969).

Randall, W. C., Szentivany, M., Pace, J. B., Wechsler, J. S., and Kaye, M. P.: Patterns of sympathetic nerve projections onto the canine heart. *Circ. Res.* 22:315-323 (1968).

Raper, C., and Wale, J.: Cardiac arrhythmias produced by interactions of ouabain and β-receptor stimulation. *Eur. J. Pharmacol.* 6:223-234 (1969).

Szentivanyi, M., Pace, J. B., Wechsler, J. S., and Randall, W. C.: Localized myocardial responses to stimulation of cardiac sympathetic nerves. *Circ. Res.* 21:691-702 (1967).

Talano, J. V., Randall, W. C., Euler, D. E., Loeb, H. S., and Gunnar, R. M.: Cardiac rhythm disturbance induced by autonomic imbalance. *Clin. Res.* 24(3):242A (1976).

Wallace, A. G., and Sarnoff, S. J.: Effects of cardiac sympathetic nerve stimulation on conduction in the heart. *Circ. Res.* 14:86-92 (1964).

Webb, S. W., Adgey, A. A. J., and Pantridge, J. F.: Autonomic disturbance at the onset of acute myocardial infarction. *Br. Med. J.* 3:89-92 (1972).

Discussion

Truex, Spear, El-Sherif, Dreifus and Lathers

DR. STANLEY GLAUSER (*Temple University School of Medicine*): Dr. Truex, from your injection studies, there appear to be collaterals between one artery and another. Why is it in the experimental situation that the mass of the necrotic tissue is depicted as being so very large?

DR. RAYMOND TRUEX (*Temple University School of Medicine*): I think the question pertains largely to injection methods and, I believe, this is where many of the complicated stories that you see in the literature arise. In the dog heart that I was referring to, or in humans, you assume that there are no large major infarcts when on examining this organ you find no evidence of fibrotic changes indicating infarct. You may see small branches between adjacent small- to medium-sized arterioles. Most of them are in the range of 40 to 80 microns in diameter. They are relatively small and they vary from heart to heart. They are also seen radiologically. Several recent publications, in the last two or three months, have demonstrated the collateral branches between adjacent coronaries with image intensifier on

149

radiograms of the heart. The secret is that these collateral branches, in most cases, are not adequate to carry and help a patient with a massive infarct survive unless a gradual occlusion occurs over a long period. For example, the person who has had left and right pinpointing branches of the coronaries practically occluded has many demonstrable collaterals. This is a slow gradual process but, if the occlusion is sudden, there is massive necrotic infarction and the collaterals cannot take care of it.

DR. JOSEPH F. SPEAR (*University of Pennsylvania, School of Veterinary Medicine*) :   I have to agree. This applies especially in the dog model where, if you try to occlude the coronary artery very slowly with an aneroid constrictor, it is very difficult to produce the kind of infarct that you can obtain with either a one-stage or two-stage acute ligation, and this is presumably the reason why.

DR. LEONARD S. DREIFUS (*Lankenau Hospital Philadelphia*) : The inference was made that, if you localize the area of automaticity by your plunge electrodes, you could approach it surgically. Yet, if you go in like this to surgically ablate it, one would usually think that you were interrupting a re-entry mechanism and not an automatic mechanism. I wonder whether this method could prove it, one way or the other?

DR. SPEAR: I think that it is very difficult to prove that an arrhythmia in an intact system is due to either a re-entrant or automatic mechanism. I believe that the data tends to support the conclusion that the late arrhythmia in the dog model is due to enhanced automaticity. There is a group in Paris who are using surgical methods to try to correct ventricular tachycardia and they feel that the tachycardias are re-entrant, and what they are doing is interrupting a re-entrant pathway. I think it becomes basically a semantic argument after a while whether it is re-entrant or automatic. It is at least confined to a very small focus.

DR. GERALD J. KELLIHER (*Medical College of Pennsylvania*) : Have you been able to use conventional microelectrode techniques to demonstrate the automaticity in those Purkinje fibers that you are presumably recording from?

DR. SPEAR: We have not, but Dr. El-Sherif and his colleagues have looked at the surviving Purkinje system in the infarct.

You can also verify *post mortem* that you were recording from an area of the Purkinje system by staining, and we used an endocardial stain routinely, following the experiments, to localize our ramifications of the Purkinje system.

DR. KELLIHER: The data seem to imply that Purkinje fibers develop automaticity 12-24 hr after acute coronary artery occlusion. Is this also the case in the acute model, or the pre-hospital phase of myocardial infarction, when the largest group of patients dies?

DR. SPEAR: We have not looked at that. Other laboratories have, and it seems like a different kind of arrhythmia. The feeling is that, perhaps, most of the ventricular arrhythmia at this stage —the acute stage—may be of a re-entrant type through the dying ventricular muscle in the infarct but, I really can not add anything to that personally.

DR. ROBERT REYNOLDS (*Medical College of Pennsylvania*): The late arrhythmia, which Dr. Spear was talking about, is presumably due to the fact that the Purkinje tissue within the subendocardial network in the infarct area is viable but depressed at this time. Could you comment, Dr. Truex, as to why this Purkinje tissue is still viable but depressed? Where does the blood supply for these Purkinje's tissues come from? Could it possibly, in part, derive from the blood supply in the ventricular cavity itself?

DR. TRUEX: That is a very good question for speculation. Actually, I think, as Dr. Spear pointed out, that, for some unknown reason, the large well-differentiated Purkinje system can resist ischemia longer than the adjacent small highly-differentiated myofibrils of the ventricular myocardium. It is purely speculation but, I think, that there is something about the inherent organelle organization of the Purkinje fiber that lets it sustain ischemic episodes better than do myocardial fibers because they are less differentiated, for one thing, and they have tremendous reserves of intra-cellular protein, etc., which is something the myocardial fiber cannot maintain due to its organization and differentiation. Also, we know that the one has a transverse tubular system and the other one does not, and this involves a whole series of transfers, the coupling reaction, what is happening to calcium and a lot of other phenomena. So, I really do not know the answer.

DR. KELLIHER: I would like to ask Dr. El-Sherif if he ever examined the role of the vagus in patients in terms of the AV conduction disturbances?

DR. NABIL EL-SHERIF (*University of Miami School of Medicine*): Well, our finding is that the vagus is important if you are dealing with AV block, and is not important if you are dealing with Purkinje blocks. As far as human data is concerned, I think this is also consistently true.

DR. SPEAR: I would like to ask Dr. Lathers a question about cause and effect. Are the nonuniform changes in neural discharge that you see after coronary occlusion caused by artificial arrhythmia? That is, if you pace the ventricle irregularly, or atrium and ventricle irregularly, do you get these kinds of effects in nerve discharge?

DR. CLAIRE M. LATHERS (*Medical College of Pennsylvania*): I have not tried pacing; however, I have induced arrhythmias, using toxic doses of ouabain and digoxin, and found a similar nonuniform neural discharge associated with these types of arrhythmias. However, as far as cause and effect are concerned, at this point I can only say that the nonuniform neural discharge is associated with these arrhythmias. Which is the cart, and which is the horse, I have not clarified yet.

DR. JAY ROBERTS (*Medical College of Pennsylvania*): For many years we have felt that there is a relationship between sympathetic discharge and arrhythmia, particularly in the case of ouabain. Since we know that calcium is necessary for the release of catecholamines from the nerve terminal, perhaps some of the protection or interactions that Dr. Dreifus referred to, might involve the secretion coupling mechanism, and may explain some of the antiarrhythmic actions of agents of this type. Since bretylium causes the release of catecholamines during its early phase of action, some of the results that were seen with this drug might have been due in part to that action; then, at a later time, when that action has ceased, you see its effects on the nerve and heart *per se*.

DR. DREIFUS: When we administer bretylium, there is a massive release of norepinephrine from the post-ganglionic fibers and, we clinically, do find a whole array of ventricular arrhythmias which could be produced by that effect. It is interesting that, for some reason, these arrhythmias do not take the patient's life. I do not know why. One would expect them to be fatal in a patient with acute infarction. When we turn to bretylium, remember, we have exhausted all of the other antiarrhythmic drugs, and the patient should be most vulnerable to arrhythmia. Now, at a later time, one cannot rule out the very positive effect of adrenergic neuron blockade as being part of the action of bretylium. However, we are still confronted by the fact that it does something to the membrane, especially with regard to its anti-fibrillatory properties, that we see in tissue bath and it produces effects which the other drugs do not. So, when you use these agents, you have to think of the total system, and here we must consider the autonomic nervous system again, since it may be on the latter that the anti-arrhythmic drugs exert their major action.

DR. EL-SHERIF: Dr. Dreifus has made an elegant presentation of the effects of antiarrhythmic drugs as we understand them right now. However, I find myself obliged to point out that in the last year, the work of our and several other laboratories has indicated one of the very nice travesties in medicine. For the last twenty years, most of the material that has been written on antiarrhythmic drugs concerned their effects on normal Purkinje or muscle cells. When we start using the same drugs in depressed cells, whether depressed by ischemia or other factors, we see surprising results. I will give one example to clarify this point. Lidocaine is classified as a type II antiarrhythmic and, when given to normal Purkinje or muscle cells, it has minimal effects on phase O of the sodium influx. However, when administered to ischemic or depressed Purkinje or muscle cells, lidocaine astonishingly not only depresses the cells further but wipes them out completely. So, it seems that the way lidocaine acts, is that it depresses already depressed muscle cells which, we think, is the basis for the re-entrant arrhythmia.

DR. DREIFUS: I would agree. In fact, the studies on the combination of procainamide and lidocaine that I presented were performed in depressed cells, and I think you have to look at the latter but also at both systems. Other drugs will wipe out all of the abnormal potentials, but unfortunately they do not always abolish arrhythmia. We can eliminate the abnormal potentials (delayed after-potentials) in depressed tissue, but then the arrhythmia keeps on returning. In other words, you may not be successful in wiping out enough to be clinically effective with your drug, without causing severe myocardial toxicity. Of course, the hemodynamic consequences of this could become disastrous. These drugs will abolish the potentials in ischemic hearts, but at what concentration and at what risk?

DR. GARRETT: I would like to ask Dr. Lathers if she knows of any experiments in which a cardioselective beta-blocking agent with minimal membrane-stabilizing effects has been used before coronary occlusion, to then observe the changes in adrenergic discharge and the arrhythmia after coronary occlusion?

DR. LATHERS: At this point, I have not used a beta-blocking agent to see if it can prevent arrhythmia or the nonuniform neural discharge associated with it. I have performed other studies, though, in which I induced arrhythmias with ouabain. Pretreatment with practolol, which meets the criteria you described, increased the dose of ouabain which produced arrhythmia and also delayed the occurrence of the nonuniform neural discharge. Practolol, as you know, is specific for cardiac beta-receptors.

DR. JUHAZ-NAGY: I would like to ask Dr. Lathers' opinion on the possible differences in this localized, discreet sympathetic discharge among the different regions of the heart, particularly in reference to its ischemic portion. It is known that ischemia excites sympathetic neural endings within the heart, which are sensitive to either the metabolic or the mechanical outcome of the ischemia. Is this the mechanism being set into motion, i.e., a positive feedback accentuating the increase in the sympathetic discharge in which the arrhythmia is both the outcome and the cause?

DR. LATHERS: First of all, data published by Dahlström in the late sixties and by Randall's group showed that, in the normal cat heart, the sympathetic innervation of the myocardium is patchy. It is predominantly found in the SA node and AV node areas, to a considerable extent in the atria, and some in the ventricle. To explain the nonuniform neural discharge which is associated with arrhythmias, you might then hypothesize that we are recording from some of the nerves that go to different parts of the heart, or to areas in ischemic as opposed to normal, undamaged regions. Therefore, I think, you can then consider the nonuniform neural discharges as being produced by differences in anatomy. Now, to come to the local ischemic damage done within the heart itself. Malliani, in 1969, first discussed the fact that when ischemic damage occurs in the cardiac tissue itself, it may excite afferents which return to the stellate ganglia, and then to the heart, via the post-ganglionic nerves—which I am recording from. So, this may be one neural mechanism that is active during the ischemic challenge. In addition, I am sure there are afferents originating in the heart, that after the ischemic damage send neural discharges back to the ganglion up to the central nervous system. Of course, there is a drop in blood pressure which occurs when the occlusion-induced arrhythmia results. It elicits some neural increase. To keep it in perspective, though, one should remember that, when we are talking about occlusion-induced arrhythmias, I am saying that it *seems* that the changes in the sympathetic nervous system are associated with these arrhythmias, but I am not ruling out changes that are taking place directly within the myocardial muscle itself, perhaps induced by the adrenal medulla, central impulses, and other factors that are all contributing to the production of the arrhythmia.

DR. TRUEX: I would also like to address my comment to Dr. Lathers. I think, perhaps, one of the confusing issues in the questions that have been asked is how did you separate sensory inputs which are running with the visceral efferents? You used the term "accelerator fibers" that you were recording from, but we have both thinly-myelinated as well as non-myelinated fibers running back with the sympathetics. First of all, how did you separate them? Is there a possibility that you may have been recording also from vasodilator fibers which were running with the sympathetics? And is there any way in which you can ascertain that the fibers that you were recording from, were coming from the ischemic area? I think this is the real essence of the questions that have been asked.

DR. LATHERS: First of all, I recorded from post-ganglionic efferent nerves going to the heart. The nerve was crushed distally to the electrode so that afferent fibers coming back from the heart would not be involved in the recording. As far as identifying where these nerves that I am recording, terminate in the heart, that I have not done, and of course it would be desirable to do so in order to complete this study.

DR. KELLIHER: On the question of automaticity, perhaps Dr. Dreifus could give us an answer. At a recent electrophysiology meeting, some data were reported which suggested that calcium iontophores, which transport this ion into the cardiac cell, increase the potassium conductance, thereby reducing automaticity. One would think that verapamil, by shutting off the calcium current, would exacerbate the late arrhythmias that Dr. Spear has identified as being due to increased automaticity. I am wondering if this is really the clinical finding with this kind of an agent, and would there not be some potential danger with such a drug?

DR. DREIFUS: I think the point is well taken. Theoretically, you are right, and that would present a serious concern. However, as it turns out, automaticity may not be the factor that causes these arrhythmias. Therefore, maybe verapamil would not adversely affect or aggravate the automatic type of arrhythmia. Dr. Watanabe and I have long held the view that, perhaps, these arrhythmias which we see could begin from an automatic beat, but then their perpetuation becomes a re-entry mechanism—a conduction problem. So, one cannot have a pure and simple system all the time. The type IV drugs, such as verapamil, lanthanum and manganese, seem to be functioning in the delayed after-potential zone and, if indeed, that is the cause of the arrhythmia, well, then it has to be a completely different phenomenon than automaticity. I must admit, we have tried to inhibit some of these arrhythmias with verapamil but have not been too successful.

DR. LATHERS: There is a paper published by Gamble and Cohn about 1972 which describes the arrhythmias they induced by coronary occlusion in the cat and then characterized the type of arrhythmia which occurred. They found that in 27 of 54 animals examined, re-entry was the predominant mechanism. In the next largest group, which included about 9 cats, both re-entry and automaticity were involved; the remaining few animals exhibited automatic arrhythmias only. So, as far as the mechanism is concerned, after occlusion-induced arrhythmias, there may be a mixture of the latter which may compound the problem.

DR. KELLIHER: I think that overlying this whole issue of what the drugs do is the fact that some people are employing a very acute model of myocardial infarction to produce arrhythmia, which is probably very similar to what happens to the patient in the pre-hospital phase, compared to the other models which are using 24- and 48-hour arrhythmias which are similar to what occurs in the patient in the coronary care unit. We are trying to correlate these studies and, as you can see today, everyone is in complete agreement as to the best drug to use for coronary-occlusion arrhythmias. That would be best summed up as five or six antiarrhythmic agents, preferably tested in normal and ischemic cells, placed into a timed-release capsule, and given to the patient immediately before he has his coronary occlusion.

Part II

MYOCARDIAL METABOLISM DURING ISCHEMIA

6

Protein Synthesis and Degradation During Ischemia

D. EUGENE RANNELS
RACE KAO
HOWARD E. MORGAN

INTRODUCTION

Maintenance of heart proteins depends upon the balance between rates of their synthesis and degradation. Reduced synthesis or increased degradation could lead to a net loss of protein. Both hypoxia (Sanders et al., 1965; Kao et al., 1974) and anoxia (Cohen et al., 1969; Jefferson et al., 1971) restricted protein synthesis in the heart and other tissues, primarily through inhibition of the ribosome catalyzed reactions of peptide-chain initiation and elongation. Similar observations were made in severely ischemic isolated perfused hearts (Kao et al., 1976a, 1976b). In other experiments, anoxia inhibited the breakdown of liver proteins (Simpson, 1953; Steinberg and Vaughan, 1956). Thus, alterations in the balance of rates of protein synthesis and degradation in the heart could contribute to irreversible loss of contractile or enzymatic proteins in oxygen-deprived tissues. It was, therefore, of interest to investigate the effects of ischemia on the balance of rates of protein synthesis and degradation and to compare these observations with those made in anoxic hearts. In the present studies, established methods of per-

161

fusion were modified to maintain a minimum coronary flow for 60 min following the development of severe ischemia. Rates of protein turnover were estimated during this period and modification of these rates was attempted by provision of insulin (Morgan et al., 1971; Rannels et al., 1975).

METHODS

Aerobic and anoxic hearts were perfused retrograde at a pressure of 60 mm Hg with Krebs-Henseleit bicarbonate buffer, containing glucose and amino acids. Aerobic buffers were gassed with 95% O_2 : 5% CO_2; anoxic buffers with 95% N_2 : 5% CO_2. Hearts were made severely ischemic by a modification of the low output, high aortic resistance method of Neely et al. (1973), as detailed previously (Kao et al., 1976b). The perfusion apparatus was based on the standard working-heart apparatus.

Following aortic cannulation, a preliminary period of retrograde perfusion was begun from a reservoir (hydrostatic pressure, 60 mm Hg) and the left atrial appendage was secured to the atrial cannula. During this period, the speed of the pump supplying perfusate to the atrial bubble trap was set to deliver 5 ml/min and the left atrial overflow was adjusted to 26 cm above the heart. A 50-min period of preliminary perfusion was allowed, during which rates of protein synthesis and degradation became dependent upon additions to the perfusate. After 45 min, electrical pacing was begun (300 beats/min). At 50 min, the tube from the reservoir was closed, left atrial inflow was opened, and recirculation of buffer was begun. No aortic outflow was allowed; thus, coronary flow was equal to the speed of the pump (5 ml/min) and aortic pressure reflected the resistance in the coronary vessels. A rapid decrease in left atrial filling pressure occurred. Perfusion under these conditions resulted in decreased coronary flow and a rapid onset of myocardial ischemia and failure: peak systolic pressure dropped about 70%; coronary flow decreased from 12 to 2 ml/min; left atrial pressure increased to 26 cm H_2O. Viability of the heart was prolonged by providing retrograde perfusion at a pressure of 20 mm Hg, supplied to both the aorta and left atrium. Twenty minutes were allowed for development of stable but reduced levels of coronary flow. Rates of protein synthesis and degradation were estimated during a subsequent 1-hr period, from 70 to 130 min of perfusion. Aerobic hearts were paced electrically to serve as controls for the ischemic preparation.

For estimates of rates of protein degradation, buffers contained 15 mM glucose, normal plasma levels of amino acids and 0.01 mM phenylalanine. In other experiments, lowering phenylalanine to this concentration, $\frac{1}{8}$ times the normal plasma level, did not affect rates of protein synthesis or degradation. Phenylalanine is not synthesized or degraded by the heart, but cycles only into and out of protein. Therefore, rates of protein degradation may be estimated by measuring the rate of dilution of the specific activity of the free phenylalanine pool and calculating the quantity of non-radioactive amino acid which would have been released from protein to account for this dilution. Net changes in the total amount of free phenylalanine, on the other hand, reflect the balance between rates of protein synthesis and degradation. In the experiments reported here, rates of protein synthesis were calculated from the difference between proteolysis and net phenylalanine release.

RESULTS AND DISCUSSION

During perfusion of aerobic hearts in the absence of insulin, rates of protein degradation increased (Rannels et al., 1975). Rates of proteolysis observed in aerobic hearts in the present experiments (Fig. 1) were within the range of those observed earlier and represented the degradation of about .93 mg of heart protein per hour. The rate of proteolysis in aerobic hearts was inhibited 60% by anoxia, while severe ischemia reduced the rate to 20% of that in control tissues (Fig. 1). Proteolysis was underestimated somewhat in these experiments as phenylalanine released from degraded protein did not mix completely with the free phenylalanine pool prior to its reincorporation into newly-synthesized proteins (Rannels et al., 1975). This restricted mixing lowered the rate of dilution of phenylalanine—specific activity. In other experiments, similar changes in the rates of proteolysis were observed during anoxia or ischemia when cycloheximide was present to prevent reincorporation.

Net release of phenylalanine from aerobic hearts suggested that the catabolic pathway predominated in these tissues (Fig. 1). Net phenylalanine release was inhibited 56 and 73% by anoxia and ischemia, respectively. When protein synthesis was calculated from

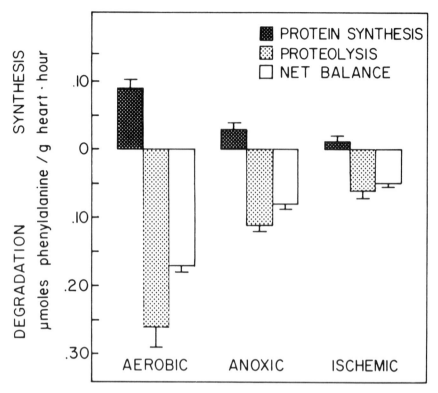

1   Effects of anoxia and ischemia on protein turnover. Hearts were perfused as described in "Methods." Content and specific activity of phenylalanine in perfusate samples were determined by amino-acid analysis, as described previously (Rannels et al., 1975). Data from paced and unpaced aerobic hearts were similar and are combined in the figure. Estimates of protein turnover were made between 70 and 130 min of perfusion, as described in the text. Each bar represents the mean and S.E.M. of at least 6 determinations.

the difference between proteolysis and net phenylalanine release, both anoxia and ischemia were found to inhibit the rate. Qualitative changes in protein synthesis, estimated in our study, correlate well with those measured directly from incorporation of [14C]phenylalanine into whole-heart protein, although the rate of synthesis is underestimated by the present method.

Inhibition of protein turnover in anoxic and ischemic hearts was accompanied by depletion of high-energy phosphate compounds, including creatine phosphate, ATP, and GTP. AMP accumulated; ADP was unchanged. Intracellular amino acids were not depleted in anoxic or ischemia hearts, although amino-acid transport has been reported to decrease in anoxic cells (Rabinovitz et al., 1955; Quastel and Bickis, 1959; Riggs and Walker, 1963). In perfused aerobic hearts, intracellular levels of most amino acids remained at or above those found *in vivo*. Only levels of glutamate declined. Anoxia and ischemia increased intracellular concentrations of leucine, isoleucine, and valine, probably by inhibition of their oxidation; both anoxia and ischemia augmented intracellular alanine. Decreases in intracellular levels of methionine and aspartate were also observed during anoxia. In other experiments, reduced rates of phenylalanine incorporation in energy-poor hearts accompanied the inhibition of ribosome-associated reactions. Inhibition of these reactions was consistent with the energy requirements of the steps of peptide-chain initiation and elongation, as observed in cell-free systems (for review, Rannels et al., 1976).

Provision of insulin to aerobic hearts reduced the rate of proteolysis by 50% (Fig. 2). Furthermore, net breakdown of protein was nearly abolished in these tissues. In anoxia or ischemia, insulin did not further inhibit protein breakdown although net proteolysis decreased somewhat when insulin was present during anoxia. In separate experiments, when reincorporation of phenylalanine into protein was blocked by addition of cycloheximide to the perfusate, similar inhibitory effects of insulin (Rannels et al., 1975) and anoxia or ischemia were observed.

Insulin had no effect on calculated rates of protein synthesis in either anoxic or ischemic tissues, although the hormone increased synthesis only modestly in aerobic hearts. Direct measurements of protein synthesis showed that insulin nearly doubled incorporation of [^{14}C]phenylalanine into protein of aerobic hearts, but had no effect in anoxic or ischemic tissues (Kao et al., 1976b).

In summary, when hearts were perfused by methods designed to produce anoxia or severe ischemia, rates of protein synthesis were inhibited. This inhibition did not appear to involve depletion of amino acids from these tissues but was linked to inhibition of the energy-dependent steps of peptide-chain initiation and elongation. Insulin did not affect rates of protein synthesis in energy-poor hearts (Kao et al., 1976b). Rates of protein degradation increased when hearts were perfused under aerobic conditions; provision of insulin prevented or reversed this increase (Rannels et al., 1975; Fig. 2). When hearts were perfused under anoxic or ischemic con-

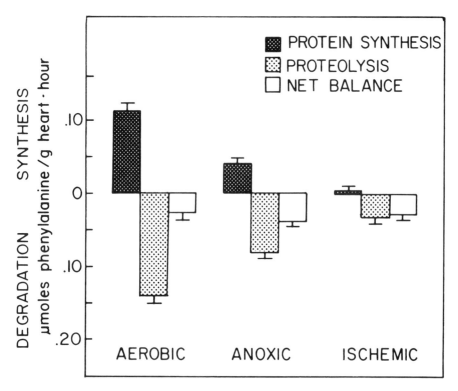

2 Effects of insulin on protein turnover in anoxic and ischemic hearts. Hearts were perfused and rates of protein turnover estimated, as described in "Methods" and Fig. 1. Each bar represents the mean and S.E.M. of at least 6 determinations.

ditions, protein degradation, as estimated from the release of free amino acids, was inhibited. Provision of insulin did not further reduce the rate of protein breakdown.

SUMMARY

In anoxic or severely ischemic perfused rat hearts, rates of protein synthesis were inhibited. This inhibition did not appear to involve depletion of amino acids from these tissues but was linked to inhibition of energy-dependent steps of the ribosome cycle. Insulin did not alter rates of protein synthesis in these energy-poor tissues. Rates of protein degradation increased during the perfusion of hearts under aerobic conditions; provision of insulin prevented or reversed this increase. Under anoxic or ischemic conditions, protein degradation, as estimated from the release of free amino acids, was inhibited. Provision of insulin did not further reduce the rate of protein breakdown.

ACKNOWLEDGMENTS

This project was supported by NIH Contract NIH-N01-HV-12499 and Grant No. HL-11534.

REFERENCES

Cohen, J., Feldman, R. E., and Whitbeck, A. A.: Effects of energy availability on protein synthesis in isolated rat atria. *Am. J. Physiol.* 216:76-81 (1969).

Jefferson, L. S., Wolpert, E. B., Giger, K. E., and Morgan, H. E.: Regulation of protein synthesis in heart muscle. III. Effect of anoxia on protein synthesis. *J. Biol. Chem.* 246:2171-2178 (1971).

Kao, R., Rannels, D. E., and Morgan, H. E.: Effects of insulin on the inhibition of protein synthesis in hypoxic, anoxic, and ischemic myocardium. *Fed. Proc.* 33:386 (1974).

Kao, R., Rannels, D. E., and Morgan, H. E.: Effects of anoxia and severe ischemia on the turnover of myocardial proteins. In *Experimental and Clinical Aspects on Preservation of the Ischemic Myocardium*, A. Hjalmarson and L. Werko, eds. University of Göteborg, Sweden (1976a), pp. 117-122.

Kao, R., Rannels, D. E., and Morgan, H. E.: Effects of anoxia and ischemia on protein synthesis in perfused rat hearts. *Circ. Res.* (1976b).

Morgan, H. E., Jefferson, L. S., Wolpert, E. B., and Rannels, D. E.: Regulation of protein synthesis in heart muscle. II. Effect of amino acid levels and insulin on ribosomal aggregation. *J. Biol. Chem.* 246:2163-2170 (1971).

Neely, J. R., Rovetto, M. J., Whitmer, J. T., and Morgan, H. E.: Effects of ischemia on function and metabolism of the isolated working rat heart. *Am. J. Physiol.* 225:651-658 (1973).

Quastel, J. H., and Bickis, I. J.: Metabolism of normal tissues and neoplasms *in vitro. Nature* 183:281-286 (1959).

Rabinovitz, M., Olson, M. E., and Greenberg, D. M.: Relation of energy processes to the incorporation of amino acids into proteins of the Ehrlich Ascites Carcinoma. *J. Biol. Chem.* 213:1-9 (1955).

Rannels, D. E., Kao, R., and Morgan, H. E.: Effect of insulin on protein turnover in heart muscle. *J. Biol. Chem.* 250:1694-1701 (1975).

Rannels, D. E., McKee, E. E., and Morgan, H. E.: Regulation of protein synthesis and degradation in heart and skeletal muscle. In *Biochemical Actions of Hormones*, Vol. IV, G. Litwack, ed. Academic Press, New York. Still in press (1976).

Riggs, T. R., and Walker, L. M.: Some relations between active transport of free amino acids into cells and their incorporation into protein. *J. Biol. Chem.* 238:2663-2668 (1963).

Sanders, A. P., Hale, D. M., and Miller, A. T., Jr.: Some effects of hypoxia on respiratory metabolism and protein synthesis in rat tissues. *Am. J. Physiol.* 209:443-446 (1965).

Simpson, M. V.: The release of labeled amino acids from proteins of rat liver slices. *J. Biol. Chem.* 201:143-154 (1953).

Steinberg, D., and Vaughan, M.: Observations on intracellular protein catabolism studied *in vitro. Arch. Biochem. Biophys.* 65:93-105 (1956).

7

Carbohydrate Metabolism During Ischemia

MICHAEL J. ROVETTO
JAMES R. NEELY

INTRODUCTION

It has been generally accepted that a reduction in the oxygen tension of myocardial tissue leads to a stimulation of glycolysis. The increased flux of glucose through the glycolytic pathway would, therefore, partially compensate for the loss of energy produced from oxidative pathways. It has also been realized that the energy derived from glycolysis in cardiac muscle is not sufficient to maintain myocardial mechanical function. The maximum amount of energy supplied by glycolysis was estimated at about only 20% of that required by the heart (Opie, 1968).

Glycolytic production of adenosine triphosphate (ATP) can be increased under hypoxic and anoxic conditions (Krause and Wollenberger, 1967; Kubler and Spieckermann, 1970; Morgan et al., 1961; Williamson, 1966). In these studies, the rate of glycolysis was observed to increase 3-4 fold over that in aerobic hearts. Insulin had only a modest stimulatory effect on the glycolysis rate in anoxic hearts perfused with 5.5 mM glucose as the substrate

(Morgan et al., 1961). Thus, hypoxia or anoxia are sufficient stimuli to increase glycolysis too close to a maximal rate.

In studies on the effect of anoxia or hypoxia on glycolysis, coronary flow was maintained at a high rate. However, experiments employing ischemic hearts also indicated that a reduction in oxygen tension, caused by decreased coronary flow, resulted in increased glucose utilization and lactate production. Brachfeld and Scheuer (1967), employing an *in situ* dog heart preparation in which ischemia was produced by cannulating and controlling blood flow in the left coronary artery, reported that glucose utilization rose during ischemia. In that investigation, samples for analysis of venous effluent concentration of glucose were drawn from the coronary sinus and, thus, the data represented uptake of glucose from both ischemic and non-ischemic tissue. On the other hand, Gudbjarnson et al. (1970) found that, in *in situ* dog hearts, the high rate of lactate production was not maintained throughout ischemia produced by ligation of a branch of the left coronary artery. More recently, we reported that the glycolytic rate in an isolated working rat heart increased only modestly in ischemia or was inhibited by it (Rovetto et al., 1973).

The purpose of our studies described below was to determine the factors which limit glycolysis during ischemia, and to explore methods that could reverse or prevent the inhibition of glycolysis.

MATERIALS AND METHODS

Perfusion Techniques

Hearts from pentobarbital-anesthetized 200-300 g male Sprague-Dawley rats were perfused by either the working-heart technique or Langendorff procedure. Unless specified differently in the figures and tables, the perfusate was Krebs-Henseleit (KH) buffer containing 11 mM D-glucose and equilibrated with 95:5%, $O_2:CO_2$, pH 7.35, at 37°C. Ischemia was produced in working hearts by either of the following methods: (1) the diastolic perfusion pressure was decreased by means of a one-way ball valve; or (2) a predetermined coronary flow was set with a variable-speed pump and the ventricular pressure development maintained by rendering the aortic outflow resistance infinite (Neely et al., 1973). A complete discussion of the apparatus and perfusion techniques can be found in Neely and Rovetto (1975). Briefly, these techniques for producing ischemia required a 60% reduction in coronary flow to bring about failure of ventricular pressure development (defined as peak systolic pressure of 30 mm Hg) in the electrically-paced heart. Failure occurred within 8 to 10 min. Without electrical pacing (300 beats/min), a decrease in coronary flow generally resulted in a failure of the hearts to maintain control aortic pressure and heart rates. However, these hearts continued to develop 60-75 mm Hg aortic pressures for long periods of time, at low heart rates. Both types of ischemic hearts have been used with similar results. In these models of ischemia, coronary flow was dependent primarily on the systolic perfusion pressure. Consequently, in ischemic hearts which exhibited pressure failure (paced hearts) as peak systolic pressure declined, coronary flow also decreased, setting up a continuous cycle of pressure and flow reductions. In order to study the effect of a constant, reduced rate of coronary flow, minimum flow was provided by constant pressure or flow perfusion. Thus, coronary flow could be set at values from 5-40% of the control rates.

Anoxia and hypoxia were produced by perfusing hearts with buffer equilibrated with 95:5% $N_2:CO_2$ and 75:20:5%, $N_2:O_2:CO_2$, respectively. Following failure of the ventricle, coronary flow was maintained by providing a constant aortic perfusion pressure of 60 mm Hg. For studies of the effect of coronary flow in anoxic hearts, the aortic hydrostatic perfusion pressure was adjusted to obtain a predetermined rate of coronary flow.

Estimation of Exogenous Glucose Utilization

Utilization of exogenous glucose was determined by the production of ^3H_2O from ^3H-2 or ^3H-5 glucose. The rate of ^3H_2O formation provides a measure of the rate of exogenous glucose flux through glycolysis (Neely et al., 1972). Fifty to 80 thousand CPM/ml of ^3H-glucose was included in the perfusate. Samples of the coronary effluent were collected without recirculation and were either distilled or placed on Dowex-1-4 resin (borate form) to remove the glucose (Clark et al., 1973). The radioactivity of the ^3H_2O in the distillates or column effluents was then determined in a liquid-scintillation spectrometer.

Biochemical Analysis

Hearts for analysis of labile compounds were quickly frozen between metal blocks precooled in liquid nitrogen. The frozen tissue wafer was powdered in a percussion mortar, maintained at the temperature of liquid nitrogen, and extracted in ice-cold 6% perchloric acid. Tissue concentrations of glycolytic intermediates, adenine nucleotides and creatine phosphate, were measured spectrophotometrically or fluorometrically in neutralized perchloric acid extracts by standard enzymatic procedures (Bergmeyer, 1963). Extracellular pH was determined by measuring the pH of the coronary effluent, without exposure to air. The distribution of ^{14}C-5-5-dimethyl-2,4,-oxazolidinedione (DMO) was used to calculate the intracellular pH (Carter, 1972), using 5-^{3}H-Sorbitol as an extracellular marker. The values for glycolytic intermediates, other compounds measured, and glucose utilization rates are all expressed per gram of dry tissue.

RESULTS

Relation between Coronary Flow and Glycolytic Rate

Glycolysis rates of anoxic and ischemic hearts are shown in Fig. 1. The total glycolytic flux was determined by the rate of exogenous glucose utilization and the rate of glycogen disappearance. Two points emerge from this figure. First, the rate of glycogenolysis was lower in ischemic than in anoxic hearts and second, the amount of exogenous glucose utilized by the ischemic hearts was less than that by those with anoxia. In fact, following ventricular failure, when coronary flow had decreased from an initial 6 ml/min to 3 ml/min or less, glycolysis was reduced to a rate below that of the aerobic working heart. The rate of glycolysis was not due to limited substrate delivery since glucose-6-PO$_4$ was elevated and less than 10% of the glucose was utilized in one pass through the heart. In addition, insulin and high perfusate concentrations of glucose caused accumulation of free intracellular glucose and failed to increase the glycolytic rate of ischemic hearts (data not shown). The data for ischemia shown in Fig. 1 were from hearts in which coronary flow was continually decreasing. In order to determine more specifically the effect of coronary flow on glycolysis, ischemia was produced and coronary flow was maintained at predetermined levels. The results of these studies are shown in Fig. 2. If coronary flow was maintained at about 2 ml/min, exogenous glucose utilization was stimulated after a lag period of 10 min. At a coronary flow rate of about 5-6 ml/min, glucose utilization was increased even further. The rate of glucose utilization was independent of workload and heart rate, and was affected only by the rate of coronary

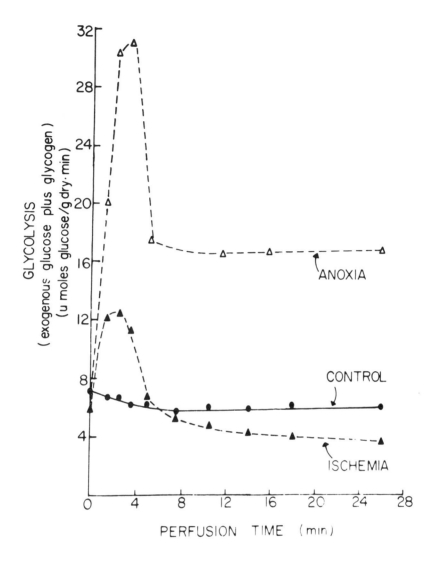

1 **The effect of ischemia and anoxia on total glucose utilization by the heart.** The hearts were perfused with Krebs-Henseleit bicarbonate buffer containing 11 mM glucose. Immediately following the samples at zero time, the hearts were made ischemic by reducing coronary flow by 60%, anoxic by switching from perfusate equilibrated with 95:5%, $O_2:CO_2$ to one equilibrated with 95:5%, $N_2:CO_2$—or continued to be perfused as aerobic working hearts (control). No provision was made for maintaining coronary flow in the ischemic hearts and, as ventricular failure ensued, coronary flow decreased and was 0.6 ml/min at the end of the perfusion period. Each point represents the sum of the rate of utilization of exogenous glucose and of glucose from endogenous glycogen. Each point represents the mean value for 8-10 hearts.

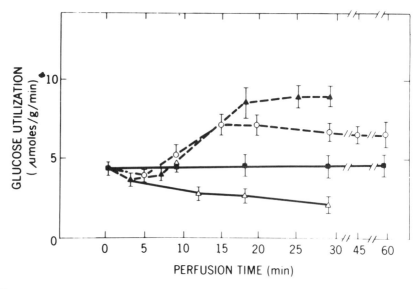

2   Utilization of exogenous glucose at different rates of coronary flow, as a function of time, in hearts perfused with buffer equilibrated with 95:5%, O_2:CO_2. The rate of glycolysis in control hearts is represented by the solid squares. In the other hearts, ischemia was initiated at zero time by decreasing coronary flow from the control rate of 14.8 to about 6 ml/min. Coronary flow was maintained at this level in one group of hearts (solid triangles), allowed to decline to about 2 ml/min and maintained at this level in a second group (open circles), or allowed to continue to decrease throughout the ischemic period in a third group (open triangles). In this last group, coronary flow was 0.6 ml/min, following 30 min of perfusion. Each point represents the mean value for 8-10 hearts. From Neely et al., 1975b. (Reproduced by permission of the American Heart Association, Inc.)

flow. The time-dependent increase in exogenous glucose utilization reflects the breakdown of glycogen and dilution of the specific activity of the ^{3}H-glucose-6-PO$_4$ pool (see Fig. 1).

Inclusion of fatty acid (1 mM palmitate) in the perfusion medium did not alter the relationship between coronary flow and the rate of glucose utilization. Although palmitate depressed the control rate of glucose utilization, during ischemia that rate still increased to about 10 μmoles/g/min, at a coronary flow rate of 5-6 ml/min (Neely et al., 1975b). Thus, in the presence or absence of fatty acid, glycolysis could be stimulated during ischemia but never

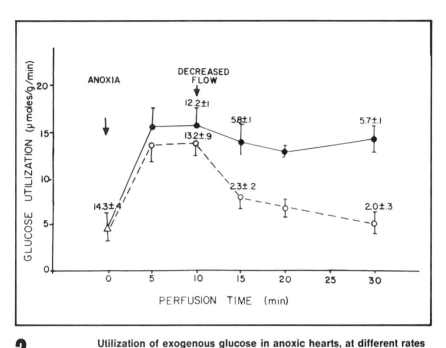

3   **Utilization of exogenous glucose in anoxic hearts, at different rates of coronary flow.** Immediately following the zero time sample, hearts were perfused with buffer equilibrated with 95:5%, N_2:CO_2. During the first 10 min of anoxic perfusion, coronary flow was maintained at a high rate by a 60 mm Hg aortic hydrostatic perfusion pressure. After 10 min, coronary flow was reduced to the level indicated by the numbers above the data points at 15 and 30 min, and anoxic perfusion continued. Each point represents the mean ± SEM for 8-10 hearts. From Neely et al., 1975a. (Reproduced by permission of University Park Press.)

increased to the rate observed under anoxic conditions, at a high rate of coronary flow.

Although the rate of oxygen consumption was depressed in the ischemic hearts and was directly proportional to coronary flow (Neely et al., 1975b), limitation of glycolysis under these conditions could have been due to oxidative metabolism rather than to coronary flow. Therefore, in order to further determine the effect of coronary flow on glycolysis, hearts were made anoxic and the rate of flow was decreased, following 10 min of perfusion—a time sufficient to achieve a maximum rate of glycolysis. These results are shown in Fig. 3. It can be seen that, at comparable rates of coronary flow, glucose utilization was limited in these hearts to about the same extent as in ischemic hearts. Thus, a reduction in coronary flow was sufficient to limit glycolysis, regardless of whether or not substrates were being oxidized.

Site of Glycolytic Inhibition

Under aerobic and anoxic conditions, phosphofructokinase is the rate-limiting step for flux of glucose through glycolysis (Williamson, 1966). In order to determine the rate-limiting enzymatic step during ischemia, tissue concentrations of glycolytic intermediates were measured at several time intervals. These results are presented in Fig. 4 as a percentage of the control values. The average coronary flow was 15, 5.3, 3.0, and 0.6 ml/min for the control, 2, 8, and 16 min ischemic hearts, respectively. The rate of glucose utilization decreased from about 6 to 3 μmoles/g/min during ischemic perfusion. In these hearts, the concentrations of the hexose phosphates, glucose-6-PO$_4$ (G6P), fructose-6-PO$_4$ (F6P) and fructose-1, 6-PO$_4$ (F, 1-6, P), were elevated at 2 min and remained so throughout the ischemic period. However, the largest changes in glycolytic intermediates were the increases in the triose phosphates, dihydroxyacetone phosphate (DHP) and glyceraldehyde-3-phosphate (G3P). These changes indicated that glycolysis was restricted by flux through glyceraldehyde-3-phosphate dehydrogenase.

Since ischemia inhibited the glycolytic rate of hearts perfused with insulin and high concentrations of glucose (Rovetto et al., 1973), it was of interest to determine the rate-limiting step in glycolysis under these conditions. Fig. 5 shows the changes in concentrations of glycolytic intermediates in hearts perfused with 22 mM glucose and 25 μunits insulin/ml perfusate. Insulin increased the concentrations of the hexose phosphates under aerobic conditions, and subsequent ischemia produced only modest changes in the level of these intermediates. However, during ischemia, the concentration of the triose phosphates rose and, by 16 min, DHP was about 300% of the control value. These data indicate that, as was the case without insulin, glycolysis was limited by the activity of glycereldehyde-3-PO$_4$ dehydrogenase.

Although these data taken alone are only suggestive of a limitation of glycolysis at the dehydrogenase step (the apparent restriction could be due to a build-up of difficult to measure products of the reaction), it can be calculated that the dehydrogenase was displaced from equilibrium during ischemia (Rovetto et al., 1975).

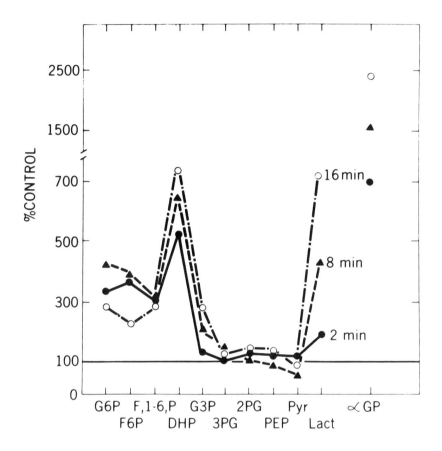

4

Effects of ischemia on tissue levels of glycolytic intermediates at various times during ichemia, when coronary flow was allowed to decline as ventricular pressure failed. Hearts were perfused with buffer containing 11 mM glucose and equilibrated with 95:5%, O_2:CO_2. Coronary flow was about 15 ml/min in control hearts, and 5, 3 and 0.6 ml/min in ischemic hearts after 2, 8 and 16 min, respectively. G6P = glucose-6-PO_4, F, 1-6-P = fructose-1,6-diphosphate, Pyr = pyruvate, αGP = α-glycerol-PO_4 F6P = fructose-6-PO_4, DHP = dihydroxyacetone phosphate, 3 PG = 3-phosphoglycerate, PEP = phosphoenolpyruvate, and Lact = lactate. Each point in the figure represents the mean value for at least 10 hearts. From Rovetto et al., 1975. (Reproduced by permission of the American Heart Association, Inc.)

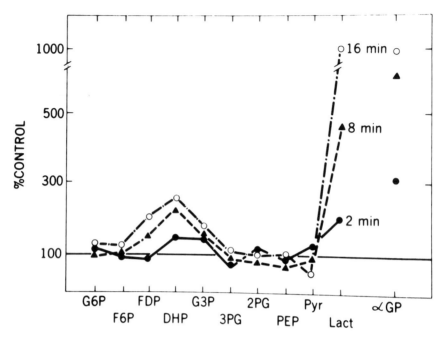

5

Effects of ischemia on glycolytic intermediates in hearts perfused with buffer containing insulin and high concentrations of glucose. Hearts were perfused in a similar manner to those represented in Fig. 4. However, the perfusate contained 25 μunits insulin per ml and 22 mM glucose. The abbreviations are the same as those in Fig. 4. Each point represents the mean value for at least 10 hearts. From Rovetto et al., 1975. (Reproduced by permission of the American Heart Association, Inc.)

These calculations were based on estimating the NADH concentration from the lactate dehydrogenase equilibrium constant, the lactate, pyruvate ratio and the measured intracellular pH.

Effect of pH, Lactate and Pyruvate on Glycolytic Rate

Two major differences between anoxia and ischemia are the concentrations of tissue lactate and the intracellular pH. Lactate concentration under anoxic conditions is about two times that of the control level, or about 6 mM. In contrast, under ischemic conditions, the concentration of lactate can increase to 35 mM or higher.

During anoxia intra- and extracellular pH remained at the control values of 7.00 and 7.25, respectively, whereas, during ischemia, these values can decrease to 6.8 (Neely et al., 1975). This latter figure represents the lowest value found (after 30 min of ischemia and at a coronary flow of 0.5 ml/min). Also, in this study, intracellular pH equaled the coronary effluent pH, at values below 6.9.

Thus, it was of interest to determine how independent changes in pH and lactate would effect glycolysis. The rates of glucose utilization under aerobic, anoxic and hypoxic conditions are shown in Fig. 6. Decreasing the perfusate pH from 7.35 to 6.75 had no effect on glucose utilization, whereas a further decrease in pH to 6.55 resulted in its reduction. At this pH, the aerobic hearts failed to continue developing aortic pressure adequate for coronary perfusion and flow was maintained by means of a pump. Decreasing the perfusate pH in hypoxic and anoxic hearts substantially reduced the rate of glucose utilization. In the hypoxic hearts, a perfusate pH of 6.8 prevented the stimulation of glycolysis, which occurred at a pH of 7.35, and, in the anoxic hearts, a similar reduction in pH resulted in an inhibition of anoxia-stimulated glucose utilization. Also, in the anoxic hearts, an elevation of pH to 7.7 did not stimulate glycolysis above that seen at a perfusate pH of 7.35.

Thus, under ischemic conditions not only is there a relationship between the rate of glycolysis and pH, but a combination of oxygen deficiency and lowered pH are capable of inhibiting glycolysis at high rates of coronary flow.

There is also an inverse relationship between the rate of glucose utilization and tissue lactate concentration in ischemic hearts and anoxic hearts perfused at a low rate of coronary flow (Rovetto et al., 1975). Fig. 7 gives the results of studies in which the perfusate pH was 7.35, and contained 20 and 40 mM lactate. In the anoxic hearts (top panel), coronary flow was maintained at 15 ml/min. Tissue lactate increased to 8 mM in these hearts perfused with buffer without added lactate and to about 30 mM with 20 mM lactate added to the perfusate. The addition of lactate prevented the increased rate of glucose utilization seen in hearts perfused without lactate. Addition of 40 mM lactate to buffer, perfusing aerobic hearts at a high rate of coronary flow, reduced the rate of glucose utilization (0 time, Fig. 7, lower panel). The tissue lactate concentration at this time was 3 and 40 mM for hearts perfused with and without lactate, respectively. Production of ischemia and maintenance of coronary flow at 4 ml/min increased the rate of glucose utilization in hearts perfused with lactate-free buffer. In contrast,

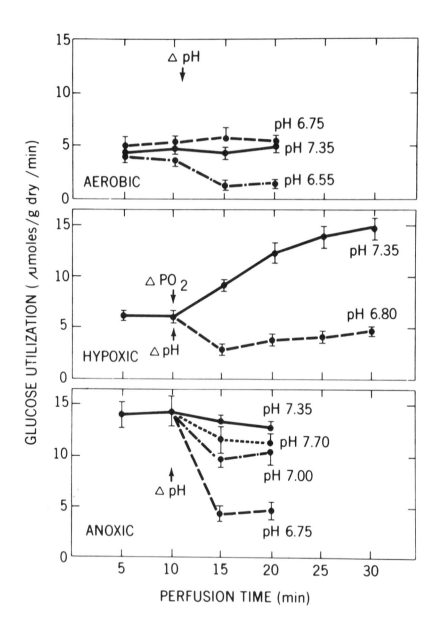

glycolysis was not changed in hearts perfused with lactate in the perfusion medium. For comparison, the glycolytic rate of hearts perfused at 1 ml/min is shown (broken line). In these hearts, tissue lactate increased to 20 mM. Here, the glycolytic rate was about the same as that in hearts receiving higher coronary flow but which were perfused with buffer containing lactate. In contrast to these results obtained with perfusate containing L(+) lactate, perfusion of anoxic hearts with 40 mM D(−) lactate did not influence the rate of glycolysis.

Fig. 8 shows the data obtained during perfusion of anoxic hearts with 20 mM pyruvate. Similar to the results with lactate, pyruvate also produced an inhibition of glycolysis in anaerobic hearts. At present, it is not clear whether pyruvate is converted to lactate and thereby inhibits glycolysis, or whether this is a direct action of pyruvate. It is also interesting to note that perfusion of anoxic hearts with lactate causes inhibition of glycolysis at glyceraldehyde-3-PO_4 dehydrogenase, which is the enzymatic step limiting glycolysis during ischemia.

---

6 **Effect of extracellular pH on exogenous glucose utilization by aerobic hypoxic or anoxic hearts.** The perfusates in all cases contained 11 mM glucose. During the first 10 min of perfusion in aerobic and hypoxic hearts, the perfusate was equilibrated with 95:5%, O_2:CO_2, and in anoxic hearts it was equilibrated with 95:5%, N_2:CO_2. The perfusate pH was 7.35 under these conditions. Coronary flow in all of these hearts was maintained between 12 and 15 ml/min. Following 10 min of aerobic perfusion, the pH of the perfusate was changed to either 6.75 or 6.55 by equilibrating it with a 70:30%, O_2:CO_2 gas mixture and adjusting the pH with HC1. The intracellular pH, as determined with DMO, was 7.01 ± 0.1, 6.70 ± .03 and 6.50 ± .05, for hearts receiving perfusate at pH 7.35, 6.75 and 6.55, respectively. In the middle panel of the figure, hypoxia was induced at 10 min by perfusing with buffer equilibrated with a gas mixture of 20:75:5%, O_2:N_2:CO_2 for pH 7.35, or a 20:50:30%, O_2:N_2:CO_2 gas mixture for a pH of 6.80. In the anoxic hearts (bottom panel) perfusion was either continued with perfusate at pH 7.35 or changed to a perfusate equilibrated with 98:1.8%, N_2:CO_2, pH 7.70, 90:10%, N_2:CO_2, pH 7.00 or 70:30%, N_2:CO_2, pH 6.75. Each curve is described by mean values from 6-12 hearts. From Rovetto et al., 1975. (Reproduced by permission of the American Heart Association, Inc.)

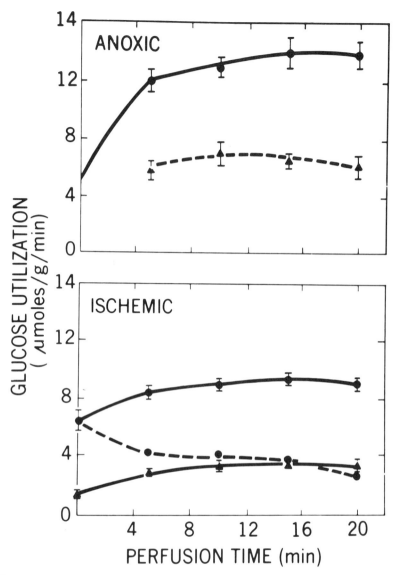

7

Effect of extracellular lactate on exogenous glucose utilization in anoxic or ischemic hearts. The perfusates contained 11 mM glucose (solid circles) or 11 mM glucose plus 20 mM lactate (broken line, top panel) or 40 mM lactate (triangles, bottom panel). Anoxia or ischemia was induced at zero time. In the anoxic hearts, coronary flow was maintained at about 14 ml/min. In the ischemic hearts, coronary flow was maintained at either 4 ml/min (solid lines) or allowed to decline to 1.0 ml/min (broken line). Each curve is described by mean values from 6 hearts. From Rovetto et al., 1975. (Reproduced by permission of the American Heart Association, Inc.)

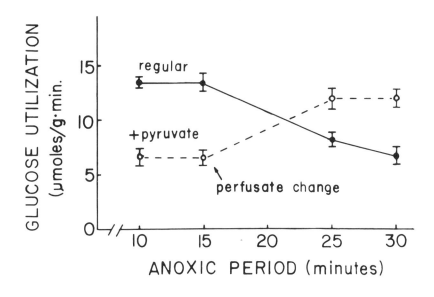

8

Effect of extracellular pyruvate on exogenous glucose utilization in anoxic hearts. Anoxia was induced at zero time and the hearts were perfused with buffer at pH 7.35, containing 11 mM glucose (solid line) or—11 mM glucose plus 40 mM pyruvate (dashed line). At 15 min, the perfusates were switched; thus, the hearts previously perfused with pyruvate were now perfused with regular buffer and vice versa. Each set of data was obtained from 8 hearts.

Attempts to Increase Glycolytic Flux during Ischemia

Although the maximum amount of ATP derived from glycolysis can only contribute about 15% of the total required for myocardial mechanical function (Neely et al., 1975), the fact that this source of ATP is not fully utilized under ischemic conditions represents a possibility for increasing the energy supply of the heart. Since both lactate and pH appear to be involved in limiting glycolytic flux decreasing the tissue lactate concentration or raising the intracellular pH are logical approaches to take in attempting to augment ATP production during ischemia.

Fig. 9 illustrates the effect of including extra buffer in the

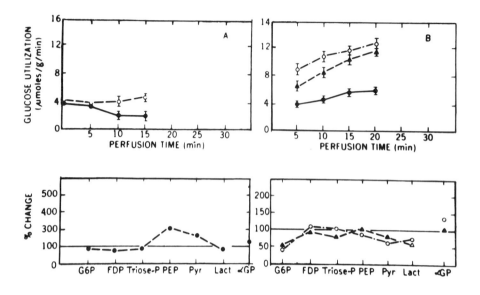

9

Effect of additional buffer capacity on glucose utilization and glycolytic intermediates in ischemic hearts. Ischemic hearts were perfused with regular Krebs-Henseleit bicarbonate buffer (solid lines), bicarbonate buffer plus HEPES (open lines) 25 mM (A) or 50 mM (B), or with bicarbonate buffer plus 50 mM tricine (B) (solid triangles). With the addition of the extra buffer to the perfusate, NaCl was left out to maintain the same osmolality. The tissue concentrations of glycolytic intermediates were measured at the end of 15 min (A) and 20 min (B), and are expressed as a percentage of the concentration in hearts perfused with regular bicarbonate buffer. The perfusates contained 11 mM glucose and ischemia was induced at zero time. In A, no attempt was made to maintain coronary flow, as ventricular failure occurred and, after 15 min, flow rates were $0.6 \pm .1$ and $1.2 \pm .2$ ml/min for regular and HEPES buffer, respectively. In B, a minimum constant aortic perfusion pressure of 30 cm H_2O was provided after ventricular failure occurred, and flow rates averaged $2.35 \pm .25$, $4.6 \pm .3$ and $4.2 \pm .3$ ml/min with regular HEPES and tricine buffers, respectively. The coronary effluent pH was 7.0 with bicarbonate buffer alone and 7.4 with the other buffers. The points represent mean values for 6 hearts. From Rovetto et al., 1975. (Reproduced by permission of the American Heart Association, Inc.)

perfusate in order to maintain cellular pH. In Fig. 9A, the perfusate contained 25 mM HEPES (hydroxyethlypiperazine ethanesulfonic acid), in addition to the 25 mM HCO_3 in the regular perfusate. Ischemia was induced at zero time, glucose utilization was measured during the subsequent 15 min, and glycolytic intermediate concentrations were determined in the tissue, following freezing at 15 min. There was no difference in the rate of decline of ventricular performance between hearts perfused with regular KH buffer and such buffer containing HEPES. However, the coronary flow of hearts perfused with the fortified buffer was higher at the end of perfusion than in hearts perfused with regular KH buffer (1.2 as compared to 0.6 ml/min). Associated with the higher rate of coronary flow in hearts perfused with HEPES was an elevated glycolytic rate, small decreases in glucose-6-PO_4, fructose-1,6-P and triose phosphate concentrations, and increased levels of phosphoenol-pyruvate and pyruvate. These results indicate a relief of inhibition of glyceraldehyde-3-PO_4 dehydrogenase.

In order to more fully determine the effect of extra buffer capacity on glycolysis, hearts were made ischemic and, following ventricular failure, a minimum coronary flow rate was provided by a hydrostatic aortic perfusion pressure of 30 cm H_2O. These hearts were perfused with regular KH buffer, or KH buffer containing 50 mM HEPES, or 50 mM tricine (N-tris-hydroxymethylmethyl glycine); the pH was 7.4 (Fig. 9B). Ischemia was produced at zero time when coronary flow was 6 ml/min; after 20 min, the latter declined to 2.4, 4.6 and 4.2 ml/min in hearts perfused with regular KH, HEPES, and tricine buffers, respectively. With maintenance of coronary flow, glycolysis rose during ischemia in the presence of all three buffers, but to a much greater extent in the hearts perfused with the fortified buffers. The increased glycolytic rate in the hearts receiving the extra buffer was associated with a 50% reduction in the concentration of glucose-6-PO_4, which suggests that flux through phosphofructokinase was enhanced by the extra buffer capacity, augmented coronary flow, or both.

In order to try to distinguish between these two possibilities, hearts perfused with regular KH buffer were rendered ischemic and coronary flow was maintained at 4 ml/min; glycolytic rates and intermediates were then measured. At this coronary flow rate, glycolysis was increased to about 8 μmoles/g/min, the concentrations of hexose, triose phosphates and lactate dropped, and pyruvate and pH rose above the levels seen at a coronary flow of 0.6 ml/min. These changes indicate that flux through glyceraldehyde phosphate dehydrogenase was increased. Also, since the rate of glycolysis was somewhat higher at comparable rates of coronary flow, when extra buffers were included in the perfusate (Fig. 9), these data indicate that increased buffering capacity, in addition to raising coronary flow during ischemia, also augmented flux through phosphofructokinase. Thus, the raised coronary flow seems to affect glyceraldehyde-3-PO$_4$ dehydrogenase, and maintenance of pH increases coronary flow and acts on phosphofructokinase.

Although maintenance of cellular pH appears to be beneficial from the standpoint of enhancing glycolytic ATP production, maximum rates (a rate comparable to the anoxic rate) of glycolysis were not obtained. Therefore, attempts were made to decrease the lactate concentration in ischemic tissue.

Providing that lactate crosses the cell membrane by simple diffusion, its efflux from ischemic tissue seems to be limited by something other than its extracellular concentration (Rovetto et al., 1973). There is an apparent 20 mM intra-extracellular concentration gradient for lactate diffusion at a coronary flow of 0.5 ml/min. Thus, agents which would increase the permeability of the cell membrane to lactate might enhance ATP production from glycolysis.

It was suggested that hyaluronidase may reduce myocardial infarct size by increasing the entry of exogenous glucose in the tissue (Maroko et al., 1972). From the data presented above, substrate supply does not appear to be the problem. However, hyaluronidase could render the membrane more permeable to lactate, which, in turn, would lead to a higher rate of glycolysis. In order to explore this possibility, hearts were made ischemic, coronary flow was maintained by constant flow perfusion and glucose utilization determined (Fig. 10). During the 20-min ischemic perfusion, the glycolytic rate was no different in the hearts perfused with hyaluronidase from that in hearts perfused with regular KH buffer. Also, the tissue lactate concentration did not differ between these two groups of hearts. In order to determine the effect of longer-term exposure to hyaluronidase, ischemic hearts were perfused at a constant pressure of 30 cm, H$_2$O for 2 hr. Initial coronary flow rates were not altered by hyaluronidase and were not different from those in hearts perfused with regular KH buffer. However, following 2 hr of ischemic perfusion, coronary flow had decreased by about 40% in hearts with regular buffer but was maintained in the presence of hyaluronidase.

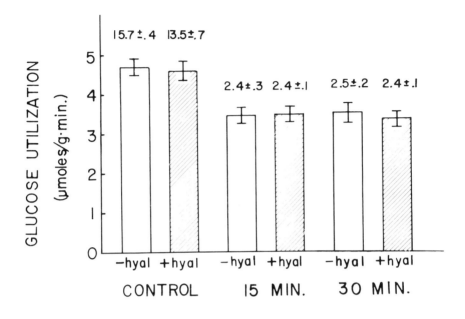

10   **Effect of hyaluronidase on glucose utilization in ischemic hearts.**
The control values were obtained, following 10 min of aerobic
perfusion as working hearts, and just prior to inducing ischemia.
Upon ventricular failure, coronary flow was provided by a constant-
flow rotary pump at about 15% of the control value. The mean
values for coronary flow $\pm$ SEM are indicated by those given above
each bar. The lengths of the bars represent the mean values for 8
hearts and the vertical lines through the means denote $\pm$ SEM.

Although the rate of glucose utilization was not significantly different in these two groups of hearts, creatine phosphate was higher
and lactate lower in the hyaluronidase-treated tissue. These findings
probably reflect the higher rate of coronary flow in hyaluronidase-
treated hearts since there was no difference in the values obtained
for hearts with the same rate of coronary flow, regardless of
whether or not hyaluronidase was present. The above results suggest that hyaluronidase does not enhance lactate efflux from the
tissue but that its beneficial effect may be exerted by preventing an
increase in coronary vascular resistance during ischemia.

DISCUSSION

The objectives of our studies were as follows: (1) to estimate the contribution of glycolysis to myocardial energy production and determine the factors which control glycolysis, and (2) to explore interventions which could possibly increase this contribution in ischemic tissue. Since coronary flow in the *in vivo* situation is probably considerably lower than under the conditions used in this investigation (the blood-perfused aerobic control coronary flow can be estimated to be about 3 ml/ml in the rat) (Neely et al., 1975a), our conditions are probably only comparable to those existing in the peripheral areas of ischemic tissue, which receive high levels of coronary flow. Thus, the findings that glycolysis was not maximally stimulated with a 60% reduction in coronary flow (6 ml/min) and that glycolysis was directly related to coronary flow during ischemia, strongly suggest that, in larger blood-perfused hearts, the contribution of glycolysis is less than maximal. In fact, in blood-perfused *in situ* pig hearts, glycolysis was stimulated only slightly during hypoxia and inhibited with ischemia (Liedtke et al., 1975).

Although at a maxmum rate of glycolysis, ATP production could only account for less than 20% of the energy needs of the tissue, this rate of ATP formation could be of considerable importance to cells which are not being supplied sufficient oxygen. Therefore, studies of the mechanism whereby glycolysis was limited or inhibited were considered important in order to achieve relief of this restriction.

During ischemia, glycolytic flux was limited at the levels of glyceraldehyde-3-PO_4 dehydrogenase, as indicated by reduced levels of intermediates prior to this step, and either no changes or decreased concentrations of intermediates beyond it. Since the NADH level increased during ischemia, it is possible that the observed results could have been due to a mass-action effect. However, when NADH concentrations are taken into account, the dehydrogenase step is displaced from equilibrium. Moreover, NADH also increases during anoxia, a condition under which glycolysis is stmulated.

Two changes which occur during ischemia that differ from those in anoxia are the large increments in H^+ and lactate concentrations. Experiments in which these parameters were varied independently indicate that either one of them can inhibit glycolysis under ischemic or anoxic conditions. Although lactate and pyruvate prevent glucose utilization under aerobic conditions presumably by acting as alternative substrates, their ability to block glycolysis during anoxia suggests that this action does not depend on oxidation. In this regard, Williamson (1965) found that pyruvate and acetate, each reduced glucose utilization under aerobic conditions, by restricting the activity of glyceraldehyde-3-PO_4 dehydrogenase and phosphofructokinase, respectively. Furthermore, fatty acids which limit glucose metabolism under aerobic conditions and, like acetate, increase citrate concentrations did not reduce glucose utilization during ischemia (Neely et al., 1975b). The mechanism whereby lactate and pyruvate limit glycolysis is not known but it does not involve a decrease in the intracellular pH since this value remained constant at 7.00 in anoxic hearts perfused with these substrates.

The effects of a raised H^+ concentration on glycolysis were not as unexpected as those of increased lactate, since the lowered pH restricted glycolysis and appeared to act through inhibition of phosphofructokinase (Delcher and Shipp, 1966; Opie, 1968). However, modest elevation of H^+ (pH 6.8) only caused inhibition when accompanied by oxygen deficiency. This observation indicates that a low pH and either a high NADH level, a reduced phosphate potential, or both, effectively inhibit glycolysis.

Since both lactate and H^+, in the presence of oxygen deficiency, lead to an inhibition of glycolysis, attempts to improve the glycolytic rate were centered around these two variables. Elevation of perfusate pH did not increase the rate of glycolysis in anoxic hearts, in the present study, nor did it elevate the rate of lactate production or oxygen consumption in hypoxic hearts (Scheuer and Stezoski, 1972). However, in this investigation, maintenance of pH did enhance glycolysis in ischemic hearts. The higher pH increased glycolysis by the following two mechanisms: The major effect of lower H^+ concentration appeared to be on the coronary vascular resistance which was reduced in the presence of extra buffer. The increased coronary flow that resulted was adequate to augment glucose utilization. The second effect seemed to be due to increased flux of glucose through phosphofructokinase and, coupled with the increased coronary flow, it elevated the rate of glycolysis over that observed at comparable rates of coronary flow in the absence of the extra buffer.

Attempts to increase cellular efflux of lactate were less successful than those to maintain pH. Although hyaluronidase appears to reduce myocardial infarct size (Maroko et al., 1972), its mechanism of action does not seem to involve a metabolic effect. Intracellular glucose concentration was not measured in the presence of hyaluronidase, but an increased rate of glycolysis—through increased substrate delivery—would not be expected. Glycolytic ATP production is limited within the pathway *per se* and increased amounts of glucose did not relieve this inhibition. Hyaluronidase also did not reduce the concentration of lactate in the tissue, except through an indirect effect on coronary flow. Thus, hyaluronidase did not increase the glycolytic rate of ischemic hearts. However, the mechanism of the protective action of hyaluronidase may, possibly, be based on preventing a rise in coronary vascular resistance and a further reduction in blood flow, as ischemia progresses.

REFERENCES

Bergmeyer, H-U.: (Ed.) *Methods of Enzymatic Analysis*, 2nd ed. Academic Press, New York (1963), pp. 1064.

Brachfeld, N., and Scheuer, J.: Metabolism of glucose by the ischemic dog heart. *Am. J. Physiol.* 212:603-606 (1967).

Carter, N. W.: Intracellular pH. *Kidney Int.* 1:341-346 (1972).

Clark, M. G., Bloxham, D. P., Holland, P. C., and Lardy, H. A.: Estimation of the fructose diphosphotase-phosphofructokinase substrate cycle in the flight muscle of *Bombus affinis. Biochem. J.* 134:589-597 (1973).

Delcher, H. K., and Shipp, J. C.: Effect of pH, pCO_2 and bicarbonate on metabolism of glucose by perfused rat heart. *Biochem. Biophys. Acta* 121:250-260 (1966).

Gudbjarnason, S., Mathes, P., and Ravens, K. G.: Functional compartmentation of ATP and creatine phosphate in heart muscle. *J. Mol. Cell. Cardiol.* 1:325-339 (1970).

Krause, E. G., and Wollenberger, P. G.: Aktivierung der Phosphorylase-b-kinase im akut ischämischem Myokard. *Acta Biol. Med. Ger.* 19:381-393 (1967).

Kubler, W., and Spieckermann, P. G.: Regulation of glycolysis in the ischemic and the anoxic myocardium. *J. Mol. Cell. Cardiol.* 1:351-377 (1970).

Liedtke, A. J., Hughes, H. C., and Neely, J. R.: Metabolic responses to varying restrictions of coronary blood flow in swine. *Am. J. Physiol.* 228:655-662 (1975).

Maroko, P. R., Libby, P., Bloor, C. M., Sobel, B. E., and Braunwald, E.: Reduction by hyaluronidase of myocardial necrosis following coronary artery occlusion. *Circulation* 46:430-437 (1972).

Morgan, H. E., Henderson, M. J., Regen, D. M., and Park, C. R.: Regulation of glucose uptake in muscle. I. The effects of insulin and anoxia on glucose transport and phosphorylation in the isolated perfused heart of normal rats. *J. Biol. Chem.* 236:253-261 (1961).

Neely, J. R., Denton, R. M., England, P., and Randle, P. J.: The effects of increased heart work on the tricarboxylate cycle and its interactions with glycolysis in perfused rat heart. *Biochem. J.* 128:147-159 (1972).

Neely, J. R., Liedtke, A. J., and Rovetto, M. J.: Relationship between coronary flow and ATP production from glycolysis and oxidative metabolism. In

Recent Advances in Studies on Cardiac Structure and Metabolism, P. E. Roy and P. Harris, eds. University Park Press, Baltimore (1975a), pp. 301-321.

Neely, J. R., and Rovetto, M. J.: Techniques for perfusing isolated rat hearts. In *Methods in Enzymology,* J. G. Hardman and B. W. O'Malley, eds. Academic Press, New York (1975), pp. 43-60.

Neely, J. R., Rovetto, M. J., Whitmer, J. T., and Morgan, H. E.: Effects of ischemia on ventricular function and metabolism in the isolated working rat heart. *Am. J. Physiol.* 225:651-658 (1973).

Neely, J. R., Whitmer, J. T., and Rovetto, M. J.: Effect of coronary blood flow on glycolytic flux and intracellular pH in isolated rat hearts. *Circ. Res.* 37:733-741 (1975b).

Opie, L. H.: Metabolism of the heart in health and disease, Part I. *Am. Heart J.* 76:685-698 (1968).

Rovetto, M. J., Lamberton, W. F., and Neely, J. R.: Mechanisms of glycolytic inhibition in ischemic rat hearts. *Circ. Res.* 37:742-751 (1975).

Rovetto, M. J., Neely, J. R., and Whitmer, J. T.: Comparison of the effects of anoxia and whole heart ischemia in isolated working rat heart. *Circ. Res.* 32:699-711 (1973).

Scheuer, J., and Stezoski, S. W.: Effect of physical training on the mechanical and metabolic response of the rat heart to hypoxia. *Circ. Res.* 30:418-429 (1972).

Williamson, J. R.: Glycolytic control mechanisms. I. Inhibition of glycolysis by acetate and pyruvate in the isolated perfused rat heart. *J. Biol. Chem.* 240: 2308-2321 (1965).

Williamson, J. R.: Glycolytic control mechanism. II. Kinetics of intermediate changes during the aerobic-anoxic transition in perfused rat heart. *J. Biol. Chem.* 241:5026-5036 (1966).

8

The Nature of Ischemic Injury in Cardiac Tissue

JOHN R. WILLIAMSON
CHARLES STEENBERGEN
TERRELL RICH
GILBERT DELEEUW
CLYDE BARLOW
BRITTON CHANCE

INTRODUCTION

Although it is well recognized that the development of myo-cardial ischemia produces changes in many biochemical parameters in the cell, the specific factors responsible for diminished mechanical performance have not yet been clearly defined. Numerous attempts have been made to study regional ischemia in dog heart by ligation of a major coronary vessel (e.g., Jennings, 1969; Opie, 1976). How-ever, in this preparation, it is virtually impossible to isolate the mechanical properties of the ischemic areas from the remainder of the normal myocardium. In addition, it is difficult to measure blood flow, metabolic fluxes and rates of energy production because of the inhomogeneity of ischemia in the affected area. Therefore, a model of ischemia was developed, in the rat heart, by uniformly decreasing flow through the coronary arteries below a level required to maintain normal myocardial function (Neely et al., 1973). An objective of this ischemia model was to maintain initially the cardiac output and systolic aortic pressure at the control level while lowering coronary flow rate. In this manner, any subsequent decline of pressure development would be the result of the ischemic process.

It has already been well documented that ischemia is associated with diminished oxygen delivery and accumulation of metabolic end products, such as H^+, CO_2, and lactate (see Opie, 1976). Previous work has indicated that respiratory acidosis has a strong negative inotropic effect (see Williamson et al., 1975a). However, the relative importance of extracellular H^+ ion changes versus those in intracellular H^+ has not been clearly established. The effects of anoxia on myocardial function and metabolism have also been studied and compared with the effects of ischemia (Rovetto et al., 1973). Ischemia has been shown to produce a greater fall of intracellular pH than anoxia in perfused rat heart (Neely et al., 1975). High-flow anoxia is produced by maintaining the coronary flow rate at its aerobic control level but reducing the arterial PO_2 to zero, which results in a homogeneously anoxic tissue. A decrease in pressure development is observed under these conditions because of the greatly diminished capacity of anaerobic energy production. Thus, either hypoxia or acidosis could be the precipitating event in the development of ischemic heart failure. However, since ATP levels in the myocardium are well maintained in the initial stages of anoxia or ischemia (8mM), it is not clear mechanistically how a deficiency of ATP production causes decreased mechanical function, since the Km values of the various ATP—requiring enzymes, associated with contraction and maintenance of ionic homeostasis, are in the region of 0.1 mM.

In this chapter, we are primarily concerned with defining the sequence and nature of ischemic changes in the intact myocardium in relation to altered mechanical and biochemical properties, and to the function of the mitochondria *in situ*. The most important finding is that graded ischemia, produced by diminishing oxygen delivery through a reduction of coronary flow, causes multiple discrete areas of anoxia in the tissue, surrounded by areas which are well oxygenated. The steep oxygen gradients in the tissue are determined by the local capillary fluid flow providing oxygen. It is suggested that the biochemical basis of this phenomenon resides in the very high affinity of cytochrome oxidase for oxygen, which makes the mitochondria able to respire at maximum rate at very low tissue oxygen tensions of about $10^{-7}M$. Consequently, the transition to the anaerobic zero-flux state at an oxygen tension of $10^{-8}M$ is very abrupt because the mitochondria are acting as an oxygen sink. The recognition of anoxic zones as the basis of tissue hypoxia clearly requires a re-evaluation of the meaning of changes in biochemical parameters measured in the bulk tissue.

EXPERIMENTAL PROCEDURES

Heart Perfusion

Hearts were perfused, using a modification of the procedure described by Neely et al. (1967). Hearts from 300-400 g male Sprague-Dawley rats were excised, and the aorta was cannulated as quickly as possible so that coronary flow would only be briefly interrupted. The pulmonary artery and left atrium were subsequently cannulated, and left atrial filling was initiated from a reservoir placed 12 cm above the left atrium. The closed-aorta preparation was achieved by clamping the aortic outflow, thus diverting the entire left ventricular output through the coronary vessels (Williamson et al., 1975a). Aortic pressure was measured by a Statham P23d pressure transducer connected to the aortic cannula, which also made connection with a 3ml air space to provide elasticity. Left ventricular pressure was measured by inserting a 23-gauge needle through the left ventricular wall and attaching it to a Statham P23b pressure transducer. Effluent pH and O_2 tension were measured in the effluent from the pulmonary artery without exposing the buffer to air.

An extracorporeal electromagnetic flowmeter connected to the pulmonary artery cannula was used to monitor coronary flow. Pyridine nucleotide fluorescence was measured with a 3-way light guide which permitted simultaneous determinations of pyridine-nucleotide fluorescence and reflected 366 nm excitation light (Chance et al., 1975). By electronically subtracting the reflectance current from the fluorescence current, the corrected fluorescence was obtained which at least partially compensated for heart movement artifacts. Hearts were paced at 250-300 beats per minute, using atrial leads.

A second perfusion apparatus was employed to induce ischemia without a simultaneous change of the systolic aortic pressure. This apparatus was a modification of that described by Neely et al. (1973) in which a 1-way check valve was placed immediately above the aortic cannula to decrease the diastolic aortic pressure and, thus, the coronary flow. A fluid reservoir was placed 85 cm above the aortic cannula so that the heart had to eject against the resistance of the check valve plus 85 cm of water. The heart was initially perfused with a bypass around the 1-way valve to provide adequate coronary flow, which essentially resulted in an open aorta, working heart preparation. Aortic pressure, left ventricular pressure, effluent pH, effluent O_2 tension, and pyridine nucleotide fluorescence were measured as in the closed-aorta preparation. Coronary flow and/or flow through the 1-way valve was measured with an extracorporeal electromagnetic flowmeter.

Interventricular septa were obtained from hearts of adult male rabbits, which were rapidly excised and rinsed in oxygenated buffer (Rich and Brady, 1974). The coronary artery was cannulated and perfusion begun. The septum was then isolated and mounted between two clamps at its base. The apex of the septum was connected to a Statham tension transducer. The perfusion rate was controlled by a Gilson peristaltic pump. Pyridine nucleotide fluorescence was measured with a 3-way light pipe, similar to that described above. Simultaneous changes in the redox state of cytochromes b and c, and in the degree of myoglobin oxygenation were measured, using dual-wavelength spectroscopy with separate light pipes (Chance et al., 1975). Arterial pH and pO_2 were also continuously monitored. The temperature of the septa was maintained at 27-28°C.

In all experiments, the basic perfusion fluid was Krebs bicarbonate buffer containing 5 mM glucose and 10^{-2} units/ml of insulin which was equilibrated with 95% O_2 and 5% CO_2 at 37° and a pH of 7.4. Respiratory acidosis was produced by increasing the percentage of CO_2 in the gas mixture, while keeping the bicarbonate concentration at 25mEq/liter. For the anoxic perfusions, N_2 was substituted for O_2 in the gas mixture. The artificial buffer solutions were prepared by replacing the $NaHCO_3$ with an equimolar amount of sodium, as either NaOH or NaCl, and adding 10 or 25 mM MES (2-N morpholino ethane sulfonic acid) (pKa 6.15), MOPS (2-N morpholino propane sulfonic acid) (pKa 7.2), HEPES (N-2 hydroxyethyl piperazine-N-2 ethane sulfonic acid) (pKa 7.55), or Tris (Tris (hydroxy methyl) aminomethane) (pKa 8.3). The artificial-buffer medium was adjusted to the required pH with HCl, and the solution was equilibrated with 100% O_2 at 37°. In all conditions, the perfusate sodium, calcium and potassium concentrations were the same.

Analytical Methods

At the end of perfusion, hearts were rapidly frozen with aluminum tongs precooled in liquid N_2. Lyophilized hearts were extracted with 6% (w/v) perchloric acid, homogenized, centrifuged, and the supernatant neutralized with 3N K_2CO_3 to pH 5-6, followed by a second centrifugation to remove precipitated KCO_4. Extracts were assayed by standard spectrophotometric and fluorometric techniques (Williamson and Corkey, 1969).

Intracellular pH was determined, using the DMO (dimethyl 2,4 oxizolidine dione) distribution method, as described by Waddell and Bates (1969). ^{3}H-Sorbitol, ^{14}C-DMO and 0.2mM carrier DMO were added to the perfusion medium. Immediately after the hearts were frozen, a sample of perfusate was collected to obtain ^{14}C and ^{3}H counts in the extracellular space. Aliquots of the PCA extracts of the lyophilized hearts and of the perfusates were mixed with Handifluor and counted in a 3-channel liquid-scintillation counter which automatically corrected for quenching.

RESULTS AND DISCUSSION

Effects of Extracellular and Intracellular pH Changes on Myocardial Contractility

The closed aorta perfused rat-heart preparation was used for the following series of experiments, since under these conditions systolic left ventricular pressure development provides a convenient monitor of cardiac work. Fig. 1 illustrates the effects of a pH 7.4 to 6.6 transition in hearts perfused either with bicarbonate buffer or different artificial buffers in replacement of bicarbonate. With the bicarbonate buffer, respiratory acidosis was produced by increasing the proportion of CO_2 in the equilibrating gas mixture from 5% to approximately 35%. As seen from Fig. 1, left ventricular pressure fell rapidly to 20% of control values, upon changing from bicarbonate buffer equilibrated at pH 7.4 to similar buffer equilibrated at pH 6.6. Other hearts were perfused with buffer containing either 10 mM Tris, 10 mM HEPES or 10 mM MOPS equilibrated at pH 7.4 with 100% O_2. At time zero, perfusion was switched to similar buffer, previously adjusted to pH 6.6 by addition of HCl (metabolic acidosis). Under these conditions, the fall of left ventricular pressure was small and relatively slow with each of the artificial buffers. Further experiments (not shown) indicated that the extent and kinetics of the left ventricular change were not appreciably affected by the buffer concentration.

A comparison of changes of systolic left ventricular pressure with changes of arterial perfusion fluid pH, using bicarbonate or

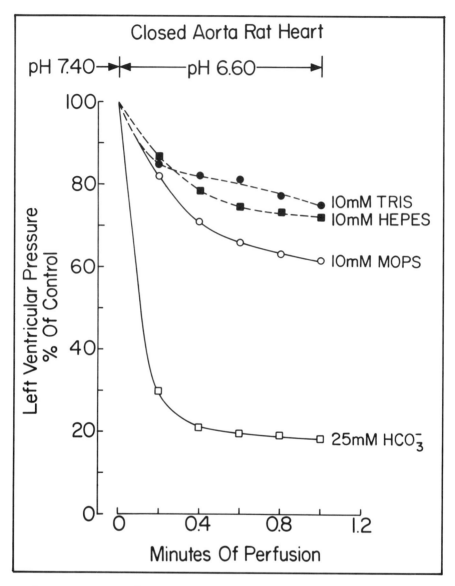

1 Comparison of the effects of respiratory (bicarbonate/CO_2) and artificial buffer acidosis on changes of left ventricular pressure in perfused rat heart.

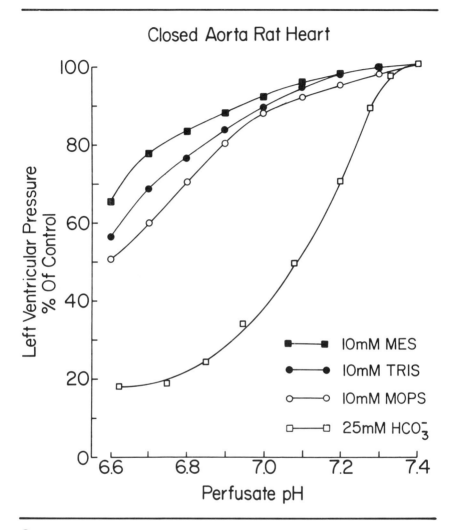

Closed Aorta Rat Heart

- ■——■ 10mM MES
- ●——● 10mM TRIS
- ○——○ 10mM MOPS
- □——□ 25mM HCO_3^-

2 Titration of pH in relation to changes of left ventricular pressure with artificial buffers and bicarbonate/CO_2 buffer.

artificial buffers, is shown in Fig. 2. In this experiment, hearts were initially perfused with each buffer at pH 7.4 for 10 to 15 min until a stable baseline of left ventricular pressure and cardiac output was achieved, and perfusion was rapidly changed to a similar buffer equilibrated at a progressively more acid pH. Left ventricular pressure was recorded after 1 min of perfusion, and perfusion was returned to pH 7.4 conditions before proceeding to the next pH transition. With the bicarbonate/CO_2 buffer, left ventricular pressure decreased rapidly at pH values below 7.3, with 50% of control pressure being reached at pH 7.1. With the artificial buffers, on the other hand, little fall of left ventricular pressure was observed until the pH dropped below 7.0 and, even at pH 6.6, left ventricular pressure was 50% to 65% of control.

The above data illustrate that extracellular pH is not the main determinant of myocardial contractility during pH transitions. Respiratory acidosis is clearly more effective than metabolic acidosis in decreasing systolic left ventricular pressure. The reason for this difference is that CO_2 is much more permeable than H^+ or the artificial buffers across the sarcolemma and rapidly equilibrates with bicarbonate to produce a greater fall of intracellular pH in respiratory than in metabolic acidosis. Fig. 3 shows that, in respiratory acidosis, there is a linear correlation between intracellular pH and coronary effluent pH over the range from pH 6.7 to 7.4, with the intracellular pH decreasing by 0.45 units per pH unit change of the effluent fluid. With 25 mM MES present as artificial buffer, the reduction in intracellular pH was only 0.22 units for a change of one pH unit in the effluent fluid.

On the basis of present and previous studies (Williamson et al., 1975a; Williamson et al., 1976), two mechanisms may be proposed to account for the diminished cardiac function induced by respiratory acidosis. The first involves an interaction of hydrogen ions with calcium ions at superficially located Ca^{2+}-binding sites on the sarcolemma (Williamson et al., 1975b). These sites are affected by changes in extracellular pH and may be responsible for a decrease of the inward calcium current during the plateau phase of the action potential. Such a change has been observed with frog atrial fibres under acidic conditions (Chesnais et al., 1975). However, the effects of acidosis on cardiac electrical activity appear complex, depending greatly on the muscle preparation, species, temperature, and ionic composition of the media (Coraboeuf et al., 1976; Tsien, 1976). Thus, while the action potential was shortened in rat heart, it was slightly lengthened in guinea-pig heart (Delahayes, 1968). Coraboeuf et al. (1976) have suggested that a lengthening of the action potential may occur if the decrease of delayed rectification K^+ conductance was greater than the combined effects of decreased inward Na^+ and Ca^{2+} currents, and decreased K^+ conductance of anomalous rectification. The decrease of K^+ conductance could be

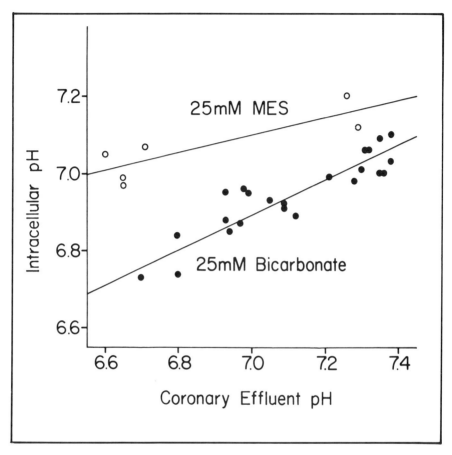

3

Correlation of intracellular pH with coronary effluent pH.

the cause of arrhythmias which develop during acidosis and ische-mia, while a decrease of Ca^{2+} current could reflect a reduction in the amount of activator calcium entering the cell per beat. Since at present, both the amount and source of activator calcium for trig-gering contraction in cardiac muscle are in dispute (Langer, 1976; Morad and Goldman, 1973), the detailed mechanism by which extra-cellular H^+ ions act on excitation-contraction coupling must remain an open question until the effects of pH changes, induced by arti-ficial buffers or respiratory acidosis on the electrical properties of the heart, are more carefully evaluated. However, it is to be expected that these changes would be mediated primarily by the extracellular H^+ concentration; they could affect tension development indirectly by modulating alterations in intracellular Ca^{2+} concentration through a possible Ca-dependent calcium-release mechanism from intracellular storage sites (Fabiato and Fabiato, 1975).

The second mechanism by which changes in pH may affect cardiac contractility has been discussed in detail by Katz and Hecht (1969), and involves an intracellular action of H^+ ions to decrease the binding of Ca^{2+} to troponin, with a resultant reduced activation of myosin ATP-ase and actin-myosin interaction. This mechanism, therefore, involves a direct effect of intracellular pH on the acto-myosin complex, and would account for the bulk of the effects of respiratory acidosis on myocardial function. It is proposed that a similar mechanism is responsible for the early effects of ischemia. Currently available evidence with glycerinated fibers from cardiac muscle (see Katz and Hecht, 1969; Ebashi, 1976) or skinned ventricular cells (Tsien, 1976) shows that a fall of pH below about 7.0 shifts the Ca^{2+} titration curves for activation of tension development or ATP-ase activity towards higher Ca^{2+} concentration, indicating a competitive interaction between H^+ and Ca^{2+} at specific binding sites. However, direct attempts to show an effect of pH on Ca^{2+} binding to purified troponin have so far been unsuccessful (Fuchs, 1974). Clearly this aspect needs to be re-examined in order to resolve the apparent discrepancies between the different types of experiments. Nonetheless, at present, the proposals of Katz and Hecht (1969) appear to afford the most useful working hypothesis to describe the link between intracellular acidosis and impaired cardiac contractility.

Effects of Ischemia on Intracellular pH and Pyridine Nucleotide Fluorescence

In order to compare directly the effects of respiratory acidosis with those of ischemia in the perfused rat heart, coronary flow through the left ventricle was restricted by placing a 1-way check valve immediately above the aortic cannula in the standard open aorta working heart perfusion. Recordings of physiological parameters obtained with this preparation are illustrated in Fig. 4. Initially, coronary perfusion was maintained with a bypass around the 1-way check valve. The bypass consisted of a second 1-way check valve with the opposite orientation. Thus, during diastole, there was retrograde flow from the aortic reservoir placed 85 cm above the

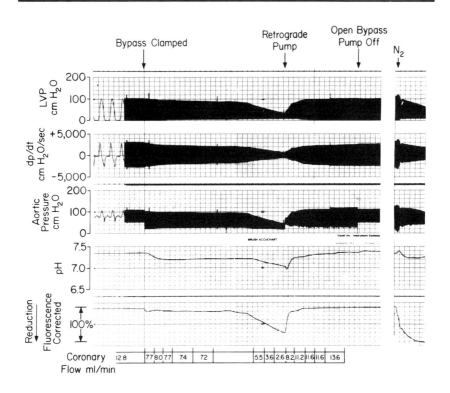

4   Model of ischemia in the perfused rat heart.

heart through the bypass to provide coronary flow. During systole, the bypass valve forced the left ventricle to eject fluid through the main check valve against an afterload of 85 cm of H_2O plus the inherent resistance of the check valve. This was made very small by use of a light metal spring in place of the teflon spring in the commercial valve. Because the entire cardiac output was forced through the main check valve during the control perfusion, there was no change in the resistance to ejection by the heart after the bypass was closed. The coronary flow under the control conditions was 12.8 ml/min, while the total left ventricular output was about 40 ml/min. Immediately upon clamping the bypass, there was little change in the systolic aortic pressure and left ventricular output. Diastolic aortic pressure decreased abruptly, since the aortic pressure could not be maintained during the relaxation phase of the beat in the absence of retrograde flow from the aortic reservoir. This caused an immediate fall in coronary flow to 7.7 ml/min and a slight decrease of the coronary effluent pH from 7.35 to 7.20. Since there were no significant changes in myocardial function immediately after the bypass was closed, the subsequent deterioration was a manifestation of the ischemic process. Left ventricular pressure and systolic aortic pressure were well maintained for about 10 min in this particular heart, after which time, heart failure developed simultaneously with hypoxia (as denoted by an increase of pyridine nucleotide fluorescence), and a further drop in the coronary effluent pH occurred. Coronary flow decreased to 2.6 ml/min, at which point retrograde aortic pumping was commenced to augment the coronary flow to about 8 ml/min. This caused an abrupt reoxidation of the pyridine nucleotides and a restoration of cardiac work. Since an immediate and complete reversal of function was achieved, it is evident that the failure was caused by impaired coronary flow. In contrast to the data presented by Opie (1976) following coronary ligation in open chested dogs, the present data indicate that the onset of hypoxia and fall in intracellular pH (as indicated indirectly from the recording of coronary effluent pH) were approximately coincident.

The correlation between coronary effluent pH and intracellular pH, measured by [14C] DMO distribution, for a series of hearts with differing degrees of ischemia, is shown in Fig. 5. The solid line is the linear regression line for respiratory acidosis taken from Fig. 3, while the data points and the dashed line refer only to ischemic hearts. It is evident that, below a coronary effluent pH of 7.2, the intracellular pH falls rapidly, and declines further in ischemia than it does with respiratory acidosis for any given decrease of effluent pH. The drop in the intracellular pH with ischemia is presumably caused mainly by the rise of intracellular pCO_2 (Khuri et al., 1975). Although a direct kinetic correlation between the decline of left ventricular pressure development and intracellular pH change is not available at present, the current data provide supportive evidence favoring the hypothesis of Katz and Hecht (1969) that ischemic heart failure is caused by a diminished intracellular pH.

In Fig. 4, it has already been illustrated that whenever oxygen delivery to the myocardium falls below the oxygen requirements for the prevailing work load, oxygen deficiency in the tissue is revealed by an increased state of reduction of the pyridine nucleotides. With

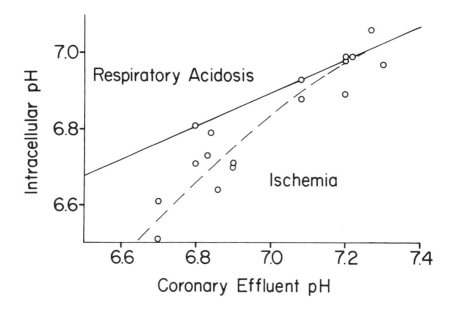

5 Comparison of intracellular pH and coronary effluent pH during ischemia.

the surface fluorometry technique, an average value of pyridine nucleotide fluorescence in the area of heart under observation (0.1 to 0.2 cm²) is recorded. A greater spacial resolution of increases in pyridine nucleotide fluorescence, over the entire surface of the heart, can be obtained by the technique of flash photography recently introduced by Barlow and Chance (1976). This technique uses xenon flash tubes, fitted with Corning 5840 filters to provide 330-380 nm excitation, and Corning 9788 plus Wratten 45 filters over the camera lens to allow transmission of NADH fluorescence in the 430-510 nm region to the camera film. Fig. 6 shows preliminary results of the application of this technique to the ischemic heart in an experiment similar to that depicted in Fig. 4. The picture taken of the control normal working heart (upper left) shows a uniform texture of the ventricular surface, indicating uniform oxygenation of the tissue and a homogeneous degree of pyridine nucleotide reduction. In the

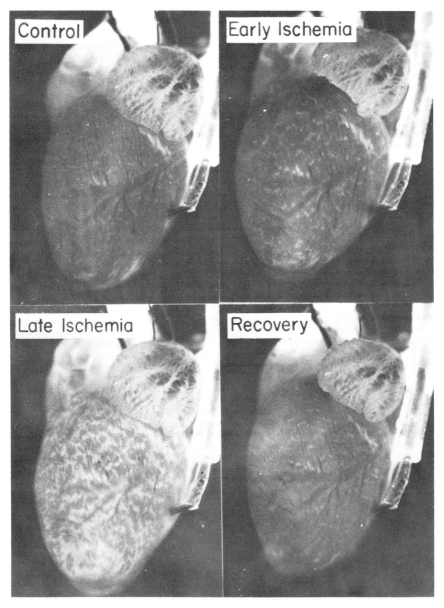

6   Xenon flash photographs of pyridine nucleotide fluorescence in normal and ischemic rat hearts.

early phase of ischemia, shortly after the 1-way valve bypass was clamped, the picture in the upper right shows a few bright spots indicative of small regions of high pyridine nucleotide fluorescence. As ischemia progressed (lower left), these areas increased in size and number, but the picture is noteworthy in illustrating a marked heterogeneity of hypoxic areas in the severely ischemic tissue. A uniform bright appearance of the heart was only obtained with zero coronary flow or complete anoxia (data not shown). The lower right picture shows that when the 1-way valve bypass was opened to restore coronary flow, the appearance of the heart was similar to that in the control situation, indicating that the hypoxic heterogeneity was reversible for short durations of ischemia. The depth of penetration of the fluorescent excitation light is estimated to be up to 0.2 mm, so that observation is made mainly of tissue in the sub-epicardial layers of cells. However, the hypoxic zones are almost certainly present through the whole wall thickness of the ventricle. As discussed in more detail below, these data indicate that tissue hypoxia, as it affects electron flux in the respiratory chain, is an all or none phenomenon. Thus, clusters of cells, in areas with oxygenation adequate to support electron transport at the rate determined by the prevailing phosphate acceptor ratio, are adjacent to other clusters of cells which are anoxic. It is evident, therefore, that tissue analyses of the intact, rapidly frozen heart during ischemia must be interpreted in relation to the demonstrated heterogeneity of the anoxic zones.

Effects of Ischemia on Tissue Metabolite Contents

Results of the total tissue content of adenine nucleotides, creatine, creatine-P and lactate, in a series of hearts with a graded severeity of ischemia, are shown in Table 1. In this experiment, the degree of ischemia was quantitated by the extent of decrease in the systolic aortic pressure, after clamping the bypass to the 1-way check valve. The arterial effluent pH fell progressively from 7.35 in control hearts to 6.90, with a 75% decrease of systolic aortic pressure, while the intracellular pH dropped from 7.03 to 6.70. The lactate content increased 10-fold. The ATP content declined by 25%, with corresponding increases of ADP and AMP. The total adenine-nucleotide content remained constant. The creatine-P content diminished by 85%, with a corresponding rise of the creatine content. The overall tissue ATP/ADP ratio fell from 6.4 to 2.3 while the creatine-P/creatine ratio dropped from 0.76 to 0.07. The final values

Table 1. Effects of graded ischemia and anoxia in perfused rat hearts

Hearts were perfused for 15 min. in Krebs-Henseleit buffer containing 5 mM glucose and 1×10^{-2} units per ml of insulin at pH 7.4; the apparatus used had a 1-way valve in the aortic outflow tract and a bypass around the valve. At time zero, the bypass was clamped. Hearts were frozen with tongs precooled in liquid nitrogen after the systolic aortic pressure fell to the desired percentage of its preischemic level. Control hearts were perfused using the closed aorta preparation. In the anoxic and anoxic-acidotic hearts, coronary flow was maintained by retrograde aortic pumping. The frozen tissue was lyophilized and then extracted with perchloric acid. ^{3}H-sorbitol was used to calculate the extracellular space, and the ^{14}C-DMO distribution between extra- and intracellular spaces was used to calculate the intracellular pH. pH_E refers to the effluent pH, and pH_I to the intracellular pH. Values shown are means of 2 hearts, or means ±SEM of 3 to 10 hearts.

Systolic Aortic Pressure	pH_E	pH_I	Lactate	ATP	ADP	AMP	CrP	Cr	$\dfrac{ATP}{ADP}$	$\dfrac{CrP}{Cr}$
					μmoles/g dry wt					
% of initial										
100	7.33	7.05 ± 0.02	2.5 ± 0.4	22.4 ± 0.7	3.44 ± 0.10	0.47 ± 0.03	29.7 ± 0.9	39.1 ± 1.5	6.5	0.76
93	7.26	7.01 ± 0.03	8.2 ± 1.2	21.0 ± 0.5	4.45 ± 0.32	0.83 ± 0.08	19.8	49.2	4.7	0.40
75	7.20	6.95 ± 0.03	20.7 ± 1.0	17.8 ± 0.8	5.67 ± 0.29	1.33 ± 0.23	13.8 ± 1.1	55.1 ± 3.5	3.1	0.25
50	7.08	6.90 ± 0.02	24.5 ± 2.6	17.7 ± 0.6	6.54 ± 0.46	1.54 ± 0.19	9.1 ± 0.3	60.8 ± 4.4	2.7	0.15
25	6.90	6.70	27.9	16.2	7.07	1.93	4.5	66.4	2.3	0.07
Anoxic Increased pCO2	7.21	6.93 ± 0.03	12.9 ± 0.8	16.8 ± 0.8	6.04 ± 0.23	1.26 ± 0.07	3.5 ± 0.6	59.4 ± 2.0	2.8	0.06
Anoxic	6.77	6.73 ± 0.01	11.4 ± 0.9	18.1 ± 0.9	6.22 ± 0.21	1.35 ± 0.05	2.4 ± 0.1	61.9 ± 3.5	2.9	0.04

with the severe ischemia (low-flow hypoxia) were similar to those obtained with fully anoxic hearts when N_2 replaced O_2 in the equilibrating gas mixture (high-flow hypoxia). However, anoxic hearts differed from the severely ischemic hearts in having a higher intracellular pH and a lower lactate content. This is because the higher coronary flow rate allows lactate to be removed more readily from the extracellular and intracellular spaces. The anoxic cells in the ischemic hearts probably have an adenine nucleotide and creatine-P content similar to that of cells of fully anoxic hearts; thus, the proportion of anoxic cells in the tissue with graded ischemia can be estimated to a first approximation from the percentage fall of the creatine-P content or the creatine-P/creatine ratio, relative to the fully anoxic hearts. The ATP/ADP ratio is a less suitable parameter for this purpose because of compartmentation of the adenine nucleotides between the cytosol and mitochondria. On this basis, it would appear that, when the systolic aortic pressure decreases to 50% of control values with ischemia, about 80% of the heart tissue is anoxic.

The tissue contents of citric-acid-cycle intermediates and reduced pyridine nucleotides with graded ischemia are shown in Table 2. Even in the earliest stage, with only a 7% fall of systolic aortic pressure, the NADH content increased 3-fold. Changes in the other intermediates were not statistically significant, except for a decline in the a-ketoglutarate content. As the severity of the ischemia increased, the pyridine nucleotides became progressively more reduced so that, when the systolic aortic pressure had declined by 75%, the NADH content was the same as in fully anoxic hearts. On the basis of NADH content, a 50% decrease of systolic aortic pressure corresponded to 78% of the total reducible pyridine nucleotides being in the reduced form, in agreement with the calculation given above. With increasing degrees of ischemia, acetyl-CoA, malate and fatty acyl-CoA levels rose, while those of citrate and a-ketoglutarate decreased. In addition, glutamate concentrations diminished, while aspartate levels increased (data not shown). Similar changes were observed in the fully anoxic tissue. The graded changes of these intermediates observed during the development of ischemia, therefore, presumably reflect an increasing proportion of the total heart which is anoxic. However, in the ischemic heart, the anoxic areas of tissue presumably have a lower intracellular pH than heart tissue subjected to high-flow anoxia.

Acidosis in anoxia has antagonistic effects of (1) decreasing energy demand, as a result of the inhibitory effect of H^+ ions on

Table 2. Effects of graded ischemia and anoxia on levels of citric acid cycle intermediates in perfused rat hearts

Hearts were perfused as described in Table 1. pH_I refers to intracellular pH. Values shown are means of 2 hearts, or means ±SEM of 3 to 6 hearts.

Systolic Aortic Pressure	pH_I	Acetyl-CoA	Citrate	α-Keto-glutarate	Malate	Oxal-acetate	NADH	Long-Chain Fatty Acyl-CoA	$\dfrac{NADH}{NAD}$
					mμmoles/g dry wt				
% of initial									
100	7.05	17 ± 3	730 ± 140	401 ± 23	320 ± 40	14	270 ± 60	68 ± 4	0.06
93	7.01	23 ± 1	510 ± 100	277 ± 17	320 ± 80	12	820 ± 90	73 ± 1	0.20
75	6.95	65 ± 5	610 ± 140	252 ± 95	700 ± 90	16	1320 ± 50	80 ± 18	0.36
50	6.90	79 ± 2	600 ± 110	175 ± 70	650 ± 100	17	1440 ± 110	78 ± 10	0.41
25	6.70	103	470	150	620	12	1850	100	0.57
Anoxic	6.93	143 ± 17	470 ± 80	118 ± 20	680 ± 90	11 ± 1	1850 ± 120	183 ± 10	0.63

contractile function, and (2) decreasing energy production because of the inhibitory effect of H^+ ions on glycolytic flux. As seen from Table 1, in the case of high-flow anoxic hearts, the tissue contents of lactate, adenine nucleotides, creatine-P and creatine were essentially the same whether the intracellular pH was 6.93 or 6.73, suggesting that the balance between energy production and utilization was similar in the two situations. In oxygen-deprived cells, citric-acid-cycle activity ceases, and the action of the various dehydrogenases is greatly diminished as a result of feedback inhibitions by the elevated reduced flavin and pyridine nucleotides. The metabolic changes observed between aerobic and anoxic tissue probably reflect the different strengths of inhibition at the dehydrogenases. Thus, flux through citrate synthase appears to be blocked prior to inhibition of acetyl-CoA production from pyruvate and fatty acids, with the result that acetyl-CoA accumulates in the steady state. A decrease in mitochondrial oxalacetate concentration caused by the elevated NADH/NAD ratio, together with a possible rise of the mitochondrial citrate level could account for inhibition of citrate synthase; on the other hand, NADH inhibition of isocitrate dehydrogenase may be responsible for the marked fall of α-ketoglutarate levels and changes in the mitochondrial citrate content (Williamson and LaNoue, 1975). The present data, however, give little information concerning possible alterations in the intracellular distribution of metabolites, except that the rise in the tissue aspartate/glutamate ratio indicates an increase in the cytosolic oxalacetate/α-ketoglutarate ratio, if equilibration of cytosolic aspartate aminotransferase is maintained.

Tissue Oxygen Gradients during Hypoxia

Changes in the oxidation-reduction state of NADH and the cytochrome respiratory pigments provide sensitive intrinsic probes for estimating tissue oxygen tensions. By combining suspensions of luminous bacteria with isolated mitochondria, it is possible to calibrate the percentage reduction of the different respiratory chain components against oxygen tension (Chance, 1976a). For half-maximum reduction of cytochrome c, the oxygen tension was 5×10^{-8}M in actively respiring pigeon heart mitochondria, which reflects the high affinity of cytochrome oxidase for oxygen. This may be contrasted with the much lower affinity of tissue myoglobin for oxygen, which has a dissociation constant of about 10^{-6}M, and a different absorption spectrum in the oxygenated and disoxygenated forms. In theory, therefore, if oxygen is supplied to anoxic tissue (defined as having an oxygen tension below $10^{-8}M$) where cytochrome oxidase is fully reduced and myoglobin fully disoxygenated, cytochrome oxidase and cytochrome c should become oxidized prior to changes in myoglobin oxygenation.

Fig. 7 shows the results of an experiment with pigeon-heart mitochondria, incubated with succinate and glutamate as substrate to which purified myoglobin was added. The mitochondrial suspension was made anaerobic by equilibration with argon gas. Oxidation of cytochrome aa_3 was monitored by measuring the absorbance change between the wavelength pairs of 605 and 620 nm, while myoglobin oxygenation was followed using wavelength pairs of 587 and 620 mm. As oxygen was titrated into the system, Fig. 7A shows that cytochrome aa_3 reacted more readily than myoglobin. Analysis of the results is best seen from the data points of Fig. 7B which shows a plot of percentage oxidation of cytochrome aa_3 against percentage oxygenation of myoglobin. A 50% oxidation of cytochrome aa_3 corresponded to only 20% oxygenation of myoglobin, suggesting that these two oxygen indicators can successfully be used to discriminate between oxygen tensions over the range from 10^{-6} to $10^{-8}M$ in an *in vitro* system.

Fig. 8 shows results of similar measurements made with a Langendorf perfused rat heart which had a small light guide inserted into the left ventricle for simultaneous optical measurements of changes of cytochrome aa_3 and myoglobin absorption (Chance, 1976b). The heart was made anoxic by perfusion with medium equilibrated with 95% N_2 and 5% CO_2, to produce full reduction of cytochrome aa_3 and disoxygenation of myoglobin. When stable baselines were achieved, the oxygen tension in the equilibrating gas mixture was raised in stepwise manner. The increases in oxygen tension in the arterial fluid were associated with incremental and simultaneous changes in cytochrome aa_3 and myoglobin absorbance (Fig. 8A). Fig. 8B shows that unlike in the experiment with isolated mitochondria, there was a strict proportionality between the percentage of oxidation of cytochrome aa_3 and the percentage of oxygenation of myoglobin, with both increasing and decreasing arterial-fluid oxygen tensions.

From the above findings, it is evident that differences in tissue oxygen tension in the range from 10^{-6} to $10^{-8}M$ cannot be distinguished in the intact tissue. Since cytochrome aa_3 is located exclusively in the mitochondria, while myoglobin may be assumed to be distributed uniformly in the cytoplasm, the results suggest that very

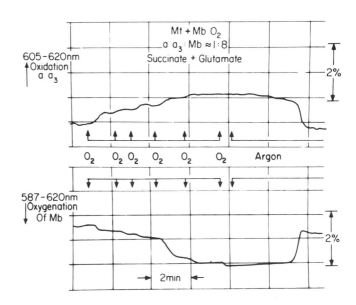

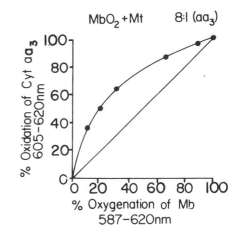

MT-N-15

7   Oxygen titration of endogenous cytochrome aa_3 absorbance changes of isolated pigeon heart mitochondria and exogenous myoglobin absorbance changes. Purified myoglobin was added to the mitochondria in a ratio of 8:1. The mitochondria suspension was made anaerobic by equilibration with argon gas.

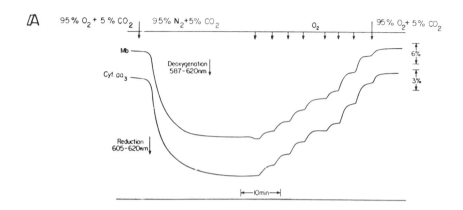

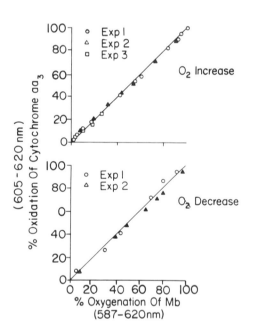

8   Effects of anoxia and oxygen titration on oxygenation of myoglobin and oxidation of cytochrome aa$_3$ in Langendorf perfused rat heart.

steep oxygen gradients of up to two orders of magnitude exist across cells in blood-free perfused heart under conditions of limited oxygen delivery. Hemoglobin has a dissociation constant of 5×10^{-4} M oxygen, hence, it is likely that similar though less steep oxygen gradients occur in the myocardium *in vivo*. These data, obtained when using direct optical techniques with the intact heart, provide additional experimental support for the concept that separate cells in the tissue, and probably also individual mitochondria, are either fully aerobic or are in the anaerobic state 5 condition. Thus, border zones of anoxia in the intact tissue may be expected to be very sharp, as directly visualized by the photographs of NADH fluorescence in Fig. 6, with the position of anoxic regions dependent on the detailed changes of localized capillary-fluid flow.

Comparison of Tissue Redox Changes between High-Flow and Low-Flow Hypoxia

The arterially perfused interventricular septum of adult rabbit hearts was used for the following experiments, since this relatively flat preparation is conveniently suited to optical measurements employing flexible light guides. The muscle is allowed to contract isometrically so that movement artifacts are minimized. Oxygen delivery to the muscle was varied either by decreasing the oxygen tension of the gas mixture equilibrated with the perfusion medium, the flow rate being held constant (high-flow hypoxia), or by decreasing the flow rate with the arterial perfusion fluid oxygen tension being held constant (low-flow hypoxia). Comparisons were made of changes in isometric tension, pyridine nucleotide and cytochrome c redox state, and myoglobin oxygenation-disoxygenation. The septa were perfused at pH 7.4 and 25° with Krebs bicarbonate medium, containing 2.5 mM Ca^{2+}, 5 mM glucose and 10^{-2} units/ml of insulin, and were stimulated at a constant rate of 90 beats/min. During the preliminary equilibration period, the perfusion rate was gradually increased with fully oxygenated medium until there was no further oxidation of any of the optically-measured parameters. The muscle in this state is defined as being 100% oxidized. Fig. 9 shows the percentage changes of the measured parameters from these control values, plotted against a common oxygen delivery rate for the high-flow hypoxia and ischemic conditions. Isometric tension and oxidation of the redox systems were well maintained at oxygen delivery rates above 4μmoles/g wet wt/min. Below this value, isometric tension began to fall, with the decrease in ten-

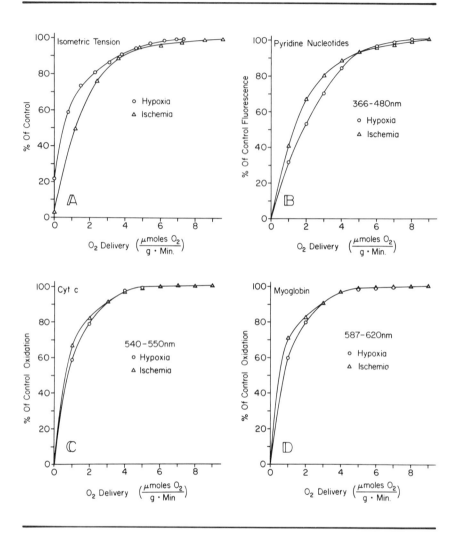

9 Effects of hypoxia and ischemia on perfused rabbit septa. Hypoxia was induced at constant coronary flow by progressively decreasing the perfusate oxygen content. Ischemia was achieved by progressively decreasing coronary flow while maintaining constant perfusate oxygen content.

sion being greater in the case of ischemia than in high-flow hypoxia at any given oxygen-delivery rate. As isometric tension diminishes, oxygen utilization also declines, while the redox state of cytochrome c indicates the balance between oxygen delivery and oxygen demand —in terms of the number of mitochondria in the tissue which are fully reduced. As the oxygen delivery rate decreased, the pyridine nucleotides and cytochrome c became progressively more reduced, and myoglobin became disoxygenated. Except for a small divergence of the pyridine nucleotide redox state, the changes were similar between high-flow hypoxia and ischemia.

Fig. 10 shows the relationship between alterations in isometric tension and oxidation of cytochrome c, both expressed as a percentage of aerobic control values, for the high-flow hypoxia and ischemic conditions, using the data presented in Fig. 9. It is clear that for any degree of tension development below 90%, cytochrome c is more oxidized in ischemia than in hypoxia. Thus, when tension development is 50% of control, cytochrome c is 73% oxidized in ischemia but only 35% oxidized in high-flow hypoxia. These data indicate that, under conditions of limited oxygen delivery, muscle contraction is more impaired in the ischemic situation than in high-flow hypoxia.

In other experiments, the septa were first made hypoxic and then ischemic at similar oxygen delivery rates (data not shown). In those experiments where the oxygen delivery rates were closely matched, the pyridine nucleotides and cytochrome c were more oxidized, and myoglobin was more oxygenated in ischemia than in hypoxia. It was also evident that, for similar levels of isometric tension development in the high-flow hypoxia to ischemia transition, the pyridine nucleotides and cytochrome c were more oxidized, whereas myoglobin was more oxygenated in ischemia than in high-flow hypoxia. Higher oxygen-delivery rates for the same levels of tension were required in ischemia as compared to high-flow hypoxia.

Direct measurements of intracellular pH have not been made with the septa preparations but, on the basis of studies with the perfused heart (Table 1), it may be predicted that the intracellular pH of the septum is lower in ischemic low-flow hypoxia than in high-flow hypoxia. Thus the data in Figs. 9 and 10 can be interpreted on the basis of a protective effect of intracellular acidosis against anoxic damage (Bing et al., 1973). For a given change in intracellular Ca^{2+} concentration during the contraction cycle, increased H^+ concentration will diminish actin-myosin interaction and ATP-ase activity, and thus decrease oxygen demand, which is

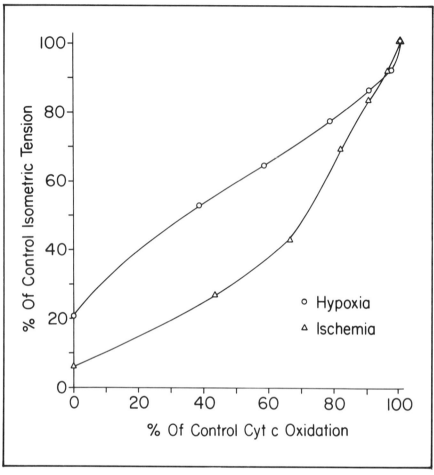

10   Comparison of isometric tension and cytochrome c oxidation during hypoxia and ischemia in perfused rabbit septa. Data from Figs. 9A and 9C are replotted at similar oxygen delivery rates. Tension and relative cytochrome c oxidation are plotted as percentage of control.

reflected by an oxidation of the steady-state redox level of cytochrome c, at a constant rate of oxygen delivery.

The data in Fig. 9 also allow an evaluation of the relationship between the percentage oxidation of cytochrome c and percentage oxidation of pyridine nucleotides and myoglobin, as oxygen delivery to the septum is decreased. The findings obtained for the situation

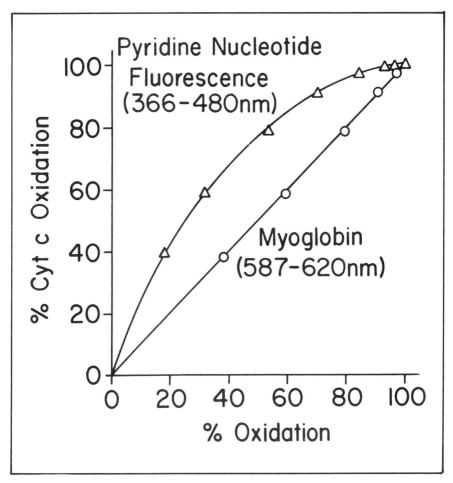

11

Comparison of pyridine nucleotide fluorescence and myoglobin oxygenation with cytochrome c oxidation in rabbit septa. Data from Fig. 9 are replotted at various oxygen delivery rate values to show the relationship between myoglobin oxygenation and pyridine nucleotide, and cytochrome c oxidation states.

of high-flow hypoxia are presented in Fig. 11. The percentage oxidation of cytochrome c was strictly proportional to the percentage oxidation of myoglobin; this is in agreement with the relationship existing between percentage oxidation of cytochrome aa_3 and percentage oxidation of myoglobin obtained with the perfused rat heart

(Fig. 8). The occurrence of very steep oxygen gradients in the contracting myocardium may, therefore, be regarded as an established phenomenon. Fig. 11 also shows that there was a different relationship between the percentage oxidation of cytochrome c and percentage oxidation of pyridine nucleotides, so that pyridine nucleotides are more readily reduced than cytochrome c as the rate of oxygen delivery is diminished. This may be due mainly to the fact that measurements of the pyridine nucleotide surface fluorescence do not distinguish between changes of NADH in the cytosol or mitochondria. Cytosolic NADH, in fact, makes a significant contribution to the overall pyridine nucleotide fluorescence signal (Williamson et al.,1973). Furthermore, the ratio of NADH/NAD increases, as the cytosolic phosphate potential (ATP/ADP x P$_i$) falls; this is a result of the link between these systems through the glyceraldehyde-3-P dehydrogenase and P-glycerate kinase reactions (Williamson, 1976).The possibility that cytosolic NADH may contribute significantly to the measured changes in pyridine nucleotides fluorescence in the intact tissue, is reinforced by the observations of Chance (1976a) on isolated mitochondria, which showed that, as the oxygen tension was decreased, cytochrome c reduction occurred prior to that of pyridine nucleotide.

The comparison of high-flow anoxia and ischemia in the arterially perfused septum further substantiates the contribution of localized anoxia and intracellular acidosis to ischemic failure. The presence of discrete anoxic zones and sharp borders between aerobic and anaerobic tissue suggests that "ischemia" is primarily a local process even when the coronary flow supplying the entire left ventricle is decreased. The vascular resistance rises under these conditions, and it seems probable that this represents a diffuse vasospasm of the coronary arterioles. Since this same type of severe vasoconstriction occurred with respiratory acidosis during the rapid transition from pH 7.4 to 6.6 in the perfused rat heart (Williamson, 1976), it is possible that local acidosis induces vasospasm, resulting in a discrete zone of anoxia. By completely shutting off flow into one capillary bed, it may be increased in others. Thus, oxygen delivery would be augmented in certain areas while becoming negligible elsewhere. Coronary-flow rate, therefore, would appear to be a poor index of the degree of ischemia in the myocardium. Further experimentation is necessary to determine the factors responsible for producing these distinct areas of adequate oxygenation or total anoxia. An understanding of such a mechanism may resolve many of the unanswered questions concerning the development of ischemic failure.

SUMMARY

The effects of ischemia on myocardial function and metabolism have been investigated in the perfused rat heart. In order to determine the relative contributions of acidosis and hypoxia, these components of ischemia were studied separately. The closed aorta preparation, with the entire cardiac output being directed through the coronary circulation, was used to study the effects of metabolic versus respiratory acidosis on pressure development and intracellular pH. Respiratory acidosis below pH 7.3 caused a rapid fall of left ventricular pressure to 20% of control values at pH 6.6. This decline of pressure development was proportional to the decrease in intracellular pH. Artificial buffer acidosis, with no CO_2 or bicarbonate in the medium, caused a much less severe decline of pressure development than respiratory acidosis at the same extracellular pH. Intracellular pH measurements indicated that respiratory acidosis produced a greater fall of intracellular pH than artificial buffer acidosis at the same extracellular pH. It is concluded that the negative inotropic effect of acidosis is caused primarily by an increased intracellular H^+ concentration, with an increased extracellular H^+ concentration having a much smaller effect.

A model of ischemia was produced by inserting a 1-way check valve in the aortic outflow tract. This had the effect of decreasing the diastolic aortic pressure and, hence, uniformly reducing flow through the coronary arteries while at the same time maintaining the systolic aortic pressure at its control level until heart failure developed after several minutes. Thus, the cardiac work load was initially unchanged but the coronary flow was diminished. This resulted in decreased oxygen delivery even though the arterial oxygen content was unchanged, and also diminished removal of metabolic end products from the tissue. When coronary flow dropped to a critical value, reduced oxygen delivery produced hypoxia, as shown by an increase of pyridine nucleotide fluorescence. Accumulation of CO_2 and lactate in the tissue produced a decrease in intracellular and coronary effluent pH. These changes were coincident with a fall of systolic aortic pressure. Hearts were rapidly frozen at various degrees of ischemic failure, according to the extent of the decline of the systolic aortic pressure. The levels of high-energy phosphate compounds fell progressively as the heart failure became more severe. Similarly, lactate accumulation and total NADH content were proportional to the degree of heart failure. Metabolic changes in the ischemic tissue were compared with those observed during high-flow anoxia at different arterial fluid pH values. The depletion of high-energy phosphate compounds during ischemia was attributed to the hypoxia which developed as a result of decreased oxygen delivery.

Use of a technique of flash photography, to excite and record changes of pyridine nucleotide fluorescence from the heart surface, revealed that tissue hypoxia during ischemia was very heterogeneous. As ischemia progressed, many small areas of high-pryridine nucleotide fluorescence, denoting anoxic zones adjacent to normoxic tissue, became apparent. Further measurements of cytochrome aa_3, cytochrome c, and myoglobin absorbance changes—as a function of altered oxygen availability—indicated an exact correspondence between oxidation-reduction changes of the cytochromes and oxygenation-disoxygenation changes of myoglobin, despite the 100-fold greater affinity of cytochrome aa_3 for oxygen compared with myoglobin. These data support the concept of the existence of very steep oxygen gradients in ischemic or hypoxic hearts, which separate regions of cells, or even single cells and mitochondria into two populations having either normal controlled respiration or zero respiration. It is suggested that altered values of tissue metabolite contents, measured during progressive ischemia of the whole heart, reflect mainly the increased proportion of fully anoxic tissue to the total tissue mass.

The effects of high- and low-flow hypoxia (ischemia) on isometric tension development, with varying rates of oxygen delivery, were investigated further using isolated arterially perfused rabbit septa; this allowed simultaneous measurements of pyridine nucleotide fluorescence, and cytochrome c and myoglobin absorbance. At any given rate of oxygen delivery to the tissue below a critical value, isometric tension fell more with ischemia than when arterial perfusion was maintained during high-flow hypoxia. The relationship between percentage change of isometric tension and percentage oxidation of cytochrome c showed that the latter was relatively more oxidized during ischemia than during high-flow hypoxia, as isometric tension fell below 90% of the fully aerobic value. Since the oxidation-reduction state of cytochrome c measured the balance between rates of oxygen delivery and demand, the data indicate that the fall of intracellular pH with ischemia causes a specific negative inotropic effect, independent of the degree of hypoxia in the tissue. The demonstration of discrete anoxic zones, surrounded by apparently well-oxygenated tissue in the myocardium of ischemic hearts exhibiting impaired contractility, raises new questions concerning the etiology of ischemic-tissue damage and possible preventive measures. The present data suggest that diminished work performance during ischemia is caused by a combination of intracellular acidosis and a highly heterogeneous decrease of functional cell mass because of the anoxic zones.

ACKNOWLEDGMENTS

This project was supported by NIH Grants HL-14461 and HL-18708, and Contract NOI-HV-52995, awarded under the Myocardial Infarction Program of the National Heart, Lung and Blood Institute.

REFERENCES

Barlow, C., and Chance, B.: Ischemic areas in perfused rat hearts: measurements by NADH fluorescence photography. *Science* 193:909-910 (1976).

Bing, O. H. L., Brooks, W. W., and Messer, J. V.: Heart muscle viability following hypoxia: protective effect of acidosis. *Science* 180:1297-1298 (1973).

Chance, B., Legallais, V., Sorge, J., and Graham, N.: A versatile time-sharing multichannel spectrophotometer, reflectometer and flurometer. *Anal. Biochem.* 66:498-514 (1975).

Chance, B.: Pyridine nucleotide as an indicator of the oxygen requirements for energy-linked functions of mitochondria. *Circ. Res.* 38 (Suppl I): 31-38 (1976a).

Chance, B.: Discussion. *Circ. Res.* 38 (Suppl I): 69 (1976b).

Chesnais, J. M., Coraboeuf, E., Sauviat, M. P., and Vassas, J. M.: Sensitivity to H^+, Li^+, and Mg^{2+} ions of the slow inward sodium current in frog atrial fibres. *J. Mol. Cell. Cardiol.* 7:627-642 (1975).

Coraboeuf, E., Deroubaix, E., and Hoerter, J.: Control of ionic permeabilities in normal and ischemic heart. *Circ. Res.* 38 (Suppl. I): 92-97 (1976).

Delahayes, J.: Etude des mouvements d'ions dans le coeur de mammifères. Thèse d'Etat, Orsay (1968).

Ebashi, S.: Calcium ions in cardiac contractility. In *Proceedings, 8th International Meeting of the International Study Group for Research in Cardiac Metabolism,* Tokyo. In press.

Fabiato, A., and Fabiato, F.: Contraction induced by a calcium-triggered release of calcium from the sarcoplasmic reticulum of single skinned cardiac cells. *J. Physiol.* (Lond.) 249:469-495 (1975).

Fuchs, F.: In *Calcium Binding Proteins,* W. Drabikowski, H. Strzelecka-

Golaszewska and E. Carafoli, eds. Elsevier Scientific Publishing Co., Amsterdam (1974), pp. 1-27.

Jenings, R. B.: Early phase of myocardial ischemic injury and infarction. *Am. J. Cardiol.* 24:753-765 (1969).

Katz, A. M., and Hecht, H. H.: The early "pump" failure of the ischemic heart. *Am. J. Med.* 47:479-502 (1969).

Khuri, S., Flaherty, J. T., O'Riordan, J. B., Pitt, B., Brawley, R. K., Donahoo, J. S., and Gott, V. L.: Changes in intramyocardial ST segment voltage and gas tensions with regional myocardial ischemia in the dog. *Circ. Res.* 8: 204-215 (1975).

Langer, G. A.: Events at the cardiac sarcolemma: localization and movement of contractile-dependent calcium. *Fed. Proc.* 35:1274-1278 (1976).

Morad, M., and Goldman, Y.: Excitation-contraction coupling in heart muscle: membrane control of development of tension. *Prog. Biophys. Mol. Biol.* 27:257-313 (1973).

Neely, J. R., Liebermeister, H., Battersby, E. J., and Morgan, H. E.: Effect of pressure development on oxygen consumption by the isolated rat heart. *Am. J. Physiol.* 212:804-814 (1967).

Neely, J. R., Rovetto, M. J., Whitmer, J. T., and Morgan, H. E.: Effects of ischemia on ventricular function and metabolism in the isolated working rat heart. *Am. J. Physiol.* 225:651-658 (1973).

Neely, J. R., Whitmer, J. T., and Rovetto, M. J.: Effect of coronary flow on glycolytic flux and intracellular pH in isolated rat hearts. *Circ. Res.* 37: 733-741 (1975).

Opie, L. H.: Effects of regional ischemia on metabolism of glucose and fatty acids. *Circ. Res.* 38 (Suppl I): 52-68 (1976).

Rich, T. L., and Brady, A. J.: Potassium contracture and utilization of high-energy phosphates in rabbit heart. *Am. J. Physiol.* 226:105-113 (1974).

Rovetto, M. J., Whitmer, J. T., and Neely, J. R.: Comparison of the effects of anoxia and whole heart ischemia on carbohydrate utilization in isolated working rat hearts. *Circ. Res.* 32:699-711 (1973).

Tsien, R. W.: Possible effects of hydrogen ions in ischemic myocardium. *Circulation* 53 (Suppl. I): 14-16 (1976).

Waddell, W. J., and Bates, R. G.: Intracellular pH. *Physiol. Rev.* 49:285-329 (1969).

Williamson, J. R.: Mitochondrial metabolism and cell regulation. In *Mitochondria: Bioenergetics, Biogenesis and Membrane Structure*, L. Packer and A. Gomez-Puyon, eds. Academic Press, Inc., New York (1976), pp. 79-107.

Williamson, J. R., and Corkey, B. E.: Assays of intermediates of the citric acid cycle and related compounds by fluorometric enzyme methods. *Methods Enzymol.* 13:434-513 (1969).

Williamson, J. R., and LaNoue, K. F.: Feedback control of the citric acid cycle. Pan-American Association of Biochemical Societies *Revista* 4:53-62 (1975).

Williamson, J. R., Safer, B., LaNoue, K. F., Smith, C. M., and Walajtys, E.: Mitochondrial-cytosolic interactions in cardiac tissue; role of the malate-aspartate cycle in the removal of glycolytic NADH from the cytosol. *Symp. Soc. Exp. Biol.* 27:241-281 (1973).

Williamson, J. R., Safer, B., Rich, T., Schaffer, S., and Kobayashi, K.: Effects of acidosis on myocardial contractility and metabolism. *Acta. Med. Scand.* (Suppl) 587:95-111 (1975a).

Williamson, J. R., Schaffer, S. W., Ford, C., and Safer, B.: Contribution of tissue acidosis to ischemic injury in the perfused rat heart. *Circulation* 53 (Suppl I): 3-14 (1976).

Williamson, J. R., Woodrow, M. L., and Scarpa. A.: Calcium binding to cardiac sarcolemma. In *Recent Advances in Studies on Cardiac Structure and Metabolism*, Vol. 5, A. Fleckenstein and N. S. Dhalla, eds. University Park Press, Baltimore (1975b), pp. 27-33.

9

Effects of Ischemia on Myocardial Fatty Acid Oxidation

JANE A. IDELL-WENGER
JAMES R. NEELY

INTRODUCTION

Fatty acids represent a major substrate for energy metabolism in cardiac muscle. Under aerobic conditions, 60 to 90% of the total oxygen consumption may be used to oxidize fatty acids (Neely and Morgan, 1974; Opie, 1969). Rates of fatty acid uptake and oxidation depend on the concentration of exogenous fatty acids and on the oxidative state of the tissue (Oram et al., 1973). At concentrations below 0.5 mM, the rate of uptake is limited by extracellular availability. At higher concentrations, the rates of uptake and oxidation are limited by the activity of the citric acid cycle. The rate of oxidation is linearly related to the rate of oxidative phosphorylation; it increases as cardiac work is elevated (Oram et al., 1973) and decreases with a reduction in oxygen supply (Neely et al., 1975). Since the rates of oxidative phosphorylation and flux through the citric acid cycle are tightly coupled (LaNoue et al., 1970), the control of fatty acid metabolism in aerobic hearts occurs secondarily to regulation of these pathways (Oram et al., 1973). Control of the pathway in oxygen-deficient hearts is not understood. The purpose of the present study was to determine the regulation of fatty acid metabolism in isolated rat hearts that were made oxygen deficient. The contribution of fatty-acid oxidation to total oxidative metabolism was determined in ischemic hearts, and rate-limiting steps of fatty-acid oxidation in ischemic and hypoxic hearts were assessed by measuring tissue levels and cellular distribution of CoA and carnitine intermediates.

METHODS

Perfusion Technique

Hearts from 200- to 250-g male Sprague-Dawley rats were excised and cannulated as described for the isolated, working rat heart (Neely et al., 1967). In the working heart apparatus, cardiac output and ventricular-pressure development can be controlled by regulating left atrial filling pressure and/or resistance of the aortic outflow tract. Coronary flow in this preparation was a function of aortic pressure and, thus, changed in direct relation to left ventricular-pressure development. Whole-heart ischemia was induced by use of a one-way valve in the aortic outflow tract, which markedly restricted coronary flow during ventricular diastole but did not influence aortic output and ventricular-pressure development initially (Neely et al., 1973). The hearts received a 10-min washout perfusion and 5 min as a working control prior to the induction of a 20-min period of ischemia. Two degrees of ischemia were established by changing the height of a minimal-flow bubble trap which bypassed the one-way valve in the cannula arrangement. This system prevented coronary flow from declining further as pressure development of the heart deteriorated.

The perfusate was Krebs-Henseleit bicarbonate buffer gassed with 95% O_2:5% CO_2 for aerobic and ischemic conditions. For hypoxia, oxygen availability was restricted by gassing the perfusate with 20% O_2:5% CO_2:75% N_2, and the flow was maintained at 15 ml/min. The buffer contained 11 mM glucose and 1.0 mM palmitate bound to 3% bovine serum albumin.

Estimation of Palmitate Oxidation and O_2 Consumption

Hearts were perfused with buffer containing 1.0 mM [U-^{14}C] palmitate. The rate of palmitate oxidation was calculated from the arterial-venous difference in $^{14}CO_2$, specific activity of the perfusate palmitate and rate of coronary flow. Coronary venous samples were collected without exposure to air. Arterial samples were obtained from the left atrial perfusate just prior to entry into the heart (Neely et al., 1967). For $^{14}CO_2$ production, samples of perfusate were injected into a stoppered, Erlenmeyer flask containing 6N H_2SO_4. The $^{14}CO_2$ released was collected in a center well containing hyamine hydroxide. After 2 hr, the wells were removed, placed in toluene scintillation fluid and counted. For determining palmitate specific activity, samples of the perfusate were acidified, exposed to air for 23 hr to remove $^{14}CO_2$ and counted. Palmitate concentration was estimated after its extraction with chloroform (Duncombe, 1963). Oxygen consumption was estimated from arterial-venous differences in perfusate PO_2, measured with a radiometer model PHM 27 blood-gas monitor.

Estimation of Tissue Levels of Metabolic Intermediates

At the end of perfusion, hearts used to determine levels of metabolic intermediates were frozen, while being perfused, with a Wollenberger clamp cooled to the temperature of liquid nitrogen. The frozen tissue was powdered in a percussion mortar, extracted in cold 6% $HClO_4$ and centrifuged at 0°C. The supernatant was neutralized with KOH and used for the estimation of tissue levels of acetyl-CoA and acetylcarnitine. The precipitate was washed with 0.6% $HClO_4$ and used for estimating tissue content of long-chain acyl-CoA and acylcarnitine derivatives.

Acetyl-CoA and acetylcarnitine were assayed fluorometrically within 1 hr after making the extracts. Acetyl-CoA was estimated by the citrate synthetase method of Herrera and Freinkel (1967). Acetyl-carnitine was determined by coupling the acetyl-CoA assay to carnitine: acetyl-CoA transferase reaction (Pearson et al., 1969). Free CoASH was determined by using the α-ketoglutarate dehydrogenase reaction (Garland et al., 1965). Coupling this reaction to the carnitine: acetyl-CoA transferase reaction provided a method of measuring free-carnitine levels (Pearson et al., 1969).

Concentrations of long-chain acyl-CoA and acylcarnitine were assayed as free CoASH and carnitine after alkaline hydrolysis of the washed 6% perchloric acid precipitates (Williamson and Corkey, 1969). Levels of CoA and carnitine derivatives were determined on homogenates and mitochondrial samples after extraction with 6% $HClO_4$, as described for frozen tissue. Total CoA and carnitine in homogenates and mitochondria were assayed as free CoASH and carnitine after alkaline hydrolysis (Williamson and Corkey, 1969).

Cellular Distribution of CoA-SH and Carnitine

To estimate cellular distribution of CoASH and carnitine in ischemic hearts, the latter were perfused as described. Two hearts were pooled for each mitochondrial preparation. After 15 min of ischemic perfusion at a coronary flow of 5 ml/min, the hearts were switched to a washout perfusion with ice cold buffer containing 180 mM KC1, 10 mM EDTA, 2 mM KCN, pH 7.3-7.4. The hearts were then quickly transferred to a beaker, rinsed in the same medium, blotted, trimmed of atria and weighed. The tissue was transferred to a beaker containing 75 mM sucrose, 225 mM mannitol, 0.1 mM EDTA, 2 mM KCN, pH 7.3-7.4, and minced (final volume was 5 ml per gram tissue). The minced tissue was transferred to a flask and homogenized on ice by means of a Polytron tissue homogenizer (PT10), with an external rheostat setting of 36% maximum and the Polytron rheostat set at full speed for two 10-sec periods. The homogenate volume was adjusted to a final volume of 10 ml per gram tissue and centrifuged at $400 \times g$ for 2 min. The supernatant from this procedure was centrifuged again at $6000 \times g$ for 10 min to spin down mitochondria. The mitochondria were resuspended in a buffer containing 0.25 M sucrose, 10 mM potassium phosphate buffer, 10 mM MOPS, 2 mM KCN, pH 7.0 and centrifuged as before. The mitochondrial pellet was resuspended in the same buffer to 4.5 ml. Levels of total CoA and carnitine, and long-chain acyl-CoA and acylcarnitine were determined on the whole-tissue homogenate and on the isolated mitochondria. For normal values, hearts were removed and mitochondria prepared as described above. Concentrations of mitochondrial metabolites were extrapolated to whole tissue levels by using a value of 60 mg mitochondrial protein per gram wet weight of heart muscle. This value was obtained using the mitochondrial marker enzymes, cytochrome oxidase, citrate synthase, and β-hydroxyacyl-CoA dehydrogenase.

RESULTS

Effect of Ischemia on Palmitate Oxidation

Myocardial-oxygen consumption is proportional to the rate of oxygen delivery over a wide range of ischemic coronary flow rates (Neely et al., 1975). Oxygen consumption and palmitate oxidation were determined at a normal coronary flow rate (15 ml/min) and at two ischemic rates (5 and 1 ml/min) of flow which result in

Table 1. Effect of ischemia on oxygen consumption
and palmitate oxidation

Condition	Coronary flow (ml/min)	Oxygen consumption (μmoles/g dry wt) per min	Palmitate oxidation (μmoles/g dry wt) per min
Control	15	38.0 ± 1.7	.78 ± .08
Ischemic	5	18.3 ± 2.0	.53 ± .05
Ischemic	1	3.1 ± 1.7	.17 ± .05

Each value represents mean ± SEM of 8-10 hearts.

ventricular failure. Control hearts consumed oxygen at a rate of 38 μmoles/min/g dry weight (Table 1). This rate was reduced to 18 and 3 μmoles/min/g dry weight when the flow declined to 5 and 1 ml/min, respectively. Oxidation of exogenous fatty acid decreased similarly as coronary flow was reduced. Oxidation of palmitate accounted for 60 and 63% of the oxygen consumption in control and ischemic hearts receiving 5 ml/min coronary flow, respectively. At the lower flow, however, fatty acid oxidation accounted for about 90% of the oxygen consumption. This data indicated that fatty-acid oxidation decreased as oxygen supply was reduced and that palmitate oxidation accounted for the majority of oxygen consumption at all rates of coronary flow.

Effect of Coronary Flow and Hypoxia on Tissue Levels on Acyl-CoA and Acylcarnitine Derivatives

In order to identify the rate-controlling steps of fatty-acid metabolism, tissue levels of acyl-CoA and acylcarnitine derivatives were measured after inducing either ischemia or hypoxia. The concentrations of acetyl-CoA and acetylcarnitine decreased while those of long-chain acyl-CoA and acylcarnitine increased (Table 2). These data, combined with reduced rates of palmitate oxidation, indicate that β-oxidation became rate-limiting for fatty-acid oxidation in ischemic hearts. This inhibition of β-oxidation appeared to be very senstive to changes in oxygen supply, since hypoxia with maintained coronary flow resulted in similar changes in CoA and carnitine derivatives as did ischemia. Thus, even a mild degree of tissue hypoxia inhibits β-oxidation and this inhibition appears to be related

Table 2. Effect of coronary flow and hypoxia on tissue levels of acyl-CoA and acylcarnitine derivatives

Condition	Coronary Flow (ml/min)	Acyl-CoA and Acylcarnitine Derivatives (nmoles/g dry wt)			
		Long-chain acyl-CoA	Acetyl-CoA	Long-chain acylcarnitine	Acetyl-carnitine
Control	12	178 ± 4	162 ± 17	1307 ± 159	2002 ± 118
Ischemic	5	346 ± 20	38 ± 6	4353 ± 265	470 ± 58
Hypoxic	15	297 ± 10	57 ± 7	3808 ± 182	477 ± 58

Each value represents the mean ±SEM for 6-7 hearts.

to a decrease in oxygen supply *per se* and not to the rate of coronary flow.

Intracellular Distribution of CoA and Carnitine

The changes in acyl-CoA intermediates during ischemia indicate inhibition of β-oxidation only if the majority of the CoA derivatives are located inside the mitochondrial matrix near the site of β-oxidation. In aerobic hearts, at least 95% of the total CoA was located in the matrix (Oram et al., 1975). However, mitochondria of ischemic tissue are known to be damaged, therefore, the long-chain acyl-CoA determined on whole tissue samples may not be inside the mitochondria. More than 95% of the whole tissue total CoA and long-chain acyl-CoA was recovered in the mitochondrial fraction (Fig. 1), indicating that mitochondria isolated from ischemic hearts perfused under these conditions do not leak CoA into the cytosol.

Since the levels of acylcarnitine derivatives change in a similar manner as the acyl-CoA derivatives, it was of interest to determine their intracellular distribution during ischemia (Fig. 1). The total, fatty acyl-, and acid-soluble (free plus acetyl-) carnitine that is associated with isolated mitochondria increases from 5, 2 and 7% in normal tissue to 38, 27 and 48%, respectively, during ischemia.

The long-chain acyl-CoA associated with the mitochondrial fraction could simply be bound to proteins on the outer mitochondrial surface and would not represent matrix CoA. To determine if this possibility did exist, mitochondria from ischemic hearts were

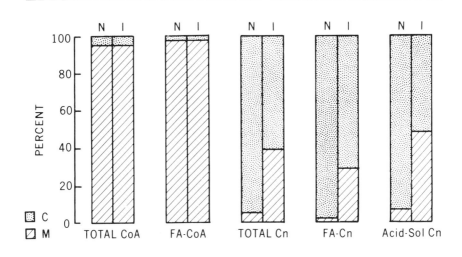

1

Distribution of CoASH and carnitine between mitochondria (M) and cytosol (C) in normal (N) and ischemic (I) heart muscle. Experimental conditions are described in "Methods."

incubated for 10 min with albumin and total CoA, long-chain acyl-CoA and free CoASH levels were determined on the mitochondria and incubation medium after 0, 5 and 10 min of incubation (Fig. 2). Mitochondrial levels of long-chain acyl-CoA decreased during incubation even though respiration was inhibited. The long-chain acyl-CoA derivatives that disappeared from the mitochondria did not show up in the incubation medium as might be expected if they were bound to the outer mitochondrial surface and available to exchange with albumin in the incubation medium. This observation suggested that ischemia activated some hydrolytic enzymes which broke down acyl-CoA esters. The decrease in mitochondrial long-chain acyl-CoA was matched by an equal molar rise in mitochondrial free CoASH indicating that the CoASH released by hydrolysis remained inside the matrix space. Very little free CoASH could be detected in the incubation medium. These data indicate that the increase in long-chain acyl-CoA in ischemic tissue occurred inside the mitochondrial matrix. Since most of the total CoA was associated with the mitochondrial fraction, it is likely that the decrease in acetyl-CoA during ischemia also occurred in the mitochondrial matrix. Thus, the

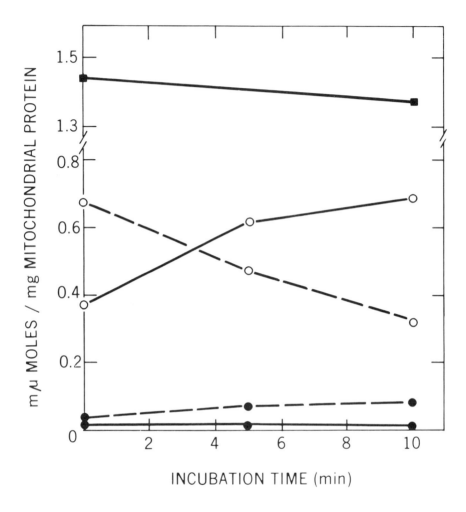

rise in levels of substrates and decrease in products of β-oxidation inside the mitochondrial matrix indicates that β-oxidation was inhibited in ischemic tissue and that this process limited the rate of fatty-acid oxidation.

DISCUSSION

The rate of β-oxidation does not appear to control the overall rate of fatty-acid utilization in aerobic hearts (Oram et al., 1973; 1975). In oxygen-deficient tissue, however, β-oxidation may limit

Levels of CoASH and long-chain acyl CoA in mitochondria from
ischemic hearts. Mitochondria were isolated from hearts perfused
under ischemic conditions (coronary flows of 4 ml/min) for 20 min
with buffer containing 11 mM glucose and 1.0 mM palmitate. The
mitochondrial suspension, containing 8.2 mg protein/ml, was
temperature equilibrated at 30°C, with stirring for 2 min. An equal
volume of buffer containing 3% BSA was added. Samples were
removed at 0 and 10 min for the determination of total CoA (solid
squares). The level of long-chain acyl CoA measured on the whole
tissue averaged 333 mμmoles/g dry weight. Of this amount, 316
mμmoles/g dry weight was recovered in the mitochondrial fraction.
Samples were removed at 0, 5 and 10 min, and centrifuged at
15,000 × g for 10 min to separate the mitochondrial (open circles)
and supernatant (closed circles) fractions. Dithiothreitol (10 mM) and
perchloric acid (6%) were added to the samples. The PCA
supernatants were assayed for free CoASH (solid lines) and the
PCA precipitates were assayed for fatty acyl CaO (dashed lines) as
described in "Methods." Protein was determined by the Lowry
et al. (1951) procedure. The CoA levels are expressed in nmoles
per mg of mitochondrial protein. Each value represents the mean
of three determinations on one preparation of mitochondria from two
hearts. The experiment was repeated five times with similar results.

2

this rate (Neely et al., 1973; Bremer and Wojtczak, 1972; Bowman,
1966). In the present study, β-oxidation seemed to be inhibited in
both hypoxic and ischemic hearts. The rise in levels of long-chain
acyl-CoA and the decrease in acetyl-CoA, in conjunction with a
slower rate of palmitate oxidation, indicated that β-oxidation was
inhibited in ischemic tissue. Similar changes in tissue levels of CoA
derivatives occurred in hypoxic hearts, indicating that this type of
oxygen deficiency also inhibited β-oxidation.

These alterations in tissue levels of intermediates can be interpreted to indicate inhibition of β-oxidation only if the changes in
CoA derivatives occurred within the mitochondrial matrix where
the β-oxidation enzymes are located. From the data presented, it
seems reasonable to assume that most of the increase in long-chain
acyl-CoA and the decrease in acetyl-CoA that occurred during hypoxic and ischemic perfusion did, in fact, take place inside the
mitochondrial matrix, indicating that β-oxidation represented the
rate-limiting process for fatty-acid metabolism. The reduced rate of
β-oxidation probably resulted from high tissue levels of reducing
equivalents. The NADH/NAD ratio increases dramatically under
these conditions (Rovetto et al., 1975), and the inability to reoxidize

FADH$_2$ would also be expected to reduce the rate of fatty acyl CoA :FAD oxidoreductase.

The accumulation of long-chain acyl derivatives may have severe consequences on the metabolism of ischemic hearts. Long-chain acyl-CoA is known to inhibit a number of enzymes. When added to the incubation of isolated mitochondria,, this acyl derivative inhibits adenine nucleotide translocase (Shug et al., 1975), and it is thought that mitochondria isolated from ischemic tissue have a reduced rate of State 3 oxygen consumption, due to the presence of high levels of acyl-CoA. Although external acyl-CoA inhibits adenine-nucleotide transport in mitochondria, it is not clear that accumulation of this compound inside the mitochondrial matrix also has such an inhibiting effect. Since nearly 100% of the acyl-CoA in ischemic hearts is inside the matrix, it is important to determine if high levels of acyl-CoA in this compartment interfere with oxidative metabolism. From the studies reported by Shug et al., 1975), mitochondria isolated from ischemic tissue, which had high levels of long-chain acyl-CoA, transported ADP at a reduced rate. ADP transport and O$_2$ consumption could be restored by incubation with albumin, which was thought to remove acyl-CoA bound to the mitochondrial surface. Levels of mitochondrial acyl-CoA were not measured and it, therefore, is not possible to interpret the data in regard to the presence of external and matrix acyl-CoA. It is possible that hydrolysis of acyl-CoA during the incubation, as occurred in the present study, lowered the level inside the matrix and removed the inhibition of adenine nucleotide translocase, whether or not albumin was present. If this were true, it would appear that acyl-CoA inhibits the translocase from the matrix as well as the cytosolic side.

The rise in matrix long-chain acyl-CoA would be expected to increase the levels of long-chain acylcarnitine in the cytosol. The whole tissue levels of acylcarnitine did rise and most of the increase occurred in the cytosolic compartment. The long-chain acylcarnitine, associated with the mitochondrial fraction, appeared to be loosely bound to the outer mitochondrial surface since it could be removed by incubation with albumin. With high levels of cytosolic long-chain acylcarnitine, the small amount of cytosolic CoASH would be expected to be largely converted to acyl-CoA. Thus, the decrease in fatty-acid activation and uptake probably resulted from lower levels of free CoASH available for activation and lower levels of carnitine as acyl acceptor in the transferase reaction.

Acylcarnitine is known to be transported into mitochondria in exchange for efflux of carnitine (Pande, 1975). Normally, only 5%

of the total carnitine present in the tissue is located inside the mito-chondrial matrix. In ischemic tissue, however, a net transfer of carnitine from cytosol to mitochondria occurs. The mechanism and significance of this increase in mitochondrial carnitine is not known at this time.

ACKNOWLEDGMENTS

This work was supported, in part, by Grant No. 5-ROI-HL-13028-07 from the National Heart and Lung Institute, NIH, and a grant-in-aid from the Pennsylvania Heart Association.

REFERENCES

Bremer, J., and Wojtczak, A. B.: Factors controlling the rate of fatty acid β-oxidation in rat liver mitochondria. *Biochim. Biophys. Acta* 280:515-530 (1972).

Bowman, R. H.: Effects of diabetes, fatty acids, and ketone bodies on tricar-boxylic acid cycle metabolism in the perfused rat heart. *J. Biol. Chem.* 241:3041-3048 (1966).

Duncombe, W. G.: The colorimetric microdetermination of long-chain fatty acids. *Biochem. J.* 88:7-10 (1963).

Garland, P. B., Shepherd, D., and Yates, D. W.: Steady-state concentrations of coenzyme A, acetyl-coenzyme A and long-chain fatty acyl-coenzyme A in rat-liver mitochondrial oxidizing palmitate. *Biochem. J.* 97:587-594 (1965).

Herrera, E., and Freinkel, N.: Internal standards in the estimation of acetyl-CoA in liver extracts. *J. Lipid Res.* 8:515-518 (1967).

LaNoue, K. F., Nicklas, W. J., and Williamson, J. R.: Control of citric acid cycle activity in rat heart mitochondria. *J. Biol. Chem.* 245:102-111 (1970).

Lowry, O. H., Rosebrough, N. J., Farr, A. L., and Randall, P. J.: Protein measurement with the Folin phenol reagent. *J. Biol. Chem.* 193:265-275 (1951).

Neely, J. R., Liebermeister, H., Battersby, E. J., and Morgan, H. E.: Effect of pressure development on oxygen consumption by isolated rat heart. *Am. J. Physiol.* 212:804-814 (1967).

Neely, J. R., Liedtke, A. J., Whitmer, J. T., and Rovetto, M. J.: Relationship between coronary flow and adenosine triphosphate production from glycol-ysis and oxidative metabolism. In *Recent Advances in Studies on Cardiac Structure and Metabolism*, Vol. 8, *The Cardiac Sarcoplasm*, P. E. Roy and P. Harris, eds. University Park Press, Baltimore (1975), pp. 301-321.

Neely, J. R., and Morgan, H. E.: Relationship between carbohydrate and lipid metabolism and the energy balance of heart muscle. *Ann. Rev. Physiol.* 36:413-459 (1974).

Neely, J. R., Rovetto, M. J., Whitmer, J. T., and Morgan, H. E.: Effects of ischemia on ventricular function and metabolism in the isolated working rat heart. *Am. J. Physiol.* 225:651-658 (1973).

Neely, J. R., Whitmer, J. T., and Rovetto, M. J.: Effect of coronary blood flow on glycolytic flux and intracellular pH in isolated rat hearts. *Circ. Res.* 37:733-741 (1975).

Opie, L. H.: Metabolism of the heart in health and disease. Part II. *Am. Heart J.* 77:100-122 (1969).

Oram, J. F., Bennetch, S. L., and Neely, J. R.: Regulation of fatty acid utilization in isolated perfused rat hearts. *J. Biol. Chem.* 248:5299-5309 (1973).

Oram, J. F., Wenger, J. I., and Neely, J. R.: Regulation of long-chain fatty acid activation in heart muscle. *J. Biol. Chem.* 250:73-78 (1975).

Pande, S. V.: A mitochondrial carnitine acylcarnitine translocase system. *Proc. Nat. Acad. Sci. USA* 72:883-887 (1975).

Pearson, D. J., Chase, J. F. A., and Tubbs, P. K.: The assay of (−)-carnitine and its 0-acyl derivatives. In *Methods in Enzymology*, Vol. 14, J. M. Lowenstein, ed. Academic Press, New York and London (1969), pp. 612-622.

Rovetto, M. J., Lamberton, W. F., and Neely, J. R.: Mechanisms of glycolytic inhibition in ischemic rat hearts. *Circ. Res.* 37:742-751 (1975).

Shug, A. L., Shrago, E., Bittar, N., Folts, J. D., and Kokes, J. R.: Acyl-CoA inhibition of adenine nucleotide translocation in ischemic myocardium. *Am. J. Physiol.* 228:689-692 (1975).

Williamson, J. R., and Corkey, B. E.: Assays of intermediates of the citric acid cycle and related compounds by fluorometric enzyme methods. In *Methods in Enzymology*, Vol. 13, J. M. Lowenstein, ed. Academic Press, New York and London (1969), pp. 434-513.

10

Adenine Nucleotide Translocase Activity During Myocardial Ischemia

EARL SHRAGO
HEI SOOK SUL

INTRODUCTION

In recent years, considerable evidence has appeared in the literature, which demonstrates that the adenine nucleotide translocase of the inner mitochondrial membrane can be modulated by long chain fatty acyl CoA esters (for review see Meijer and van Dam, 1974, and Shrago et al., 1976). These observations are important for at least two reasons: (1) Long chain fatty acyl CoA esters are the only known natural effectors of the adenine nucleotide translocase; (2) a natural effector of the adenine nucleotide translocase would influence the central role of this transport protein in cellular metabolism, in terms of regulating oxidative phosphorylation and coordinating the intra and extramitochondrial ATP/ADP ratios or the phosphate potential of the cell (McLean et al., 1971). In tissues such as the myocardium where the mitochondrial oxidation of fatty acids accounts for the major source of energy (Neely and Morgan, 1974), an important effect of long chain acyl CoA esters at the site of the adenine translocase might be anticipated.

The mitochondrial metabolism of long chain fatty acids involves

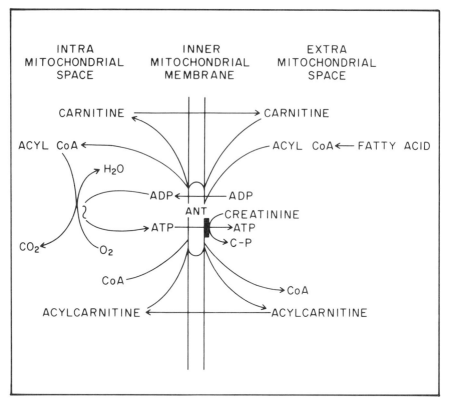

1 Interrelation of fatty acid oxidation and adenine nucleotide translocation at the inner mitochondrial membrane.

a number of critical steps not the least of which is their transport to the site of β-oxidation (Fritz and Marquis, 1965). The long chain fatty acid, which is first acylated to its CoA derivative on the outer mitochondrial membrane, is then transacylated on the outer side of the inner mitochondrial membrane to the carnitine ester by the acyl carnitine transferase enzyme. The acyl carnitine penetrates the inner membrane, possibly by a carrier system whereby carnitine is concurrently translocated from the intra- to the extramitochondrial space (Pande, 1975). On the inner side of the inner membrane, the acyl carnitine ester is again transacylated via a second acyl carnitine transferase to the acyl CoA for subsequent β-oxidation. Fig. 1, which schematically illustrates the transport of the acyl CoA to the site of β-oxidation, is designed to draw attention to the close association of this metabolic sequence with the translocation of adenine nucleotides and the synthesis of high energy phosphate esters.

Previous results obtained from a number of laboratories have shown that low concentrations of long chain acyl CoA esters can reversibly inhibit the adenine nucleotide translocase of liver (Shug et al., 1971, Lerner et al., 1972, Vaartjes et al., 1972) and heart mitochondria (Pande and Blanchaer, 1971, Harris et al., 1972, Shug and Shrago, 1973). The inhibition is specific for the acyl CoA ester in that free fatty acids and carnitine esters are not in themselves inhibitory. Addition of L-carnitine to the reaction medium, which allows for the transacylation of the acyl CoA to the acyl carnitine derivative, reverses the inhibition by the long chain acyl CoA.

Inhibition of adenine nucleotide translocation leads to a decrease in the synthesis of intramitochondrial ATP. Moreover, the ATP synthesized cannot be effectively exchanged with ADP for transport to the extramitochondrial space. As shown in Fig. 1, the mitochondrial creatine phosphokinase isozyme of myocardium is located on the outer side of the inner membrane and acts essentially as an ATP trap for the synthesis of creatine phosphate (Jacobus and Lehninger, 1973). Therefore, inhibited translocation would lead to a decrease in the level of creatine phosphate, as well as ATP depleting the energy requirements necessary for muscle contraction in the cytosol. Recent *in vivo* studies (Shug et al., 1975) have demonstrated a decrease in adenine nucleotide translocase activity, concomitant with an increase in tissue long chain acyl CoA esters in the dog heart subsequent to experimental coronary occlusion.

The present communication is intended to amplify and extend the knowledge of the mechanism by which long chain acyl CoA esters inhibit adenine nucleotide translocase activity and influence myocardial metabolism. From such information, it may be possible to gain better insight into appropriate measures which might protect the ischemic myocardium.

METHODS

Rat and guinea pig heart mitochondria were prepared according to the procedures used in this laboratory (Sul et al., 1976). Adenine nucleotide translocase activity was measured by the forward and back exchange techniques of Pfaff and Klingenberg

(1968), with slight modification as previously described (Lerner et al., 1972). Procedures for ^{14}C malate loading and transport were essentially the same as those described by Robinson (1971), as carried out in this laboratory (Shrago et al., 1974). ATP and ADP were determined in guinea pig heart mitochondria, using a luciferase enzyme system after first converting ADP to ATP with phosphocreatine and creatine kinase. Creatine phosphate formation was determined in guinea pig heart mitochondria according to Jacobus and Lehninger (1973). Long chain acyl CoA esters were isolated and determined by the method of Williamson and Corkey (1969). Protein was determined by the biuret reaction (Gornall et al., 1949). All reagents were of the highest grade commercially obtainable.

RESULTS

Initial experiments, carried out with liver mitochondria, indicated that only those acyl CoA esters which were carnitine dependent for their oxidation caused inhibition of adenine nucleotide translocation (Lerner et al., 1972; Shrago et al., 1974). In terms of myocardial metabolism this may be a significant observation since fatty-acid oxidation by heart mitochondria is 100% carnitine dependent (Neely and Morgan, 1974). The results shown in Fig. 2 indicate that isolated-heart mitochondria respond in a similar manner as liver mitochondria. Octanoyl CoA which is not carnitine dependent for its oxidation is not inhibitory while significant inhibition of the adenine nucleotide translocase occurs with low concentrations of the longer chain acyl CoA esters. The K values for myristoyl CoA, palmitoyl CoA and oleoyl CoA were calculated from double reciprocal plots and found to be 0.35 μM, 0.65 μM and 0.75 μM, respectively. These kinetic studies were carried out with intact rat-heart mitochondria which, therefore, contained some endogenous adenine nucleotides. It is, thus, likely that the true K for each acyl CoA is somewhat lower.

The inhibition of adenine nucleotide translocation by long chain acyl CoA esters is specific in that the carnitine derivatives and free fatty acids are not inhibitory. The results in Fig. 3 show that the addition of carnitine to the reaction mixture is able to overcome the inhibition of palmitoyl CoA by promoting its enzymatic conversion to palmitoyl carnitine. Since L-carnitine is the actual substrate for the acyl carnitine transferase enzyme, the concentrations of D, L-carnitine used in these experiments are somewhat higher than necessary to overcome the inhibition of palmitoyl CoA.

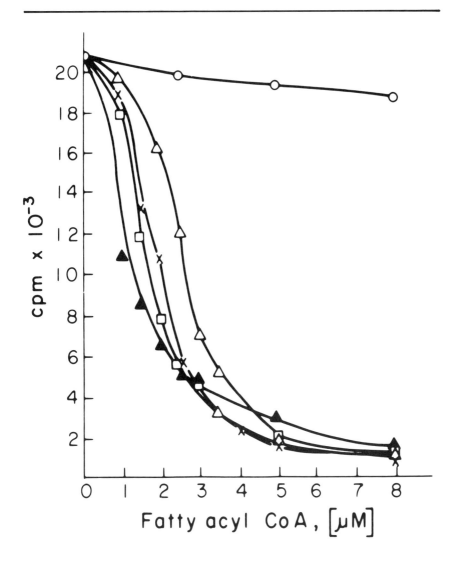

2

Concentration effect of various long chain acyl CoA esters on the adenine nucleotide translocase of rat-heart mitochondria. After preincubation of 0.85 mg mitochondrial protein with acyl CoA ester for 4 min at ice temperature, the reaction was initiated by the addition of 35,000 cpm [^{14}C] ADP and terminated in 1 min with 25 μM atractylate. Octanoyl CoA, o—o—o; palmitoyl CoA, $\triangle$—$\triangle$—$\triangle$; oleoyl CoA, x—x—x; myristoyl CoA, □—□—□; lauryl CoA, ▲—▲—▲.

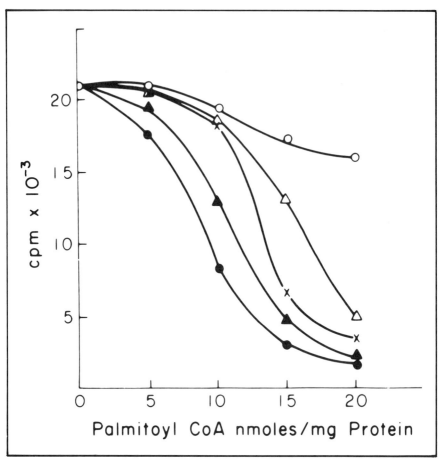

3 Effect of carnitine on the inhibition of adenine nucleotide translocation by palmitoyl CoA in rat-heart mitochondria. The experiment was carried out as in Fig. 2, except the reaction was run at 28° to permit maximum enzymatic activity of the palmitoyl carnitine transferase. D, L-carnitine 5 mM o—o—o; 1mM △—△—△; 0.1 mM x—x—x; 25 μM, △—△—△; no carnitine, o—o—o.

From what is known about mitochondrial compartmentation and selective permeability of the inner membrane, it seems likely that the inhibition by the acyl CoA ester occurs at the outer side of the inner mitochondrial membrane. The carnitine acyl transferase enzyme I, located on the outer side of the inner mitochondrial membrane, catalyzes the transacylation of the impermeable acyl CoA to the acyl carnitine and, thereby, accounts for the reversal of the inhibition by carnitine. The acyl carnitine derivative can then be transported across the membrane to the matrix side of the mitochondria. It is apparent, therefore, that reconversion here to the acyl CoA might also contribute to inhibition of adenine nucleotide translocation at the inner side of the inner membrane. The site of preferential inhibition by the acyl CoA esters has been further investigated and the results shown in Fig. 4. When isolated mitochondria are incubated with palmitoyl carnitine, the pattern of inhibition varies considerably, depending upon whether or not free CoA is added to the reaction mixture. With only endogenous CoA, there is minimal inhibition of the adenine nucleotide translocase and even this is completely eliminated in the Nagarse-treated mitochondria, which apparently removes any endogenous CoA outside of the inner membrane. In the presence of added CoA, however, there is a marked inhibition of the adenine nucleotide translocase. Since CoA cannot traverse the inner membrane, the results are interpreted to demonstrate that inhibition occurs when palmitoyl carnitine, in the presence of CoA, is converted to palmitoyl CoA on the outer side of the inner membrane by acyl carnitine transferase I. The fact that palmitoyl carnitine alone, which can penetrate the inner mitochondrial membrane, did not produce inhibition was good indication that its reconversion to palmitoyl CoA in the matrix would not cause inhibition of adenine nucleotide translocation. Additional evidence is provided by the results shown in Table 1 where mitochondrial acyl CoA levels were determined, following incubation with palmitoyl carnitine. If it can be assumed that the acyl CoA which accumulated, without addition of free CoA, was that within the matrix, the results strongly suggest that the inhibitory site of the adenine nucleotide translocase is only on the outer side of the inner membrane. It is recognized, however, that such assumptions are somewhat clouded by incomplete knowledge regarding the actual compartmentation of the accumulated acyl CoA esters, as well as endogenous adenine nucleotides which might compete effectively to prevent the inhibition.

Certain monovalent cations possess the ability to interfere with the inhibition of adenine nucleotide translocation by long chain acyl CoA esters (Duszynski and Wojtczak, 1975). Fig. 5 gives the results of a representative experiment showing that when increasing concentrations of K^+ are added to the incubation media, this successfully diminishes the inhibition by palmitoyl CoA. The effect is

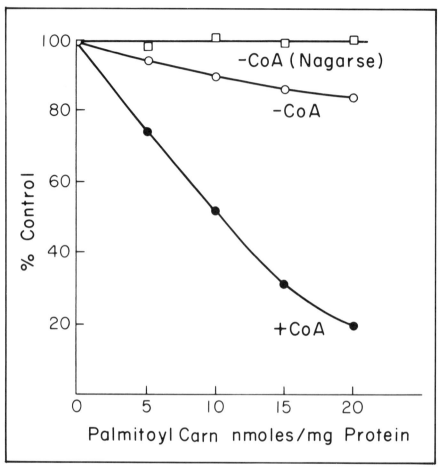

4 Effect of free CoA on the adenine nuclotide translocase of rat-heart
mitochondria, as a function of palmitoyl carnitine. Intact or Nagarse-
treated mitochondria were preincubated in 250 mM sucrose, 4 mM
Tris pH 7.4, 1 mM EDTA and 1 mM KCN for 4 min at 28°. The
reaction was then cooled to ice temperature and run as in Fig. 2.
The concentration of CoA was 1 mM.

not specific for K^+, however, in that some other monovalent cations,
such at Na^+, act in a similar manner. These findings, which should
be compared with those data in Fig. 2 where the basal medium
contains 75 μM KCl, suggest an effect of ionic strength on the
reaction.

Table 1. Accumulation of long chain acyl-CoA esters in heart
mitochondria incubated with palmitoyl carnitine

Acyl-CoA was isolated and assayed in rat-heart mitochondria, following their incubation with
palmitoyl carnitine, by the method of Williamson and Corkey, (1969). The concentration of
CoA was 1 mM.

Palmitoyl carnitine added (nmoles/mg protein)	Acyl-CoA accumulated (nmoles/mg protein)	
	-free CoA	+CoA
0	0.48 ± 0.14	0.42
10	1.22 ± 0.30	1.82
20	1.77 ± 0.28	3.65

The inhibition of adenine nucleotide translocase by long chain acyl CoA esters and the reversal by carnitine and monovalent cations represents a complex interaction of membrane-bound enzymes. Palmitoyl carnitine transferase is inhibited by its substrate, palmitoyl CoA, and, in fact, the K_m and K_i of the enzyme for palmitoyl CoA are rather similar (Bremer and Norum, 1967). Furthermore, a rise in ionic strength increases palmitoyl carnitine transferase activity (Brosnan and Fritz, 1971; Wood, 1973). Any change in activity of the palmitoyl carnitine transferase would be reflected in the degree of inhibition of the adenine nucleotide translocase by palmitoyl CoA. Thus, the results shown in Fig. 5, as well as in Fig. 3, may be more directly related to the fall in palmitoyl CoA concentration between the inner and outer mitochondrial membrane, produced by promoting its enzymatic conversion to palmitoyl carnitine.

It has been observed that, in liver, the tricarboxylate or citrate-carrier system, like the adenine nucleotide translocase, is also inhibited by long chain acyl CoA esters, whereas the malate carrier remains unaffected (Halperin et al., 1972; Shug and Shrago, 1973a). Fig. 6 shows the effects of palmitoyl CoA and K^+ on malate transport. The data are somewhat difficult to interpret since the degree of inhibition by palmitoyl CoA depends upon the assay used. The forward exchange, which is a measure of the uptake of radioactive malate, indicates significant inhibition by palmitoyl CoA which is offset by the addition of K^+ to the incubation mixture. However, when mitochondria preincubated with radioactive malate are allowed to exchange with external cold malate (back exchange, as

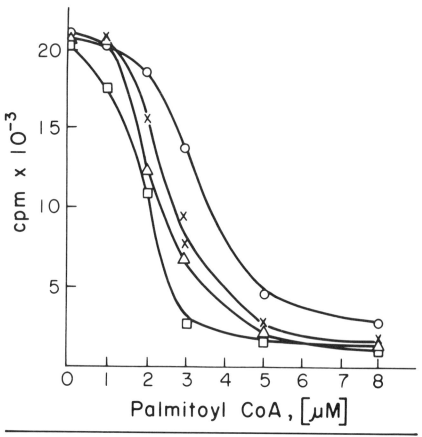

5 Effect of K+-ion concentration on the inhibition of rat-heart adenine nucleotide translocase by palmitoyl CoA. Experimental conditions were similar to those in Fig. 2. Tonicity of the reaction medium was maintained by adding sucrose in place of KC1. KC1, 100 mM, o—o—o; 20 mM, x—x—x; 10 mM, △—△—△; no KC1, □—□—□.

shown in the insert), palmitoyl CoA is ineffective as an inhibitor, whether or not K+ is present. This discrepancy is not observed when the two assay procedures are used to measure the adenine nucleotide translocase and, since the back exchange is a more specific assay reflecting actual *in vivo* conditions, the results suggest that acyl CoA esters do not affect the malate exchange. Therefore, the

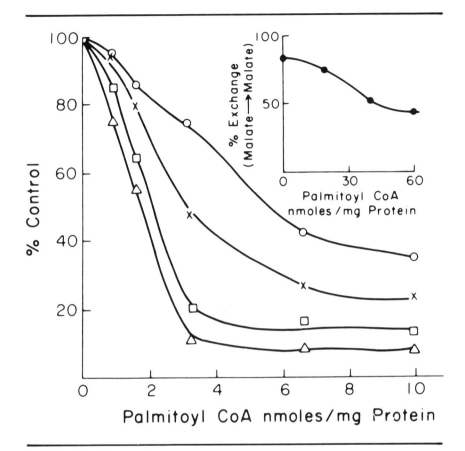

6 Effect of palmitoyl CoA and K+ ions on malate transport in rat-heart mitochondria. Mitochondria were incubated in 25 mM Tris pH 7.4, 1 mM EGTA, and rotenone, antimycin and oligomycin 1 mg/ml, with either KCl or sucrose for 1 min at ice temperature. The reaction was initiated by adding [^{14}C] malate and terminated by 10 mM mersalyl. KCl 100 mM, o—o—o; 50 mM, x—x—x; 25 mM, □—□—□; no KCl, △—△—△. Back exchange, using mitochondria preloaded with [^{14}C] malate, and allowed to exchange with 1.0 mM nonradioactive malate (insert).

ability to transport reducing equivalents into heart mitochondria—via the malate aspartate shuttle—is apparently not impeded by long chain acyl CoA esters.

Inhibition of ADP and ATP transport across the inner mito-chondrial membrane should be reflected by appropriate changes in

Table 2. Effect of palmitoyl CoA on mitochondrial
adenine nucleotides

Adenine nucleotides (ATP, ADP) were determined following incubation of guinea pig heart mitochondria by the procedure described in "Methods." The concentration of palmitoyl CoA was 20 μM or 7 nmoles/mg protein.

ADP added (μM)	nmoles Adenine nucleotides/mg protein					
	Control			Palmitoyl CoA		
	ATP	ADP	ATP/ADP	ATP	ADP	ATP/ADP
0	3.00	2.16	1.38	3.88	1.32	2.98
5	3.19	3.36	0.93	5.11	2.18	2.34
20	3.40	4.08	0.83	5.04	0.96	5.27

the ATP/ADP ratios of the mitochondrial and cytosol compartments. Adenine nucleotides were determined in mitochondria isolated from guinea-pig hearts, incubated with and without palmitoyl CoA (Table 2). The results indicate that palmitoyl CoA is able to effectively increase the intramitochondrial ATP/ADP ratio, presumably by impeding the external transport of the ATP synthesized during oxidative phosphorylation. The inability of ATP to be transported also affects the synthesis of creatine phosphate, as illustrated in Fig. 1. Creatine phosphate formation by guinea-pig mitochondria incubated with ADP as an energy source is shown in Table 3. It can be seen that the synthesis of creatine phosphate increased with rising concentrations of ADP; the latter is transported into the mitochondria, phosphorylated and then transported out again as ATP. Both palmitoyl CoA and atractylate, which inhibit the transport system, also prevent synthesis of creatine phosphate from ATP. The inhibition by palmitoyl CoA is overcome by the addition of carnitine which promotes a transacylation of the inhibitory acyl CoA to the carnitine ester. Similar observations have been made by Shug and coworkers, 1975, using beef-heart mitochondria.

DISCUSSION

Fatty acids are the preferred substrate of the myocardium, and the oxidation of the long chain fatty acids in this tissue is completely carnitine dependent. There is considerable, though admittedly, in-

Table 3. Effect of long chain acyl-CoA esters on
creatine phosphate formation

Creatin phosphate was determined following incubation of guinea pig heart mitochondria by the procedure described in "Methods."

ADP added (μM)		10	20	40	100
			nmoles Creatine phosphate formed/mg protein		
Control		207	271	336	423
Palmitoyl CoA	15 μM	119	190	233	245
Palmitoyl CoA	30 μM	103	139	214	190
Palmitoyl CoA + D, L-carnitine	15 μM 5 μM	207	239	353	382
Palmitoyl CoA + D, L-carnitine	30 μM 5 μM	205	291	336	401
Atractylate	10 μM	78	98	79	76

conclusive evidence that fatty acids may be deleterious to the ischemic myocardium (Kurien et al., 1969). Based on both *in vitro* and *in vivo* evidence, a hypothesis has been proposed which states that, during myocardial ischemia, a decrease in tissue oxygenation prevents optimum oxidation of fatty acids and permits a critical increase of intracellular long chain acyl CoA esters. The resultant inhibition of the adenine nucleotide translocase causes an immediate interruption of energy production and disruption of the ATP/ADP ratio or phosphate potential of the cell. Even if a sudden drop in total ATP is not observed experimentally, the compartmentation of the adenine nucleotides has been so modified as to decrease the ATP/ADP ratio and diminish the synthesis of creatine phosphate. Such a sequence of biochemical events could account for the impairment of muscle contraction and related clinical manifestations during myocardial infarction.

An important counterpart of this hypothesis is that the lesion produced by the long chain acyl CoA esters at the site of the adenine nucleotide translocase is a biochemical one and—potentially reversible. Strong consideration can, therefore, be given to clinical modes of intervention which would protect and promote the survival of

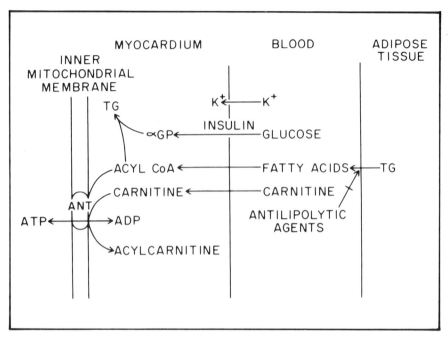

7 Mechanisms by which various therapeutic agents might interact to protect the ischemic myocardium, by preventing inhibition of adenine nucleotide translocation. See text for details.

the ischemic myocardium. The diagram in Fig. 7 is used to illustrate the possible effectiveness of various forms of therapy. First, carnitine itself, which is a natural product of the body and can be easily administered, may, by promoting the conversion of long chain acyl CoA esters to the acyl carnitine derivatives, relieve the inhibition at the translocase site. Antilipolytic agents, which inhibit lipolysis in peripheral adipose tissue and lower serum fatty acids, have been shown by Oliver and coworkers (Rowe et al., 1975) to reduce morbidity and mortality during the early stages of myocardial infarction. Though not always dramatically effective, the clinical usefulness of a glucose-insulin-potassium solution has been attributed to the fact that it facilitates ATP production through anaerobic glycolysis. However, in addition, sufficient glucose might be converted to glycerol-3-phosphate to react with the long chain acyl CoA esters in the synthesis of triglyceride. In fact, increased triglyceride formation has been observed in the dog heart following experimental coronary occlusion (Scheuer and Brachfeld, 1966). Potassium might also be effective in overcoming the inhibition of long chain acyl CoA esters. The possibility that a combination of L-carnitine and a glucose-insulin-potassium infusion might provide a superior form of therapy should be considered. Further studies are also indicated to determine whether other physiological or pharmacological agents may effectively mediate adenine nucleotide translocation and/or prevent its inhibition by long chain fatty acyl coenzyme A esters.

SUMMARY

The translocation of adenine nucleotides across the inner mitochondrial membrane plays an important role in myocardial metabolism. It is postulated that inhibition of the translocase during myocardial ischemia is due to a critical increase in long chain acyl CoA esters. The inhibition which can be modified by the addition of carnitine and K^+ ions has been partially localized to the outer side of the inner mitochondrial membrane. A disassociation between the mitochondrial and cytosolic ATP/ADP ratios, as well as decrease in creatine phosphate synthesis which is shown to occur subsequent to an inhibition of the translocase, would be detrimental to normal myocardial metabolism and function during ischemia.

ACKNOWLEDGMENT

This study was supported by U.S Public Health Service Grant No. GM-14033.

REFERENCES

Bremer, J., and Norum, K. R.: Mechanism of substrate inhibition of palmitoyl co-enzyme A: Carnitine palmitoyl transferase by palmitoyl co-enzyme A. *J. Biol. Chem.* 242:1744-1748 (1967).

Brosnan, J. T., and Fritz, I. B.: The oxidation of fatty acyl derivatives by mitochondria from bovine fetal and calf hearts. *Can. J. Biochem.* 49: 1296-1300 (1971).

Duszynski, J., and Wojtczak, L.: Effect of metal cations on the inhibition of adenine nucleotide translocation by acyl CoA. *FEBS Lett.* 50:74-78 (1975).

Fritz, I. B., and Marquis, N. R.: The role of acyl carnitine esters and carnitine palmitoyl transferase in the transport of fatty acyl groups across mitochondrial membranes. *Proc. Natl. Acad. Sci. USA* 54:1226-1233 (1965).

Gornall, A. G., Bardawell, C. J., and David, D. D.: Determination of serum proteins by means of the biuret reaction. *J. Biol. Chem.* 177:751-766 (1949).

Halperin, M. D., Robinson, B. H., and Fritz, I. B.: Effects of palmitoyl CoA on citrate and malate transport by rat liver mitochondria. *Proc. Natl. Acad. Sci. USA* 69:1003-1007 (1972).

Harris, R. A., Farmer, B., and Ozawa, T.: Inhibition of the mitochondrial adenine nucleotide transport system by oleoyl CoA. *Arch. Biochem. Biophys.* 150:199-209 (1972).

Jacobus, W. E., and Lehninger, A. L.: Creatine kinase of rat heart mitochondria. *J. Biol. Chem.* 248:4803-4810 (1973).

Kurien, V. A., Yates, P. A., and Oliver, M. F.: Free fatty acids, heparin and arrhythmias during experimental myocardial infarction. *Lancet* 2:185-187 (1969).

Lerner, E., Shug, A. L., Elson, C., and Shrago, E.: Reversible inhibition of adenine nucleotide translocation by long chain fatty acyl co-enzyme A esters in liver mitochondria of diabetic and hibernating animals. *J. Biol. Chem.* 247:1513-1519 (1972).

McLean, P., Gumaa, K. A., and Greenbaum, A. L.: Long chain acyl CoA, adenine nucleotide translocase and the coordination of the redox states of the cytosolic and mitochondrial compartments. *FEBS Lett.* 17:345-350 (1971).

Meijer, A. J., and van Dam, K.: The metabolic significance of anion transport in mitochondria. *Biochem. Biophys. Acta* 346:213-214 (1974).

Neely, J. R., and Morgan, H.: Relationship between carbohydrate and lipid metabolism and the energy balance of heart muscle. *Ann. Rev. Physiol.* 36:413-459 (1974).

Pande, S. V.: A mitochondrial carnitine acyl carnitine translocase system. *Proc. Natl. Acad. Sci. USA* 72:883-887 (1975).

Pande, S. V., and Blanchaer, M. D.: Reversible inhibition of mitochondrial adenosine diphosphate phosphorylation by long chain acyl CoA esters. *J. Biol. Chem.* 246:402-411 (1971).

Pfaff, E., and Klingenberg, M.: Adenine nucleotide translocation of mitochondria. 1) Specificity and control. *Eur. J. Biochem.* 6:66-79 (1968).

Robinson, B. H.: Transport of phosphoenolpyruvate by the tricarboxylate transport system in mammalian mitochondria. *FEBS Lett.* 14:309-312 (1971).

Rowe, M. J., Neilson, J. M. M., and Oliver, M. J.: Control of ventricular arrhythmias during myocardial infarction by anti-lipolytic treatment using a nicotinic acid analogue. *Lancet* 1:295-300 (1975).

Scheuer, V., and Brachfeld, N.: Myocardial uptake and fractional distribution of palmitate 1-^{14}C by the ischemic dog heart. *Metabolism* 15:945-954 (1966).

Shrago, E., Shug, A., and Elson, C.: In *Regulation of Cell Metabolism by Mitochondrial Transport Systems in Gluconeogenesis: Its Regulation in Mammalian Species*, R. W. Hanson and M. J. Mehlman, eds. John Wiley and Sons, Inc., Somerset, N. J. (1976), pp. 221-238.

Shrago, E., Shug, A. L., Elson, C., Spennetta, T., and Crosby, C.: Regulation of metabolite transport in rat and guinea pig liver mitochondria by long chain fatty acyl co-enzyme A esters. *J. Biol. Chem.* 249:5269-5274 (1974).

Shug, A. L., Koke, J. R., Folts, J. D., and Bittar, N.: Role of adenine nucleotide translocase in metabolic change caused by ischemia. In *Recent Advances in Studies on Cardiac Structure and Metabolism*, Vol. 10, *The Metabolism of Contraction*, P. E. Ray and G. Rana, eds. University Park Press, Baltimore (1975), pp. 365-378.

Shug, A. L., Lerner, E., Elson, C., and Shrago, E.: The inhibition of adenine nucleotide translocase by oleoyl CoA and its reversal in rat liver mitochondria. *Biochem. Biophys. Res. Commun.* 43:557-563 (1971).

Shug, A. L., and Shrago, E.: A proposed mechanism for fatty acid effects on energy metabolism of the heart. *J. Lab. Clin. Med.* 81:214-218 (1973a).

Shug, A. L., and Shrago, E.: Inhibition of phosphoenolpyruvate transport via tricarboxylate in adenine nucleotide carrier systems of rat liver mitochondria. *Biochem. Biophys. Res. Commun.* 53:659-665 (1973b).

Shug, A. L., Shrago, E., Bittar, N., Folts, J. D., and Kokes, J. R.: Long chain fatty acyl CoA inhibition of adenine nucleotide translocation in the ischemic myocardium. *Am. J. Physiol.* 228:689-692 (1975).

Sul, H. S., Shrago, E., and Shug, A. L.: Relationship of phosphoenolpyruvate transport, acyl CoA enzyme A inhibition of adenine nucleotide translocase and calcium ion efflux in guinea pig heart mitochondria. *Arch. Biochem. Biophys.* 172:230-237 (1976).

Vaartjes, W. J., Kemp, A. Jr., Souverijn, J. H. M., and Van Den Bergh, S. J.: Inhibition by fatty acyl esters of adenine nucleotide translocation in rat liver mitochondria. *FEBS Lett.* 23:303-308 (1972).

Williamson, J. R., and Corkey, B. E.: Assays of intermediates of the citric acid cycle and related compounds by fluorometric enzyme methods. *Methods Enzymol.* 13:437-440 (1969).

Wood, J. M.: Effect of ionic strength of the activity of carnitine palmityltransferhse I. *Biochem.* 12:5268-5273 (1973).

Discussion

Rannels, Rovetto, Williamson, Neely and Shrago

DR. STEPHEN ROBINSON (*Hahnemann Medical College*): I have a question concerning the effect of the degree of acidosis on coronary flow. Is there a differential effect of acidosis on coronary flow?

DR. JOHN R. WILLIAMSON (*Johnson Research Foundation*): Yes. In those experiments where the acidosis was mixed with ischemia, something occurs that we do not understand at all; namely, as Dr. Rovetto mentioned, there is an increase in coronary resistance at some critical decrease in pH, and there is supposed to be a decreased vascular resistance—but the opposite happens. So that in our experiments at the lower pH, there was some ischemia involved as well. Recovery was always very good, even with prolonged periods of acidosis, but there was a period of arrhythmias before the hearts would beat properly and develop proper output, and this period was longer, the more severe the acidosis.

DR. ROBERT B. JENNINGS (*Duke University Medical Center*): Dr. Williamson, I would like you to discuss the following proposition relative to CO_2. It seems to me that in low-flow ischemia *in vivo*, where one converts from aerobic to anaerobic metabolism, and there is excess lactate production, any excess CO_2 should be derived from the lactate interacting with bicarbonate in the plasma. There should be virtually no CO_2 production from mitochondrial metabolism, and there is very little pentose phosphate metabolic capacity in myocardium under aerobic or anaerobic conditions. So, the CO_2 that does appear should come from the reaction of lactate and buffer.

DR. WILLIAMSON: That may be so, if you are referring more to total ischemia. Of course, if there is any oxygen, CO_2 will be produced and with diminished flow it will not be removed from the system. I was concentrating on the partial ischemic situation. I think you are probably right, that as fixed acids build up, the intracellular bicarbonate must fall to help the CO_2 rise. In our own data with different degrees of ischemia and graded acidosis, the contribution of increased lactate was not very great.

DR. JOHN SPITZER (*Louisiana State University Medical Center*): Dr. Williamson, I would like to know how deep into the tissue one can investigate the nucleotide process, and how do you explain the patchiness of ischemia?

DR. WILLIAMSON: The depth of penetration has not been measured precisely. I estimate it at something like 0.2 to 0.4 mm, thus, it is epicardial surface. To explain the patchiness, I think, the mitochondria have this very high capacity for absorbing oxygen, and so what you are seeing is the whole of the capillary system from its arterial to its venous end. The border zone or the area in between, which we are trying to tie in with the myoglobin and cytochrome oxidase indicators, is very sharp, thus there is not much distance between capillaries where oxygen tension is between 10^{-4} to 10^{-8} moles. We would like to think of this as mitochondria either turned on or turned off.

DR. EUGENE BRAUNWALD (*Harvard Medical School*): I would like to make one comment that deals with this issue of the very sharp border. I think it depends on how one defines a border, the size of the population of cells that one studies, and how uniform the ischemia might be. In the rat hearts that you showed, the degree of uniformity was probably great, because you diminish flow to the entire heart. In the dog heart or in the pig heart, in which a coronary vessel is occluded, it is possible to demonstrate an enormous gradient of flows in different segments of cardiac tissue, and a very wide spectrum of segmental mechanical performances. There is really a good correlation in any given heart between the extent of reduction of blood flow and the extent of mechanical dysfunction. From these considerations, the way I would interpret your findings is that, in any small portion of myocardium, there will be a fraction of cells that are totally ischemic, and a fraction that might be perfectly normal, and that what we gross physiologists have defined as a border zone might be 50% normal cells and 50% knocked out, and a more severe zone might be 25% remaining and 75% knocked out. This still allows for the concept that part of the cells are functioning and part are not, and I wonder if you would comment on that.

DR. WILLIAMSON: I think you have summarized it extremely well. I agree completely. Perhaps Clyde Barlow, who pioneered this methodology, would like to say something since he has done more work with total ischemia.

MR. CLYDE BARLOW (*Johnson Research Foundation*): A profused rabbit heart is the biggest heart I have worked on. If you occlude a coronary artery of such a heart, there is a very sharp boundary with almost no gray zone between normal and ischemic tissue.

DR. FRANKLIN HULL (*Wayne State University*): How do you correlate the increase in CO_2 content in the ischemic heart with the observations you have talked about today. The question was raised earlier as to whether there would be sufficient mitochondrial oxidative capacity in serious ischemia to generate much CO_2. I heard information presented several years ago in which CO_2 electrodes were used to measure the rise in pCO_2. However, I do not recall how rapidly that occurred.

DR. WILLIAMSON: Very fast. It is in minutes (or as fast as you can reasonably measure) but I think this whole problem which Dr. Jennings raised needs a bit more experimentation and thought.

DR. JENNINGS: I was simply saying that, I think, it is more likely that the CO_2 comes from the lactate reacting with the bicarbonate buffer, than it does from any metabolic reaction.

I would like to comment also on the border zone. I believe, there is a very sharp border zone of ischemia in myocardium, which can be shown by cyanosis, by nucleotide fluorescence, by electrocardiographic changes, and by microspheres, but I think the point is, that inside that sharp border between ischemic and normal-functioning myocardium, there are graded degrees of ischemia which probably are a reflection of flow and, perhaps, oxygen content.

DR. WILLIAMSON: I hate to let this pass. I don't know what graded degrees of ischemia mean.

DR. JENNINGS: You would use the term high-flow ischemia or low-flow ischemia.

DR. WILLIAMSON: At the mitochondrial level, do you criticize the hypothesis that mitochondria are either on or off?

DR. JENNINGS: I agree that they are on or off. I don't know how much on, and how much off.

DR. WILLIAMSON: So, it is a statistical problem in the tissue.

DR. D. EUGENE RANNELS, JR. (*Hershey Medical Center*): My question is sort of related. How many mitochondria do you need in any one cell to have that cell working, as opposed to not working? Secondly, I think it is worthwhile remembering that our technique of looking at mitochondrial function basically involves centrifugational procedures where only good mitochondria are in the pellet and the bad ones are left behind. We make our judgment on whether that cell is good or not on the basis of the collected mitochondria, but we may be excluding all the bad mitochondria and just getting the good ones. Therefore, I think that is a very difficult and complex problem, and I do not believe there is an answer to it at this time.

DR. WILLIAMSON: I think it could be resolved by working with isolated heart cells that do beat—if one can picture whether a mitochondrion is good or bad in the cell. I believe this is a problem worth working on.

DR. STEVEN BASKIN (*Medical College of Pennsylvania*): Dr. Shrago, I noticed that you had a number of differences between some of the biochemical parameters you measured in your mitochondria. Have you performed comparative studies among mitochondria from hearts of various species? There are differences in physiological responses of different hearts, to either pharmacological agents or other interventions. Can some of the effects that you see be due to the source of mitochondria?

DR EARL SHRAGO *(University of Wisconsin)*: The physiological studies that we have conducted, have only been in the dog. The biochemical studies seem to be consistent in rat, guinea pig, and beef heart, probably rabbit heart, although we have not performed enough of them to be certain. We have not seen any differences among the animals we have used for *in vitro* investigations and we have employed only the dog for *in vivo* studies. The pig would probably be a good model, I would think.

DR. WILLIAMSON: Dr. Michael Kohn of Garfinkle's group has some interesting data on computer simulation of adenine nucleotide compartmentation. Could he tell us about it since it is very relevant to the topic of ischemia.

DR. MICHAEL KOHN *(University of Pennsylvania)*: Our problem has been to obtain an idea of the distribution of adenine nucleotides in the cells of the profused rat heart. We now have a computer model which is consistent with observed flux rates, substrate and product concentrations, and other criteria we have used for testing it. From this model and parallel models for cardiac metabolic pathways, it has been possible to determine that approximately 85% of the AMP is located in the mitochondria under normal conditions, whereas about 75% of the ADP is bound to actin.

DR. HULL: I have a question for Dr. Neely. If one perfuses the ischemic rat heart with acetate, how does this affect the levels of long-chain acyl CoA that are generated? Specifically, when perfusing with acetate, to what extent will it compete with long-chain fatty acyl CoA formation? A second question and that to Dr. Shrago. Have you conducted any such studies to see to what degree the acetate might offset the ischemia-induced changes in adenine nucleotide translocase activity?

DR. JAMES R. NEELY *(Hershey Medical Center)*: In the normal aerobic heart, acetate competes very effectively. In the ischemic heart, I am not sure how well it competes; we have not performed this type of study. Pyruvate does compete to some extent, and lowers the level of long-chain acyl CoA, compared to what you see with long-chain fatty acids alone. In regard to your last question of how you might lower long-chain acyl CoA, and the last slide that Dr. Shrago showed, which indicated carnitine added to the blood would increase the tissue level of carnitine and perhaps lower long-chain acyl CoA (as one mechanism to account for the beneficial effect of carnitine), it seems to me for that to be beneficial one has to also provide a means of disposing of the long-chain acyl carnitine that is formed. If you put in carnitine, it would be expected to lower fatty acyl CoA temporarily but, as long as fatty acids are entering the tissue, that effect should be very transient and, unless you provide a means of washing out the long-chain carnitine that is formed, or eliminate it by some other means, it probably would not represent a long-term beneficial effect. Perhaps Dr. Shrago would like to comment.

DR. SHRAGO: I think I would have to agree, unless acyl carnitine gets into the mitochondria where it does not do any harm when it is reconverted to acyl CoA. Any substrate which would use up extra matrix ATP or CoA, so fatty acids would not be activated, would be helpful in lowering acyl CoA levels. We have suggested that glucose may work by synthesizing enough a-glycerol phosphate, so that the acyl CoA would be converted to a triglyceride. One might conceive of other mechanisms that could lower ATP or CoA levels, and thereby leave the fatty acids floating around, tied to their binding protein and possibly not causing any problem. However, we have not carried out any experiments to test any other interventions than the one I showed.

DR. MURTHY (*Squibb Institute for Medical Research*): Dr. Shrago, was the effect of carnitine in decreasing ST segment elevation due to a decreased heart rate or was it the result of a biochemical change produced by carnitine?

DR. SHRAGO: That is a good question. What makes us concerned is the possibility of carnitine acting at the translocase site, rather than somewhere else, which would lower the heart rate. We do not know. Hopefully, we shall be able to obtain some answers to this question with further experiments.

DR. KATHRYN LaNOUE (*Hershey Medical Center*): Dr. Shrago, what was your translocase assay? Did it show smaller nucleotide pools on the inside of the mitochondria?

DR. SHRAGO: We have been proceeding from the premise that the nucleotide pool on the outside of the inner membrane does not amount to much. As far as the concentration inside the mitocondria is concerned, I do not know the answer.

DR. WILLIAMSON: Dr. Neely, is there any difference in the function of ischemic hearts when they are perfused with fatty acids as substrates, as opposed to glucose? You have shown that fatty acyl CoA is higher when fatty acids are the substrates.

DR. NEELY: If there is a difference in performance when high levels of fatty acids are present in the rat heart, it is very minor. We have not been able to see an appreciable difference in pressure development or heart rate during ischemia with fatty acids, as opposed to ischemia with glucose. The story may be quite different in a pig heart, where we do have some evidence that providing substrate other than the long-chain fatty acids does improve function and survival, but again, this may be related to something other than just the availability of the fatty acids.

11

Salvage of Ischemic Myocardium*

EUGENE BRAUNWALD

INTRODUCTION

Ischemic heart disease represents the most common serious health problem of contemporary Western Society. It has been estimated that in this country alone, more than 675,000 patients die each year from ischemic heart disease and its complications; approximately 1,300,000 patients develop myocardial infarction; and countless more suffer from congestive heart failure secondary to ischemic myocardial damage. Acute myocardial infarction, thus, remains the most common cause of in-hospital deaths in this country, indeed, in the Western World. In-hospital deaths in patients with acute myocardial infarction result mainly from primary arrhythmias and from pump failure (Harnarayan et al., 1970). While fatalities due to arrhythmias have been reduced by modern monitoring techniques and more vigorous prophylaxis and treatment, the death rate following mechanical failure, manifested by car-

---

* The A. N. Richards Lecture delivered before the Physiological Society of Philadelphia, May 6, 1976.

diogenic shock and/or pulmonary edema, is still very high. These syndromes have been found to be associated with larger infarctions than those exhibited by other patients who succumbed to myocardial infarction, but who did not die as a consequence of pump failure (Page et al., 1971; Sobel et al., 1972). In addition, the prognosis in patients with larger infarcts is distinctly worse than it is in those with smaller ones (Sobel et al., 1972).

It had long been assumed that the myocardium in the vascular territory of a totally obstructed coronary artery rapidly develops ischemia and that only a brief interval elapses before the damage becomes irreversible. Since it is now apparent that clinical prognosis following infarction depends directly on the quantity of residual viable, normally functioning myocardium, these widely held assumptions have taken on fresh significance. It would appear that if only one could effectively limit tissue damage after coronary occlusion, pump failure and its consequences might be averted. Basic to any consideration of this problem is the progression of myocardial ischemic injury, following coronary artery occlusion. In studies of experimentally-induced infarcts in animals, myocardial tissue supplied by an occluded vessel does not show an essentially homogeneous area of necrosis. Rather, in the aftermath of occlusion, the affected myocardium is likely to manifest a region of central necrosis, surrounded in patchy fashion by a substantial amount of abnormal but still viable tissue. Moreover, this ischemic zone may increase in size for some time, while the necrotic zone remains relatively small. Indeed, according to certain studies, the ischemic zone may continue to enlarge for up to 18 hr after occlusion (Cox et al., 1968); thereafter, the region of central necrosis expands rapidly at the expense of ischemic tissue. The absence of a clear demarcation between normal and necrotic tissue, on histological examination of human hearts at autopsy, has been noted repeatedly, and it appears likely that the progression from ischemic damage to necrosis follows a time course in man similar to that in experimental animals. Death from cardiogenic shock may now be viewed as the end-result of a vicious cycle (Fig. 1) (Braunwald, 1976). Coronary obstruction causes myocardial ischemia that impairs myocardial contractility and ventricular performance which, in turn, reduces arterial pressure and, therefore, coronary perfusion pressure, leading to further ischemia and extension of necrosis, until, in most cases, death occurs. There is some evidence that stasis in the smaller arteries and arterioles distal to a major proximal occlusion can result in secondary microvascular obstruction, further impairing myocardial perfusion.

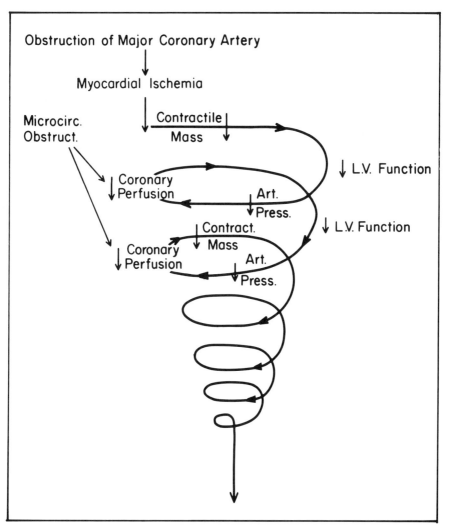

1 Diagram depicting the sequence of events in the vicious cycle in which coronary artery obstruction leads to cardiogenic shock and progressive circulatory deterioration.

Accordingly, a treatment which could decrease the extent of tissue death in the myocardium and, by this mechanism, diminish the frequency of intractable cardiogenic shock and pulmonary edema would be extremely useful, not only by reducing immediate mortality, but also by leaving the patient who had suffered a coronary occlusion with more viable myocardium. Such a patient would be expected to be less likely to develop chronic heart failure and would have a greater reserve of functioning myocardium, should another coronary occlusion occur.

There is considerable evidence to suggest that factors which influence myocardial oxygen demands may aggravate or alleviate symptoms of myocardial ischemia. For example, in patients with angina and hyperthyroidism, treatment of the hypermetabolic state, and the associated reduction of myocardial oxygen needs, is often associated with relief of angina (Somerville and Kevin, 1950). Also, diminishing myocardial oxygen requirements by beta-adrenergic blockade (Wolfson et al., 1966) or carotid sinus nerve stimulation (Braunwald et al., 1967) decreases symptoms of myocardial ischemia. Conversely, treatment of hypothyroidism or the development of tachycardia—factors that augment myocardial oxygen needs—increase the frequency and severity of myocardial ischemia in patients with coronary artery disease. The importance of the decreased availability of oxygen is apparent in cases where arterial hypotension and acute anemia may cause infarction in patients with coronary artery disease, in the absence of coronary occlusion.

The above-mentioned clinical observations suggested to us that the ultimate size of a myocardial infarct is not irrevocably determined by the site of coronary occlusion, but might be modified by other factors (Braunwald, 1967). We then proposed that when coronary occlusion occurs, the survival of the cardiac tissue normally perfused by the obstructed vessel depends on the balance between oxygen available to that segment of myocardium and its oxygen requirements; thus, we felt that the survival of the patient with coronary occlusion could, in large measure, hinge on the balance between the supply of and demand for myocardial oxygen (Braunwald et al., 1969).

Our approach to this problem extended from a consideration of the determinants of myocardial oxygen consumption, and how they are altered by some of the common interventions and drugs employed in the treatment of patients with acute myocardial infarction. These studies were based on the premise that an increase in myocardial oxygen requirement will, if other factors remain constant, tend to enlarge the area of ischemia and—ultimately of necrosis—whereas reducing myocardial oxygen consumption will tend to have the opposite effect.

DETERMINANTS OF THE HEART'S OXYGEN CONSUMPTION

The determinants of myocardial oxygen consumption have been reviewed elsewhere (Braunwald, 1969, 1971), but will be briefly summarized here. It has been known for many years that the total metabolism of the arrested, quiescent heart represents only a small fraction of that of the working organ. Thus, while the oxygen consumption of the beating mammalian heart ranges from 3 to 15 ml/min/100 g of left ventricle, the oxygen consumption of the heart arrested with excess potassium is only about 1.3 ml/min/100 g. Since the quantity of oxygen required for electrical activation of the heart is approximately 0.5% of the total O_2 consumed by the normally contracting organ (Klocke et al., 1966), this difference between the arrested and beating heart results almost exclusively from its contractile activity.

In studies where the relative effects of aortic pressure, stroke volume and heart rate on the oxygen consumption of the isolated supported heart were determined, a close relation between myocardial oxygen consumption and the so-called tension-time index (TTI), that is, the area beneath the left ventricular pressure pulse per minute, was demonstrated (Sarnoff et al., 1958). It was then emphasized that the tension of the myocardial wall is a more definitive determinant of myocardial energy utilization than is the developed pressure (Rodbard et al., 1964), and that myocardial wall tension is a direct function of the radius and intraventricular pressure, and is inversely related to ventricular wall thickness. Evidence was later provided from our laboratory that, in addition to developed tension, the peak velocity of contraction of the myocardium, reflecting the contractile or inotropic state of the heart, is also a major determinant of myocardial oxygen consumption (Ross et al., 1965; Sonnenblick et al., 1965). The basal metabolism of the organ, the activation of the heart, maintenance of the active state and shortening against a load, all contribute to the heart's oxygen demands, but less so than the principal determinants, i.e., tension, contractility and frequency of contraction (Braunwald, 1969, 1971).

It was proposed that, since the blood supply to the ischemic zone surrounding the infarct is markedly reduced, the survival of this tissue may depend on its oxygen consumption. According to this

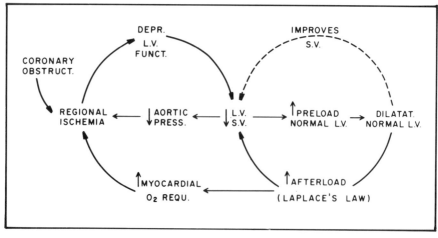

2
Schema showing changes in circulatory regulation in ischemic heart disease. DEPR. L.V. FUNCT., represents depressed left ventricular function; S.V. stroke volume; DILATAT. dilatation; and O₂ REQU. oxygen requirements. Solid lines produce or intensify the effect, whereas a broken line diminishes it. (From Braunwald et al., 1974. Reproduced by permission of the **New England Journal of Medicine**.)

concept, with occlusion of a coronary artery at any specific site, if the oxygen consumption of the myocardium were stimulated by factors, such as increased rate, tension and/or contractility, the viability of the ischemic border zone may be reduced and the size of the infarct enlarged. Furthermore, such an unfavorable alteration in the relationship between myocardial oxygen supply and demand could impair the contractile function of the ischemic myocardium at the margin of the infarct. This depression of left ventricular function could then result in enlargement of this chamber which, in accordance with Laplace's Law, will produce an increase in tension development at any level of ventricular pressure (Braunwald, 1974). A rise in tension, in turn, leads to even higher levels of oxygen consumption, which could impair myocardial function further and, thus, bring about the vicious cycle of cardiogenic shock already referred to (Fig. 2).

ASSESSMENT OF ISCHEMIC INJURY

In order to study the effects of various physiological and phar-macological interventions on the myocardium, following coronary occlusion, methods for recording myocardial ischemic injury and for predicting the subsequent development of myocardial necrosis had to be developed. Since it has long been appreciated that myocardial ischemia produces changes in the ST segment, it was natural to attempt to utilize this portion of the electrocardiogram as an index of ischemic injury (Braunwald and Maroko, 1976). The electro-physiological bases of changes in the ST segment in myocardial ischemia have not been completely clarified, but it has been postu-lated that, following repolarization of normal tissue, the resting membrane potential of ischemic cells is lower than that of normal cells, and that for this reason a "current of injury" flows across the boundary between the normally polarized region and the ischemic zone. According to this concept, the current disappears when the entire heart is depolarized during excitation and the elevated ST segment really results from a depressed TQ segment (Nahum et al., 1943). It has also been suggested that ST segment elevation may occur as a result of failure of the injured area to depolarize during excitation (Eyster et al., 1938); this produces a current flow during depolarization across the boundary between the partially polarized, injured region and the depolarized normal zone. A closely related possible mechanism of ST segment elevation is an altered wave form of the transmembrane action potential of ischemic tissue, with loss of the normal plateau portion, so that current flows between such an area and normal tissue during inscription of the action potential (Samson and Scher, 1960; Cohen and Kaufman, 1975).

It is likely that alterations in the permeability of myocardial-cell membranes—which modify ion transport and, thereby, alter the magnitudes of the resting potential, the transmembrane potential inscribed during the plateau of the action potential, and the voltage time course of repolarization—represent the ultimate cause of the ST segment shift during acute myocardial ischemia. However, it is critical to recognize that factors other than ischemia can also affect the ST segment. These changes in the electrical activity of non-ischemic cells include, but are not limited to, alterations in pH and ion concentrations, temperature changes, drugs, such as quinidine

and digitalis, intraventricular conduction defects, sympathetic stimulation of the heart and epicardial injury due to pericarditis
(Braunwald and Maroko, 1976).

In 1949, Wegria first reported on the correlation in experimental animals between changes in the ST segment of the electrocardiogram and coronary blood flow (Wegria et al., 1949). Reduction in flow by two-thirds, or more, always produced marked ST
segment changes, while minor fluctuations occurred when coronary
blood flow was decreased by between one-third or two-thirds of control; no alterations were noted when coronary flow was diminished
by less than one-third. Becker et al, (1973) measured regional myocardial perfusion with radioactive miscrospheres and correlated the
results with epicardial electrograms. ST segments were substantially
elevated in most, though not all, sites overlying low-flow zones.

The relation between ST segment changes and myocardial metabolism has been examined in several studies. When global ischemia
of the left ventricle was produced, ST segment changes occurred almost simultaneously with the first biochemical indices of ischemia,
i.e., decrease in myocardial lactate extraction, and efflux of K^+ from
the heart (Scheuer and Brachfeld, 1966). In a correlation of epicardial ST segment changes with metabolic alterations in the underlying myocardium, after occlusion of the anterior descending
coronary artery in dogs, Karlsson found that biopsies of the myocardium subjacent to sites with epicardial ST segment elevations
showed lactate accumulation, as well as depletion of ATP and creatine phosphate (Karlsson et al., 1973), reflecting anaerobic myocardial metabolism. Sayen et al. (1961), using polarographic measurements of intramyocardial oxygen tension, found that ST segment
elevations in the epicardial electrocardiogram promptly followed reduction of oxygen tension below 65% of control. More recently,
Angell et al. (1975) compared the magnitude of ST segment elevations in surface electrograms with the intramyocardial oxygen tension in the subjacent tissue recorded by means of platinum-iridium
electrodes. The ST map correlated closely with the oxygen tension
as the latter was varied by altering coronary perfusion pressure.
Also, Khuri and associates (1975) varied coronary blood flow and
recorded myocardial PO_2 and PCO_2, using a mass spectrometer.
When regional ischemia was produced, epicardial ST segment elevations correlated with changes in myocardial gas tensions. However,
intramyocardial ST segments proved to be more sensitive than those
recorded from the epicardium.

We have noted consistently, in the open-chest anesthetized dog,

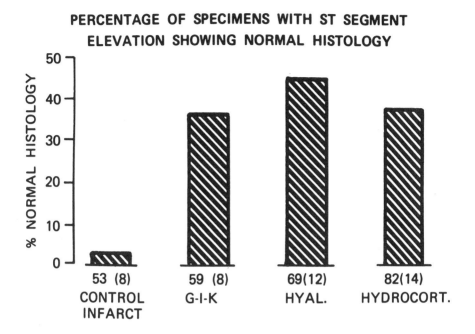

PERCENTAGE OF SPECIMENS WITH ST SEGMENT ELEVATION SHOWING NORMAL HISTOLOGY

3 Comparison of the effect of treatment on histology in areas with ST segment elevations over 2 mV. First column: control group; Second column: glucose-insulin-potassium (GIK) group; Third column: hyaluronidase group; Fourth column: hydrocortisone group. Note that in all three treatment groups more than one third of sites that were expected to show early signs of myocardial infarction were spared. (From Maroko and Braunwald, 1973. Reproduced by permission of **Annals of Internal Medicine**.)

that epicardial ST segment elevation recorded shortly after occlusion of the left anterior descending coronary artery, or one of its major branches, is an excellent predictor of the loss of myocardial viability, as judged by the depletion of cardiac creatine phosphokinase (CPK) activity in the subjacent myocardium, and by its histological and electronmicroscopic appearance 24 hr (Maroko et al., 1971, 1972e; Maroko and Braunwald, 1973; Khuri et al., 1975) or one week later (Ginks et al., 1972) (Fig. 3). A linear inverse correlation was demonstrated between the log of myocardial CPK activity and the degree of local ST segment elevation (Fig. 4) (Maroko et al., 1971;

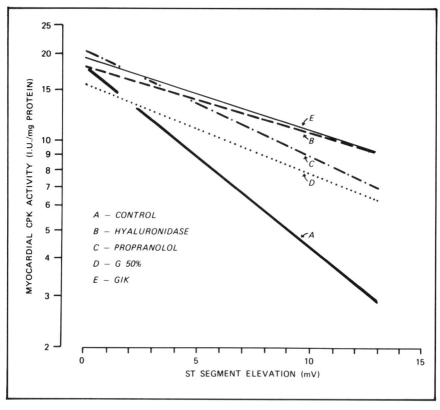

4

Relationship between ST segment elevation 15 min after occlusion and log of CPK activity from the same specimens, obtained 24 hr later. Line A: control group (occlusion alone). Fifteen dogs, 101 biopsies. Line B: hyaluronidase (13 dogs, 94 biopsies). Line C: propranolol. Line D: glucose 50% (6 dogs, 46 biopsies). Line E: glucose-insulin-potassium infusion (13 dogs, 96 biopsies). All interventions started 30 min following coronary artery occlusion, i.e., 15 min after the epicardial mapping. There is a statistical difference ($P < 0.01$) between the slope of line A and the slopes of the other lines showing less CPK depression after treatment. (From Maroko and Braunwald, 1973. Reproduced by permission of **Annals of Internal Medicine**.)

Maroko and Braunwald, 1973). In the absence of an intervention, myocardial CPK activity has always been found to decrease 24 hr after sustained occlusion whenever epicardial ST segment elevation exceeds 2 mV 15 min following occlusion. However, the epicardial ST segment measurement has a serious limitation in that is rela-

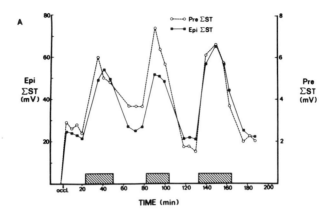

5

An example of the correspondence between the Epicardial ΣST and Precardial ΣST as ischemic injury following coronary artery occlusion was varied during intermittent intravenous infusions of isoproterenol (shaded rectangle). During the first and second infusions, isoproterenol was administered at the rate of 0.17 ug/kg/min; during the third infusion isoproternol was given at the rate of 4.0 ug/kg/min following an i.v. bolus of 1 mg/kg of propranolol. Time, in minutes following coronary occlusion.

tively insensitive to the more extensive subendocardial ischemic damage.

It was also observed, using multiple precordial electrodes in the dog, that changes in myocardial ischemic injury, as measured by ST segment elevations, parallel those found in the epicardium (Muller et al., 1975) (Fig. 5), and that both precordial and epicardial ST segment changes occurring soon after coronary occlusion predict myocardial CPK activity measured 24 hr later. The exact relation between precordial and epicardial ST segment elevation varied for each dog but, in general, the precordial electrocardiogram was less sensitive than the epicardial EKG in detecting ischemia (Muller et al., 1975). This approach has been extended to precordial electrocardiograms in the closed-chest pig (Capone et al., 1975).

It is clear from the experimental studies that, in the absence of other changes capable of influencing the ST segment (e.g., electrolyte concentration, drugs, intraventricular conduction defects, sympathetic stimulation, and pericarditis), the latter's elevation, recorded directly at a given epicardial site, reflects ischemia of the subjacent myocardium; it has also become evident that when such

Table 1. Interventions that increase myocardial injury
following coronary artery occlusion

A. INCREASING MYOCARDIAL OXYGEN REQUIREMENTS

   1. Isoproterenol
   2. Digitalis (in the non-failing heart)
   3. Glucagon
   4. Bretylium tosylate
   5. Tachycardia
   6. Hyperthermia

B. DECREASING MYOCARDIAL OXYGEN SUPPLY

   1. Directly

      a. Hypoxemia
      b. Anemia

   2. Through collateral vessels - reducing coronary perfusion pressure

      a. Hemorrhage
      b. Sodium nitropusside
      c. Minoxidil

C. DECREASING SUBSTRATE AVAILABILITY - HYPOGLYCEMIA

---

elevation is present 15 to 20 min after the onset of a permanent coronary occlusion, some degree of myocardial damage will be encountered 24 hr or later—unless a favorable intervention is inter-
posed. In our studies, reviewed below, interventions designed to
minimize myocardial ischemic damage, upon coronary occlusion,
were considered efficacious if 24 hr following the coronary event,
treated subjects revealed significantly *less* morphological damage
and reduction in CPK activity—for any degree of ST segment elevation seen shortly after the occlusion—than did untreated controls.

EFFECTS OF ALTERING MYOCARDIAL OXYGEN BALANCE

Using the technique of recording epicardial ST segments, it
was found that a variety of interventions (Table 1), notably those
which raise myocardial oxygen consumption, such as isoproterenol
(Fig. 6), digitalis, glucagon, bretylium tosylate, and pacing-induced
atrial tachycardia, all augment the severity and extent of myo-

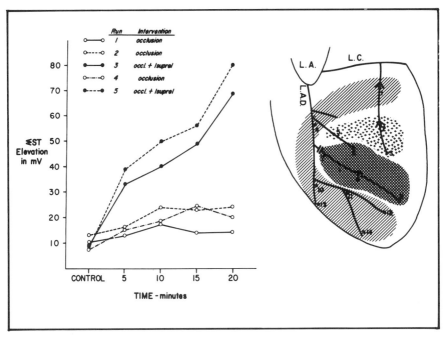

6

Effects of occlusion alone and occlusion after the infusion of isoproterenol (0.25 ug/kg/min). Right panel: Schematic rpresentation of the anterior surface of the heart. The coronary arteries and branches, and sites of epicardial electrograms are marked. LAD = left anterior descending coronary artery; LA = left atrial appendage; LC = left circumflex coronary artry. Cross-hatched area: area of injury after 15 min of occlusion. Stippled area: increase of area of injury when the occlusion was performed under the influence of isoproterenol. Lined area: area that showed no ST segment elevation under any circumstances. Left panel: ∑ST in the same experiment after three simple occlusions and after two occlusions under the influence of isoproterenol. Time = minutes after occlusion. (From Maroko et al., 1971. Reproduced by permission of **Circulation**.)

cardial injury (Maroko et al., 1971). More recently, Redwood and associates (1972), employing subepicardial electrodes, studied the influence of atropine-induced tachycardia in conscious dogs and found a comparable increase in myocardial injury, as reflected in ST segment elevations. Similarly, Shell and Sobel (1973), using serum CPK disappearance curves as an index of myocardial damage, have shown that pacing-induced atrial tachycardia results in raised serum CPK activity after each increment in heart rate.

Table 2. Interventions that reduce myocardial injury
following coronary artery occlusion

A. DECREASING MYOCARDIAL OXYGEN REQUIREMENTS
  1. Propranolol*
  2. Practolol
  3. Digitalis (in the failing heart)
  4. Counterpulsation

    a. Intra-aortic balloon*
    b. External*

  5. Nitroglycerin*
  6. Decreasing afterload in patients with hypertension*
  7. Reducing intracellular free fatty acid levels

    a. Antilipolytic agents – beta-pyridyl carbinol
    b. Lipid-free albumin infusions
    c. Glucose-insulin-potassium* (presumed)

B. INCREASING MYOCARDIAL OXYGEN SUPPLY

  1. Directly

    a. Coronary artery reperfusion*
    b. Elevating arterial pO_2*
    c. Thrombolytic agents
    d. Heparin* (presumed)

  2. Through collateral vessels

    a. Elevation of coronary perfusion pressure by methoxamine, phenylephrine
       (Neosynephrine), or norepinephrine
    b. Intra-aortic balloon counterpulsation*
    c. External counterpulsation*
    d. Hyaluronidase*

  3. Increasing plasma osmolality

    a. Mannitol
    b. Hypertonic glucose

C. AUGMENTING ANAEROBIC METABOLISM (PRESUMED)
  1. Glucose-insulin-potassium*
  2. Hypertonic glucose
  3. L-Carnitine
  4. Sodium dichloroacetate

D. PROTECTING AGAINST AUTOLYTIC AND HETEROLYTIC PROCESSES
   (PRESUMED)
  1. Corticosteroids*
  2. Cobra venom factor
  3. Aprotinin

*Intervention has been applied to patients

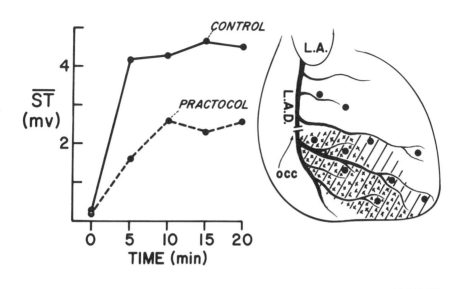

7   Left: average ST segment elevations in all sites (ST) at various times after occlusion; control occlusion [solid line]; occlusion after practolol [dashed line]. Right: diagram of the heart showing the site of occlusion [occ.], the area with ST segment elevation 15 min after control [diagonal lines] and after treatment [crosshatched lines] [LA = left atrial appendage; LAD = left anterior descending coronary artery.] (From Libby et al., 1973b. Reproduced with permission of **Cardiovascular Research**.)

If these interventions in fact, increase infarct size by augmenting myocardial oxygen requirements, the opposite should be achieved with methods that reduce myocardial oxygen consumption (Table 2). Thus, two beta-adrenergic blocking agents, propranolol (Maroko et al., 1971) and practolol (Libby et al., 1973b), which exert such an effect, were investigated and found to decrease myocardial injury after coronary artery occlusion (Figs. 7 and 8). Using histological techniques, Sommers and Jennings (1972) also observed smaller infarctions following coronary occlusion after pretreatment with propranolol. Moreover, in recent experiments in our laboratory, Kloner and coworkers [in press] have shown that beta-adrenergic blockade reduces not only ischemic injury of myocardial cells

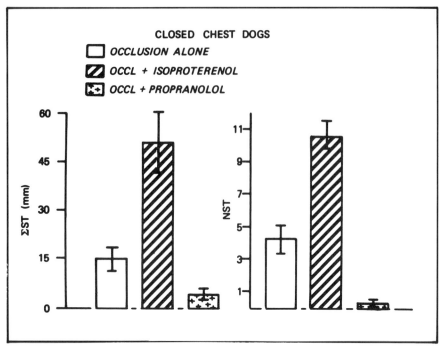

8 Changes in average ΣST (left panel) and average number of sites with ST elevations (NS-T) (right panel) 15 min after occlusion alone (bars at left), after occlusion during infusion of isoproterenol (middle bars) and after occlusion after administration of propranolol (bars at right) in closed-chest dogs. (From Maroko et al., 1972c. Reproduced by permission of **American Journal of Cardiology**.)

but also minimizes microvascular injury. Thus, in untreated dogs, following coronary occlusion, electronmicroscopy showed swollen myocardial cells as well as endothelial gaps, blebs and swelling. All of these changes were decreased in propranolol-treated dogs.

Experiments by Mueller and associates (1970), in patients with acute myocardial infarction, demonstrated that while the infusion of isoproterenol resulted in either increased lactate production or a shift from lactate extraction to production, the administration of propranolol shifted lactate production to extraction, or increased lactate extraction (Mueller et al., 1974). Thus, these clinical observations, which show the detrimental metabolic effect of isoproterenol and the beneficial action of propranolol, also support the hypothesis that myocardial oxygen consumption is important in determining the extent of myocardial tissue damage from ischemia.

Subsequently, the effects of digitalis on the magnitude of ischemic injury were investigated in the failing heart (Watanabe et al., 1972). Digitalis may reduce myocardial oxygen consumption in the latter by lowering wall tension caused by the shortening of the ventricular radius; this overrides the rise in myocardial oxygen consumption, resulting from increases in contractility. Thus, in the failing heart, digitalis reduced myocardial ischemic injury after coronary occlusion, even though the opposite effect had been observed in the non-failing heart (Maroko et al., 1971).

To study the importance of the oxygen supply to the ischemic myocardium, either hemorrhagic hypotension or arterial hypertension were induced after coronary occlusion (Maroko et al., 1971). Arterial hypotension increased the area of myocardial ischemic injury, while raising arterial pressure by infusions of methoxamine or neosynephrine reduced that area. In these experiments, the effect of arterial pressure on coronary blood flow and, therefore, on myocardial-oxygen delivery appeared to be more important than the changes produced in myocardial oxygen demand as a result of altering wall tension. Moreover, the inhalation of 40% oxygen significantly diminished electrocardiographic evidence of acute myocardial ischemic injury as well as the extent of subsequent myocardial necrosis (Maroko et al., 1975c); the inhalation of 10% oxygen had the opposite effect (Fig. 9) (Radvany et al., 1975b).

The consequences of altering the balance between oxygen supply and demand by causing a redistribution of coronary blood flow were also studied with minoxidil and sodium nitroprusside, two potent vasodilators (Chiariello et al., 1976; Radvany et al., 1975a). Despite a marked increase in blood delivery to the nonischemic myocardium, the regional blood flow—both to the border zone and to the center of the ischemic zone—declined with either drug. This caused an increase in ischemic injury, showing the detrimental effect of this type of intervention. On the other hand, nitroglycerin was found to redistribute the flow to the ischemic area, thereby reducing myocardial damage (Chiariello et al., 1976).

Another more direct method of preserving myocardial cells would be to increase oxygen supply by restoring blood flow to the obstructed vessel (Maroko et al., 1972d). This method is not only of theoretical importance, but is the basis of the surgical restoration of blood flow in patients with acute or impending myocardial infarction. Using the same method as that employed for the studies al-

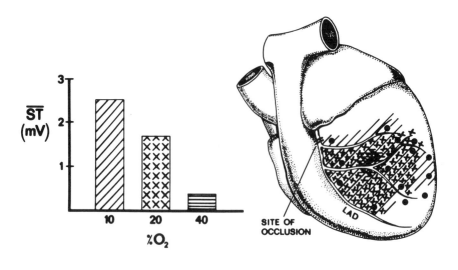

9

An example of the effects of hyperoxia and hypoxia on acute myocardial ischemic injury. Right panel: schematic representation of the heart and its arteries. The section with diagonal lines represents the area of ST segment elevation following coronary occlusion with FIO_2 of 0.10. The cross-hatched section represents the area of injury FIO_2 of 0.20. The section with horizontal lines represents the area of injury with FIO_2 of 0.40. Left panel: Average ST segment elevation (ST) 15 min following occlusion with FIO_2 of 0.10 (diagonal lines), with FIO_2 of 0.20 (cross-hatched bar) and with FIO_2 of 0.40 (horizontal lines).

ready discussed, and reperfusing the coronary artery 3 hr after occlusion, it was found that there was an acute and abrupt fall in ST segment elevation after the release of occlusion. Creatine phosphokinase activity and histological appearance, both 24 hr (Maroko et al., 1972d) and 7 days later (Ginks et al., 1972), showed preservation of extensive portions of the myocardium otherwise expected to have lost their viability. In addition, ventricular function was investigated, using radioopaque beads implanted in the inner third of the left ventricular wall (Ginks et al., 1972), and the paradoxical movements of the ventricle, which were present after coronary occlusion, ceased or were reversed half an hour after reperfusion.

Thus, not only was there an anatomical reduction in myocardial damage but the ultimate aim of restoring viable, normally functioning myocardium was achieved. It should be noted, however, that preliminary reports from several investigators, employing different methods for assessing the viability of myocardial tissue after coronary artery reperfusion and after variable time intervals from the onset of coronary artery occlusion, have shown conflicting findings. Indeed, in some studies, reperfusion actually caused a hemorrhagic infarct, larger than would have been expected from simple coronary occlusion (Bresnahan et al., 1974). Presumably, ischemic damage to the microvasculature can produce extravasation of blood during reperfusion. Despite these deleterious results in some experiments, the clear-cut demonstration, in others, of myocardial salvage atfer several hours of ischemia indicate the clinical potential of such attempts.

Another series of related experiments was performed using intra-aortic balloon counterpulsation (Maroko et al., 1972a). This intervention has the advantage of reducing the heart's need for oxygen while simultaneously increasing its supply (Braunwald et al., 1969). As anticipated, this procedure also strikingly decreased myocardial ischemic injury (Fig. 10).

These experiments, taken as a group, showed that the balance between myocardial oxygen supply and demand is an important factor in determining infarct size after coronary occlusion. They suggest that tachycardia or arterial hypotension, or both, in a patient with an acute coronary occlusion might extend the size of the ischemic zone, further impairing left ventricular function, and thus create a vicious cycle. They also point to the potentially deleterious effects of administering positive inotropic agents, such as isoproterenol, digitalis glycosides, or glucagon, to patients with acute myocardial infarction without heart failure. All of these positive inotropic agents augment myocardial oxygen demands in the non-failing heart but do not necessarily exert such an effect in the presence of heart failure (Mueller et al., 1974).

EFFECTS OF GLUCOSE-INSULIN-POTASSIUM

Investigations into the relationship between myocardial energy requirements and supply were subsequently extended to anaerobic myocardial metabolism. Normally, the heart derives almost all of its energy from the oxidation of various substrates in the Krebs

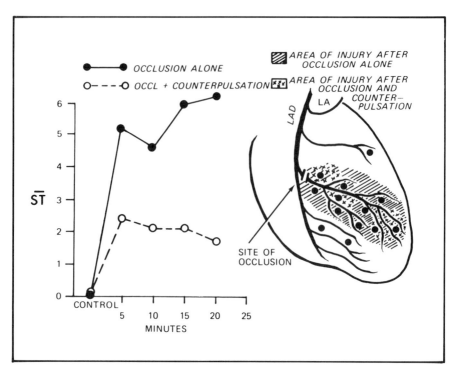

10

Effects for aortic balloon counterpulsation.
Left panel: average ST segment elevation (ST) during occlusion alone (closed circles) and during occlusion with counterpulsation (open circles). Right panel: schematic representation of the heart, with circles indicating sites where epicardial electrocardiograms were obtained. The area of ischemic injury after occlusion alone (ST > 2 mv) is depicted by the striped area and—during occlusion with counterpulsation—by the stippled area. Note the reduction of the injured zone by counterpulsation. LA = left atrial appendage; LAD = left anterior descending coronary artery. (From Maroko et al., 1972a. Reproduced by permission of **Circulation**.)

cycle; however, in the absence of oxygen, the myocardium has the capacity to derive significant quantities of energy from anaerobic glycolysis (Ballinger and Vollenweider, 1962). Experiments were therefore conducted to determine whether anaerobic glycolysis could provide sufficient energy to limit the extent of myocardial necrosis after coronary occlusion. It was reasoned that if the size of a myocardial infarct depends on the balance between the availability and the demand for the various compounds involved in energy production, then the anatomical and functional integrity of cardiac muscle might be preserved by increasing anaerobic glycolysis. Accordingly, the effects of the infusion of glucose-insulin-potassium and of hypertonic glucose alone were examined (Maroko et al., 1972e). We found that when administration was begun 30 min after coronary occlusion, glucose-insulin-potassium substantially decreased the quantity of necrosis, as reflected by creatine phosphokinase activity and histological as well as electronmicroscopic (Sybers et al., 1973) appearance 24 hr later. A number of sites in the myocardium that were otherwise expected to develop necrosis, as predicted by ST segment elevation 15 min after occlusion, demonstrated normal CPK activity 24 hr later, as a consequence of the glucose-insulin-potassium administration. Furthermore, sites that were in the center of distribution of the occluded vessel and were anticipated to show very low CPK activity 24 hr later, exhibited only moderate reduction. This lesser depression of CPK activity was reflected in an altered regression line between the ST segment 15 min after occlusion and the CPK activity 24 hr later (Fig. 4). Histologically, 36% of biopsies expected to show signs of myocardial infarction 24 hr following occlusion were normal, substantiating the protective effect of the glucose-insulin-potassium mixture (Figs. 3 and 12). The beneficial action of hypertonic glucose alone was similar to, but somewhat less marked than that of glucose-insulin-potassium.

EFFECTS OF HYALURONIDASE

Since hyaluronidase increases diffusion through the extracellular space and may, thereby, facilitate delivery of substrates to ischemic cells, its influence on the size of experimentally produced infarcts was explored (Maroko et al., 1972b). It was found in dogs with coronary occlusion that, after the administration of this enzyme, both the extent and magnitude of ST segment elevation were considerably reduced (Fig. 12). In related experiments, hyaluronidase, when administered one-half hour after coronary artery occlusion, decreased the depression of CPK activity, predicted on the basis of ST segment elevation, and also reduced the size of the infarct, as evaluated histologically (Figs. 3 and 4). The sparing of CPK activity was similar in magnitude to that observed with glucose-insulin-potassium, as discussed above; in 45% of biopsies,

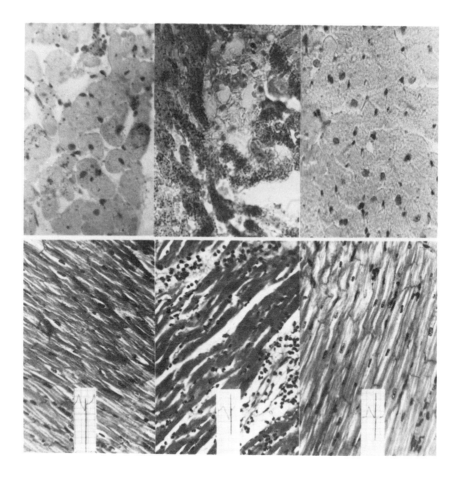

histological examinations expected to show signs of myocardial infarction were normal as the result of hyaluronidase administration.
In order to quantify directly the effects of the enzyme on infarct
size after 2 and 21 days, without relying on electrophysiological
measurements, the left coronary artery was occluded in two groups
of rats: they were either controls or received hyaluronidase shortly
after coronary occlusion (Maclean et al., 1976a). Infarct size was
determined by planimetric measurements of histological sections of
serial slices of the left ventricle: after 2 days, infarct size averaged
43% of the left ventricle in control rats and significantly less, i.e.,
only 25%, in the hyaluronidase-treated rats, while after 21 days,
infarct size was 38% in control rats and only 26% in the treated

11 Effect of glucose-insulin-potassium.
Representative photomicrographs from hematoxylin and eosin
sections (upper row, reduced from × 100) and oil red O fat-stained
sections (lower row, reduced from × 160). Inserts in the panels on
the upper row are epicardial ECG tracings made 15 min after
occlusion from the same site from which the section shown in the
photomicrograph was obtained. Left panels: H & E and oil red O
stained sections obtained from a site without ST segment elevation.
The myocardial fibers are intact with oval nuclei and contain
numerous cross-striations. No fat granules are present within the
individual fibers. The middle panels are photomicrographs obtained
from a site with ST segment elevation from dogs with occlusion
alone. There is extensive fragmentation of the myocardial fibers
and loss of the cross striations. The myocardial nuclei are pyknotic
and exhibit karyolysis, while an extensive polymorphonuclear cell
infiltrate lies within the interstitial spaces. Oil red O rat demonstrate
the presence of numerous massive fat granules within the cytoplasm
of most of the myocardial fibers undergoing ischemic necrosis.
Right panels: photomicrographs obtained from a site with ST
segment elevation of the same magnitude as that in the middle
column in a dog which had received GIK infusion. The myocardial
fibers are intact with normal cross-striations present. There is no
evidence of fragmentation of the fibers or any cellular infiltrate
within the interstitial spaces. Glycogen stains of this section
demonstrated the presence of normal amounts of glycogen within
the myocardial fibers. Oil red O stain resembles the section observed
in the control animal (lower left panel) although an occasional
small fat granule is present within a myocardial fiber. (From
Maroko et al., 1972e. Reproduced by permission of **Circulation**.)

---

animals. In the second group of rats, infarct size was calculated
from total left ventricular creatine phosphokinase depression: after
2 days, infarct size averaged 50% of the left ventricle in the untreated animals and only 24% in the hyaluronidase-treated rats.
Therefore, this enzyme clearly protects the ischemic myocardium
from evolving to an irreversible phase of injury and subsequent
necrosis. An important aspect of this investigation was the observation that myocardial tissue, otherwise destined to undergo necrosis,
was permanently salvaged.

The precise mode of action of this enzyme in reducing infarct
size is not known. However, it has been suggested that its action is
based on its ability to depolymerize hyaluronic acid (Meyer, 1947;
Hechter, 1950), to increase capillary permeability (Szabo and Magyar, 1958) and, thereby, to facilitate the transport of energy-

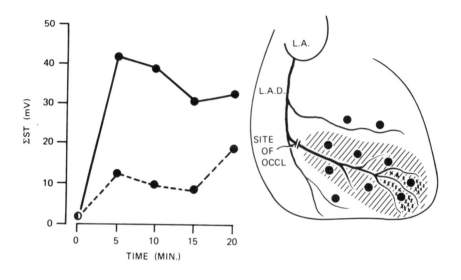

12

An example of the effect of hyaluronidase administration on the sum
of ST segment elevations (ΣST). Right: schematic representation of
the heart. Shaded section = area of ST segment elevation 15 min
following occlusion alone; cross-hatched section = area of ST
segment elevation 15 min following occlusion alone; cross-hatched
section = area of ST segment elevation 15 min following occlusion
preceded by hyaluronidase administration. L.A. = left atrium; L.A.D.
= left anterior descending coronary artery; SITE OF OCCL. = site
of occlusion; closed circles = sites where epicardial
electrocardiograms were obtained. Left: comparison between the
sum of ST segment elevation (ΣST) in the same animal after the
two occlusions. Continuous line = ΣST just before and after the
control occlusion; broken line = ΣST just before and after occlusion
with hyaluronidase pretreatment; TIME = minutes after occlusion.
(From Maroko et al., 1972b. Reproduced by permission of
Circulation.)

producing substances from the blood stream—through the inter-
stitium—to the myocardial cells. Using histochemical techniques and
staining for hyaluronic acid (Alcian green and colloidal iron), it
was observed that 24 hr after coronary occlusion the quantity of
positively-stained material in the interstitial space in the center of

the infarct is clearly reduced by hyaluronidase. This observation is consistent with the hypothesis that this agent acts through its depolymerizing capabilities, and demonstrates that hyaluronidase reaches the center of distribution of an occluded coronary artery. Such action could be significant in the presence of coronary occlusion, when nutrients must be transported through longer extravascular pathways, than when the coronary arteries are patent.

In other studies designed to study the mechanism by which hyaluronidase decreases myocardial injury after coronary artery occlusion, myocardial blood flow was determined using radiolabeled microspheres (Askenazi et al., 1976). Mean arterial pressure, heart rate, cardiac output and flow in the nonischemic myocardium, both in the control (untreated) and the hyaluronidase-treated dogs, were similar 15 min and 6 hr after occlusion. Fifteen minutes following occlusion, the flow to the ischemic myocardium in the two groups of dogs was similar. After 6 hr, flow in the ischemic zone fell in the untreated dogs. In contrast, hyaluronidase-treated dogs showed no fall in flow after 6 hr. Thus, salvage of ischemic myocardium by hyaluronidase may be explained by its beneficial effect on collateral blood flow to the injured area.

To obtain a further understanding of its mechanism of action, the nonperfused myocardium was examined by electron microscopy 3 hr following coronary occlusion [Kloner et al., 1976]. Morphometric analysis in untreated rats showed that 80% of myocardial cells and 49% of microvasculature suffered ischemic damage, while in hyaluronidase-treated rats only 50% myocardial cells and 24% of the microvasculature exhibited ischemic changes. Thus, hyaluronidase protects the myocardium in the early phase of ischemia and also diminishes the damage to the microvasculature, which may result in improved collateral flow.

Hyaluronidase offers several potential advantages, compared with other interventions which reduce infarct size after experimental coronary occlusion: (1) Its application is simple and does not require any special equipment, as does intra-aortic balloon counterpulsation; (2) it does not depress cardiac contractility or cause hypotension, as does propranolol; (3) it does not have the intrinsic property of changing ST segments as does glucose-insulin-potassium, and thus electrocardiographic monitoring may be employed for determining the extent and severity of ischemic injury; (4) most importantly, hyaluronidase has had wide clinical use and its toxicity is extremely low. Allergic reactions are rare (0.08%), generally occurring only after frequent exposure and may be avoided if a skin test is performed. Finally, in terms of effectiveness in reducing myocardial necrosis in the dog after coronary occlusion, hyaluronidase compared favorably with other procedures, such as propranolol and glucose-insulin-potassium.

ANTI-INFLAMMATORY INTERVENTIONS

Following the initial damage caused directly by ischemia, many additional factors are responsible for myocardial cell injury. These include an increase in capillary permeability, interstitial edema, leukotaxis, phagocytosis and nonspecific damage to cell membranes. Presumably, the boundary of the necrotic zone is defined not only by the ischemic stimulus *per se*, but also by many other influences that may result either in definite irreversible destruction or the sparing of these cells in the border zone.

Therefore, the effects of interventions that can limit these reactions have been examined. The activation of the complement system, which may occur during ischemic damage, releases leukotactic factors and may be responsible for increases in capillary permeability and interstitial edema, and complement may contribute substantially to the injury of cell membranes. Accordingly, the action of cobra venom factor, a protein that enzymatically cleaves C3 and thus inhibits the action of the complement system, has been investigated (Maroko and Carpenter, 1974; Maroko and Braunwald, 1976). Also, the effects on infarct size of aprotinin, an inhibitor of the kallikrein system, have been studied, since activation of that system also may enhance leukotaxis, capillary permeability, interstitial edema and proteolytic activity (Diaz and Maroko, 1975). Moreover, the effects of pharmacological doses of glucocorticoids, which may stabilize lysosomal and other cellular membranes, were also examined (Libby et al., 1973a). All three of these interventions, i.e., cobra venom factor, aprotinin and glucocorticoids, were shown to be beneficial, substantially limiting the extent of myocardial ischemic injury after experimental coronary artery occlusion in the dog. Preliminary studies in the rat model have also demonstrated the effectiveness of the above agents (Maclean et al., 1976). It may be postulated that by limiting the organism's inflammatory responses to ischemic injury, additional damage to myocardial cells is avoided and thus the cells with only reversible injury may recover, since the development of the collateral circulation occurs relatively soon following the ischemic stimulus provided by coronary occlusion.

EFFECTS OF DELAYED INTERVENTIONS

The direct clinical application of the interventions discussed above for limiting infarct size might be confined to patients who had experienced an infarct while under observation in hospital or those who might be treated for impending myocardial infarction, unless these interventions howed effects for several hours after coronary occlusion. There are some scattered data in the literature, indicating that isoproterenol, propranolol, methoxamine, phenylephrine, norepinephrine (Maroko et al., 1971), the combination of glucose-insulin-potassium and propranolol (Maroko et al., 1972e), hydrocortisone (Libby et al., 1973a), and intra-aortic balloon counterpulsation (Maroko et al., 1972a) can change the extent and severity of myocardial ischemic injury when administered 3 to 6 hr after coronary occlusion. However, more systematic studies were recently carried out with hyaluronidase (Hillis et al., 1976b). When the enzyme was given 20 min, 3 or 6 hr after coronary occlusion, myocardial salvage was reflected by less CPK depletion for any degree of ST segment elevation than was observed in control (untreated) dogs. However, this effect decreased progressively and when hyaluronidase was administered 9 hr after occlusion, it produced no detectable results, suggesting irreversible injury at that time.

CLINICAL OBSERVATIONS

One of the most formidable barriers to the clinical application of the information obtained in the laboratory is the lack of a suitable technique to assess the efficacy, or its lack, of these interventions designed to protect injured but potentially salvageable myocardium in patients. The ideal technique would have to be: (1) safe and non-invasive; (2) capable of predicting the extent of necrosis to be expected if no interventions were employed; (3) capable of assessing the extent of necrosis that actually develops; (4) capable of providing the data in items 2 and 3 accurately and in quantitative terms, i.e., in grams; (5) effective if applied immediately upon the patient's admission, so that the intervention under study can be promptly performed, since delay in treatment may be expected to reduce the population of injured cells that are salvageable; (6) relatively simple, easy to apply, and inexpensive, so that its use would not be limited to specialized centers; and (7) applicable to all patients with acute myocardial infarction. Items 2 and 3 are of particular importance, since they would allow each patient to be used as his own control.

One such technique is based on examining the rate of resolution of ST segment elevation in precordial leads. The interpretation of how rates of resolution of ST segment elevations are altered in patients by various modes of treatment will ultimately require correlation with other measurements of the size of the damaged region. One measure of this kind that is readily available clinically is the QRS complex. A reduction in the electromotive force of the epicardial R wave within 4 hr of experimental coronary occlusion was first demonstrated by Wilson and his associates (1933). Later, it was shown that a decrease in epicardial R wave voltage was found at sites in which ischemia produced a mixture of viable and necrotic myocardium, as determined by histological examination (Shaw et al., 1954).

To apply this method clinically, we would propose to use the precordial ST segment early after the onset of the clinical event as a predictor of the ultimate fate of the tissue, in a manner analogous to the epicardial ST segment in the experimental animal. This precordial ST segment, recorded soon after the onset of symptoms, may then be compared to the changes in the QRS complex that occur subsequently, such as the development or deepening of Q waves and the reduction of R waves; these changes in the QRS complex could then be employed in a manner analogous to the alterations in CPK activity, or histological appearance of the myocardium subjacent to the epicardial electrode in the experimental animal.

Recent experiments in our laboratory have confirmed the existence of a very close correlation between changes in the QRS complex of epicardial leads and of myocardial CPK activity (Hillis et al., 1976a). In these studies, unipolar electrograms, recorded from 10 to 16 epicardial sites in open-chest dogs before occlusion and 15 min and 2 hr thereafter, were analyzed for ST segment elevation and changes in Q and R waves. Transmural myocardial specimens were obtained 24 hr after occlusion from the same sites at which the EKGs had been recorded. Both in control and in the hyaluronidase-treated dogs, the development of Q waves, the fall in R waves, and their combination ($\triangle R + \triangle Q$) at 24 hr correlated well with the final depression of myocardial creatine phosphokinase activity. In addition, ($\triangle R + \triangle Q$) also correlated well with the extent of necrosis present on histological examination (Fig. 13). From these investigations, it is concluded that: (1) Q wave development and R wave fall, 24 hr after occlusion, accurately reflect myocardial necrosis, as estimated by CPK activity and histological appearance; (2) ST segment elevation 15 min after occlusion predicts subsequent changes in Q and R waves; (3) hyaluronidase and propranolol, agents shown by a variety of other techniques to reduce myocardial necrosis following coronary artery occlusion, can be detected by a diminution in the changes in QRS morphology (i.e., less Q wave development and smaller fall in R wave voltage).

This method of electrocardiographic mapping can be adapted for clinical use by utilizing ST segment elevation in the precordial leads, when the patient is first admitted to he Coronary Care Unit, as a predictor of the ultimate fate of the myocardium—in a manner analogous to that of the epicardial ST segment in the experimental animal. The evolution of the QRS complex in those leads which demonstrate initial ST segment elevation can then be compared in a control and a treated group of patients. These precordial QRS changes can be used in place of alterations in CPK activity and the histological appearance of myocardial specimens (Askenazi et al., 1975).

The analysis of changes in the QRS complex, if applied to multiple precordial leads, potentially fulfills five of the seven aforementioned criteria for assessing the efficacy of interventions designed to protect the ischemic myocardium. Although it is *not* capable of expressing the mass of infarcted myocardium in quantitative terms, and its use is restricted to patients with anterior or lateral transmural myocardial infarctions, this method: (1) is safe and atraumatic; (2) can predict the extent of necrosis to be expected at a time when much of the myocardial injury is still in a reversible phase (ST segment elevations); (3) is capable of assessing the extent of necrosis that actually develops (QRS changes); (4) can be applied immediately and need not delay therapy; and (5) is simple to employ, easy to interpret, and inexpensive. These advantages support the use of precordial QRS mapping for clinical studies of interventions designed to limit infarct size in man.

In view of the apparent lack of toxicity of hyaluronidase and the impressive experimental results with this agent, a pilot study was undertaken to examine its effectiveness in patients with acute myocardial infarction (Maroko et al., 1975b). Twenty-four patients who had suffered a typical transmural myocardial infarction, as determined by history, enzyme changes and electrocardiographic criteria, were investigated. The 11 patients who did not receive hyaluronidase served as control subjects and the 13 patients who

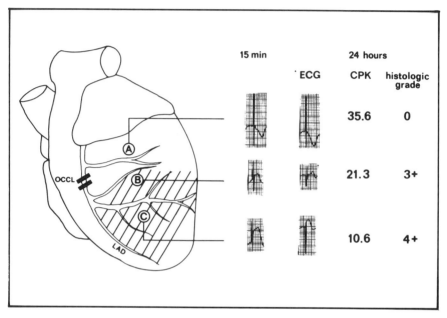

	15 min	24 hours		
	ECG	ECG	CPK	histologic grade
A			35.6	0
B			21.3	3+
C			10.6	4+

13

Panel A: Left Side: A schematic representation of the heart and its arteries. The left anterior descending coronary artery (LAD) was occluded at its midportion (occl). The shaded area represents the zone of ST segment elevation 15 min after occlusion. Right Side: Examples of epicardial electrograms, myocardial CPK values (in IU/mg protein), and histologic grades from a control dog. Site A (from nonischemic myocardium) exhibited no ST segment elevation at 15 min. At 24 hr it had no changes in QRS configuration and normal CPK activity, and it appeared normal histologically. Site B (border zone) showed moderate ST_{15m} while at 24 hr there was a significant Q wave and partial loss of R wave voltage. The CPK activity was moderately depressed, and the histologic section was graded 3+ (51-75%) necrosis. Site C (center of the ischemic zone) had marked ST_{15m} and at 24 hr it demonstrated a total loss of R wave with a QS complex. The myocardial CPK activity was greatly depressed, and the histologic section was graded 4+ (>75%) necrosis.

received the drug constituted the experimental group. Although these patients were not assigned to one of the two groups in a randomized manner and the design of the study was not blind, there was no attempt to preselect the subjects on the basis of the severity of their disease. All patients had acute myocardial infarction in-

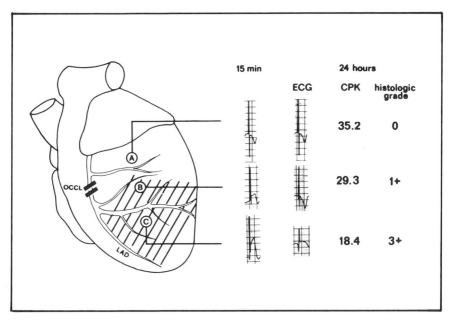

Panel B: Examples of epicardial electrograms, myocardial CPK
activity, and histologic grades in a dog which received hyaluronidase
20 min after occlusion. Site A (from nonischemic myocardium)
exhibited no ST segment elevation at 15 min, and at 24 hr there
were no changes in QRS configuration. The myocardial CPK was
normal, and the specimen appeared normal histologically. Site B
(border zone) showed moderate ST_{15m}; at 24 hr, the specimen did
not exhibit the expected loss of CPK activity, was graded 1+ (1-25%
necrosis) histologically, and did not show extensive changes in QRS
configuration, indicating that hyaluronidase acted to reduce necrosis
in the border zone. Site C (center of the ischemic zone) had marked
ST_{15m} while at 24 hr the QRS configuration and CPK activity were
moderately altered; the histologic section was graded 3+ (51-75%
necrosis). Note, in comparing Sites B and C in this figure with
those in Panel A, that for similar degrees of ST segment elevation,
hyaluronidase reduces necrosis, as measured electrically (QRS
complex), biochemically (CPK activity), and histologically. (From
Hillis et al., 1976a. Reproduced by permission from **Circulation.**)

volving the anterior or lateral walls of the left ventricle, and the
onset of chest pain occurred less than 8 hr before the beginning of
the study. Patients more than 75 years of age and others, with disease of kidney or liver, pregnancy, neoplasms or infections, were
excluded. Patients received hyaluronidase, 500 National Formulary

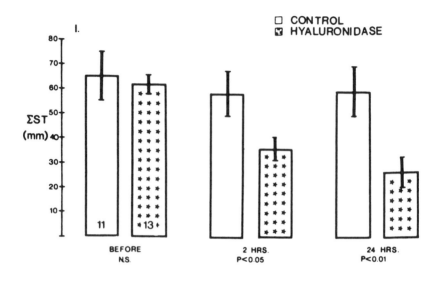

14

Panel I: the sum of ST segment elevations (ΣST) in controls and in hyaluronidase-treated patients at zero time (before treatment), and at 2 and 24 hr after treatment. Note that before treatment both groups had similar values of ΣST. However, in the treated group ΣST dropped significantly more rapidly than in the control group.

units/kg intravenously in a bolus injection, followed by identical additional doses at 2 and 6 hr, and then every 6 hr, until 42 hr after the initial administration.

The precordial electrocardiograms were recorded with 35 unipolar leads (Maroko et al., 1972c). The precordial leads were in a fixed position in a blanket covering the precordium, distributed in five rows of seven electrodes each. Average levels of ΣST and of the number of electrodes showing ST elevations greater than 1 mm (NST), before administration of hyaluronidase in this group, were not statistically different from values in the control group. However, at all times after treatment with hyaluronidase, average ST and NST were significantly lower ($P < 0.05$) than in the control group (Figs. 14 and 15).

The results of this investigation showed that the reduction in

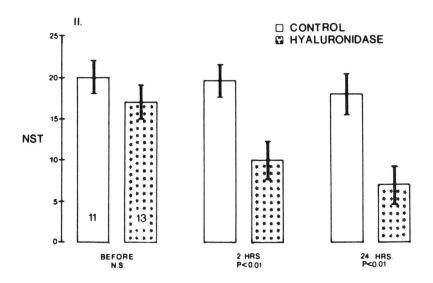

Panel II: number of electrodes showing ST segment elevations exceeding 1 mm (NST) in control patients and in hyaluronidase-treated patients at zero time (before treatment), and at 2 and 24 hr after treatment. Note that before treatment both groups had similar values of NST. However, in the treated group NST dropped significantly more rapidly than in the control group. (Maroko et al., 1975c. Reproduced with permission of **Annals of Internal Medicine**.)

the magnitude and extent of ST segment elevations was greater in the group treated with hyaluronidase than in the controls, at various times during the 24 hr after treatment. This more rapid decline in the electrocardiographic indices of injury was already evident 2 hr after drug administration. Also, although several patients in the untreated control group demonstrated an increase in ST segment elevation in sequential electrocardiograms, suggesting an extension of the infarction, this situation did not occur in any of the hyaluronidase-treated patients. Therefore, on the basis of studies on experimentally-produced coronary occlusion, we suggest that this decrease in acute myocardial ischemic injury resulting from hyaluronidase administration may reflect a reduction in the quantity of myocardium that eventually becomes necrotic.

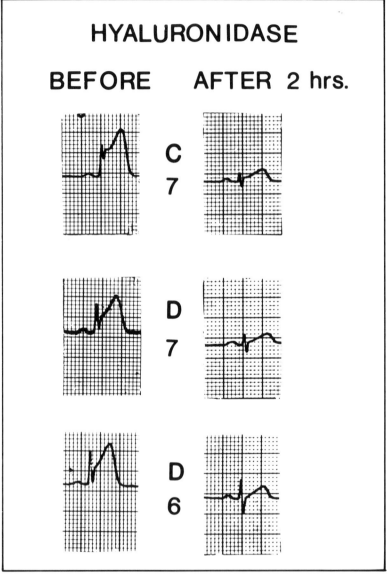

HYALURONIDASE

BEFORE   AFTER 2 hrs.

C 7

D 7

D 6

15 Three enlarged leads from a 35-lead precordial map in a patient with acute myocardial infarction, showing ST segment elevations in these leads before hyaluronidase administration (left), and the striking reduction in ST segment elevation 2 hr after its administration (right). (From Maroko et al., 1975c. Reproduced by permission of **Annals of Internal Medicine**.)

In a subsequent study, which is still in process and is being carried out in a separate group of patients, the effects of a similar regimen of hyaluronidase administration on the development of Q waves in 35 precordial electrocardiographic leads was examined (Maroko et al., 1975a). Preliminary results indicate that, in 43 control (untreated) patients with acute anterior myocardial infarction, significant changes in the QRS complex indicative of myocardial necrosis developed within five days in 73.5% of leads, with ST segment elevation of 0.15 mv or more. Also, the sum of R wave heights (ΣR) fell by 71.4% in these leads within the same time interval. In 42 hyaluronidase-treated patients, these two indices were both reduced significantly, to 59.6% and 55.0%, respectively (P < .05).

When considered together, the observations on the effects of hyaluronidase on the extent of myocardial necrosis in dogs (Maroko et al., 1972b) and rats (Maclean et al., 1976) with experimentally produced coronary occlusion, the two pilot clinical trials demonstrating the effects of this agent on the rate of resolution of abnormally elevated precordial ST segments (Maroko et al., 1975b), and the development of electrocardiographic changes indicative of necrosis in the QRS complex (Maroko et al., 1975a), all suggest that this agent may be effective in reducing the quantity of myocardium that eventually becomes necrotic after coronary occlusion. In view of its low level of toxicity and ease of administration, it is evident that expanded and rigorous clinical trials with hyaluronidase should now be undertaken.

A number of other pilot studies in patients with acute myocardial infarction have supported the hope that a significant portion of the myocardium can be salvaged by speedy intervention—within several hours after the clinical event (Table 2). A number of agents, including propranolol (Gold et al., 1974), oxygen (Madias et al., 1976), nitroglycerin (Borer et al., 1975; Flaherty et al., 1975; Come et al., 1975), and glucose-insulin-potassium (Russell et al., 1976), appear to be efficacious in limiting ischemic injury in patients whose therapy is begun within a few hours after the onset of symptoms. Although the results of these pilot studies are encouraging and exciting, the overall clinical utility of interventions designed to limit myocardial necrosis can be assessed only through carefully and rigorously conducted clinical trials.

Recognition of the importance of the mass of myocardium undergoing necrosis as a crucial determinant of prognosis, and the efforts to preserve ischemic tissue may drastically alter the therapeutic approach to acute myocardial infarction. Rather than simply maintaining the patient's vital signs, the physician's efforts may now be directed toward preserving the myocardium as well as maintaining perfusion of peripheral organs. However, these two objectives may sometimes conflict. In the first hours following the onset of the clinical event, while the ultimate size of the infarct is not yet established, myocardial preservation might be given the highest priority. Later on, once the size of the infarct has become fixed and, should heart failure supervene, it may be more appropriate to stimulate the heart with positive inotropic agents and reduce afterload, i.e., to employ interventions that may increase infarct size if given at an earlier time.

Recent observations by Reid et al. (1974) suggest that significant extensions of myocardial necrosis occur during apparently uneventful convalescence in a large proportion of patients with acute myocardial infarction. Also, in many patients previously classified as having acute myocardial infarction, tissue damage occurs in a slow, "stuttering" manner, rather than abruptly, a condition that might more properly be termed "subacute infarction." These considerations greatly expand the scope of what can be accomplished by techniques to prevent myocardial necrosis, since the interventions designed to limit infarct size could then be applied prophylactically, when they are most likely to be effective. The interesting observation by Cox et al. (1976) that the incidence of ventricular arrhythmia is a function of the size of the infarct, adds yet another dimension to the benefit that can potentially be derived from protection of jeopardized myocardium.

It is not possible, at present, to identify the specific procedure likely to be the most effective in reducing infarct size. Indeed, there may not be a single treatment; rather, it seems more likely that, in the future, patients will be carefully but rapidly subdivided and categorized according to their clinical, electrocardiographic, hemodynamic and, perhaps, coronary arteriographic findings, and the intervention will be tailored appropriately. For example, in hypertensive patients, afterload reduction may be effective; in patients without any evidence of myocardial depression, cardiospecific beta-adrenergic blockade may be the treatment of choice; in normotensive or hypotensive patients with pump failure, circulatory support may be in order. All patients with acute infarction, regardless of their hemodynamic state, may benefit from the administration of an anti-inflammatory agent, such as aprotinin, or from a drug, such as hyaluronidase.

Acute myocardial infarction continues to be the most common cause of death in the United States today, and of those patients who survive the infarct, the quantity of viable, contractile myocardium with which they are left is critical to their well being. Considering the frequency of ischemic heart disease, the potential benefits from interventions designed to salvage ischemic tissue, and the encouraging preliminary results obtained thus far, continued intensive research in this field appears to be especially desirable.

ACKNOWLEDGMENT

The important contributions of Dr. Peter R. Maroko to this work are gratefully acknowledged.

This project has been supported, in part, by Contract N01-HV-5300 from the Division of Heart and Vascular Diseases, National Heart, Lung and Blood Institute, NIH.

REFERENCES

Angell, C. S., Lakatta, E. G., Weisfeldt, M. L., and Shock, N. W.: Relationship of intramyocardial oxygen tension and epicardial ST segment changes following acute coronary artery ligation: Effects of coronary perfusion pressure. *Cardiovasc. Res.* 9:12-18 (1975).

Askenazi, J., Dye, R., Hubbard, F., Lesch, M., Braunwald, E., and Maroko, P. R.: Prediction by ST segment elevations of electrocardiographic necrosis in patients with acute myocardial infarction. *Circulation* 52 (Suppl. II): 423 (Abstr.) (1975).

Askenazi, J., Hillis, L. D., Diaz, P. E., Davis, M. A., Braunwald, E., and Maroko, P. R.; Mechanism of reduction of myocardial injury by hyaluronidase. *Am. J. Cardiol.* 37:118 (Abstr.) (1976).

Ballinger, W. F., II, and Vollenweider, H., Anaerobic metabolism of the heart. *Circ. Res.* 11:681-685 (1962).

Becker, L. C., Ferreira, R., and Thomas, M., Mapping of left ventricular blood flow with radioactive microspheres in experimental coronary artery occlusion. *Cardiovasc. Res.* 7:391-400 (1973).

Borer, J. S., Redwood, D. R., Levitt, B., Cagin, N., Bianchi, C., Vallin, H., and Epstein, S. E.: Reduction in myocardial ischemia with nitroglycerin or nitroglycerin plus phenylephrine administered during acute myocardial infarction in Man. *N. Engl. J. Med* 293: 1008-1012 (1975).

Braunwald, E.: The pathogenesis and treatment of shock in myocardial infarction: Topics in clinical medicine. *John Hopkins Med. J.* 121:421-429 (1967).

Braundwald, E.: Thirteenth Bowditch Lecture. The determinants of myocardial oxygen consumption. *Physiologist* 12:65-93 (1969).

Braunwald, E.: Control of myocardial oxygen consumption. Physiologic and clinical considerations. *Am. J. Cardiol.* 27:416-432 (1971).

Braunwald, E.: Regulation of the circulation. *N. Engl. J. Med.* 290:1124-1129; 1420-1425 (1974).

Braunwald, E. (Ed.) : Symposium on protection of the ischemic myocardium. *Circulation* 53 Suppl. III) : 1-217 (1976).

Braunwald, E., Covell, J. W., Maroko, P. R., and Ross, J., Jr.: Effects of drugs and of counterpulsation on myocardial oxygen consumption. *Circulation* 40 (Suppl. IV) : 220-228 (1969).

Braunwald, E., Epstein, S. E., Glick, G., Wechsler, A., and Braunwald, N. S.: Relief of angina pectoris by electrical stimulation of the carotid sinus. *N. Engl. J. Med.* 277:1278-1283 (1967).

Braunwald, E., and Maroko, P. R.: (Editorial) ST segment mapping—Realistic and unrealistic expectations. *Circulation* 54:529-532, 1976.

Bresnahan, G. F., Roberts, R., Shell, W. E., Ross, J., Jr., and Sobel, B. E.: Deleterious effects due to hemorrhage after myocardial reperfusion. *Am. J. Cardiol.* 33:82-86 (1974).

Capone, R. J., Most, A. S., and Sydlik, P. A.: Precordial ST segment mapping: A sensitive technique for the evaluation of myocardial injury. *Chest* 67: 577-582 (1975).

Chiariello, M., Gold, H. K., Leinbach, R. C., Davis, M. A., and Maroko, P. R.: Comparison between the effects of nitroprusside and nitroglycerin on electrocardiographic ischemic injury during acute myocardial infarction. *Circulation.* 76:766-773 (1976).

Cohen, D., and Kaufman, L. A.: Magnetic determination of the relationship between the ST segment shift and the injured current produced by coronary artery occlusion. *Circ. Res.* 36:414-424 (1975).

Come, P., Flaherty, J. T., Weisfeldt, M. L., Greene, L., Becker, L., and Pitt, B.: Reversal of the beneficial effects of intravenous nitroglycerin in patients with acute myocardial infarction by phenylephrine. *N. Engl. J. Med.* 293:1003-1007 (1975).

Cox, J. L., McLaughlin, V. W., Flowers, N. C., and Horan, L. G.: The ischemic zone surrounding acute myocardial infarction: Its morphology as detected by dehydrogenase staining. *Am. Heart J.* 76:650 (1968).

Cox, J. R., Jr., Roberts, R., Ambox, H. D., Oliver, C., and Sobel, B. E.: Relations between enzymatically estimated myocardial infarct size and early ventricular dysrhythmia. *Circulation* 53 (Suppl. I) : 150-155 (1976).

Diaz, P. E., and Maroko, P. R.: The effects of aprotinin on myocardial ischemic injury following experimental coronary artery occlusion. *Clin. Res.* 23:108A (Abstr.) (1975).

Eyster, J. A. E., Meek, W. J., Goldberg, H., and Gilson, W. E.: Potential changes in an injured region of cardiac muscle. *Am. J. Physiol.* 125:717-728 (1938).

Flaherty, J. T., Reid, P. R., Kelly, D. T., Taylor, D. R., Weisfeldt, M. L., and Pitt, B.: Intravenous nitroglycerin in acute myocardial infarction. *Circulation* 51:132-139 (1975).

Ginks, W. R., Sybers, H. D., Maroko, P. R., Covell, J. W., Sobel, B. E., and Ross, J., Jr.: Coronary artery reperfusion. II. Reduction of myocardial infarct size at one week after the coronary occlusion. *J. Clin. Invest.* 51: 2717-2723 (1972).

Gold, H. K., Leinbach, R. C., and Maroko, P. R.: Reduction of myocardial injury in patients with acute infarction by propranolol. *Circulation* 50 (Suppl. II): 33 (Abstr.) (1974).

Harnarayan, C., Bennett, M. S., Pentecost, B. L., and Brewer, D. B.: Quantitative study of infarcted myocardium in cardiogenic shock. *Br. Heart J.* 32: 728-736 (1970).

Hechter, O.: Mechanisms of spreading factor action. *Ann. N. Y. Acad. Sci.* 52:1028-1040 (1950).

Hillis, L. D., Askenazi, J., Braunwald, E., Radvany, P., Muller, J. E., Fishbein, M. C., and Maroko, P. R.: Use of changes in the epicardial QRS complex to assess interventions which modify the extent of myocardial necrosis following coronary artery occlusion. *Circulation.* 54:591-598 (1976a).

Hillis, L. D., Maroko, P. R., Braunwald, E., and Fishbein, M. C.: Influence of the time interval between coronary artery occlusion and the administration of hyaluronidase on myocardial salvage. *Circulation* 54: (Suppl. 2) 627 (1976b) Abstr.

Karlsson, J., Templeton, G. H., and Willerson, J. T.: Relationship between epicardial ST segment changes and myocardial metabolism during acute coronary insufficiency. *Circ. Res.* 32:725-730 (1973).

Khuri, S. F., Flaherty, J. T., O'Riordan, J. B., Pitt, B., Brawley, R. L., Donahoo, J. W., and Gott, V. L.: Changes in intramyocardial ST segment voltage and gas tension with regional myocardial ischemia in the dog. *Circ. Res.* 37:455-464 (1975).

Klocke, F. J., Braunwald, E., and Ross, J., Jr.: Oxygen cost of electrical activation of the heart. *Circ. Res.* 18:357-365, 1966.

Kloner, R. A., Fishbein, M. C., Cotran, R. S., Braunwald, E., and Maroko, P. R.: Effect of propranolol on microvascular injury after experimental coronary artery occlusion. *Circulation.* 54:766-774, 1976.

Kloner, R. A., Fishbein, M. C., Maclean, D., Braunwald, E., and Maroko, P. R.: Effect of hyaluronidase on myocardial ultrastructure following coronary artery occlusion in the rat. *Circulation* 54: Suppl. 2:345 (1976) Abstr.

Libby, P., Maroko, P. R., Bloor, C. M., Sobel, B. E., and Braunwald, E.: Reduction of experimental myocardial infarct size by corticosteroid administration. *J. Clin. Invest.* 52:599-607 (1973a).

Libby, P., Maroko, P. R., Covell, J. W., Malloch, C. I., Ross, J., Jr., and Braunwald, E.: Effect of practolol on the extent of myocardial ischemic injury after experimental coronary occlusion and its effects on ventricular function in the normal and ischemic heart. *Cardiovasc. Res.* 7:167-173 (1973b).

Maclean, D., Fishbein, M. C., Maroko, P. R., and Braunwald, E.: Drug-induced alterations in myocardial infarct size. Direct quantitation of infarction following coronary artery occlusion in the rat. *Science* 194:199-200 (1976a).

Maclean, D., Maroko, P. R., Fishbein, M. C., Carpenter, C. B., and Braunwald, E.: Reduction of infarct size up to 21 days after coronary occlusion in the rat. *Circulation* 54 (Suppl. 2) 628 (Abstr) (1976b).

Maroko, P. R., Askenazi, J., Tavazzi, L., Muller, J. E., Distante, A., Salerno, J., Radvany, P., Libby, P., Luepker, R., Bobba, P., and Braunwald, E.:

Effects of hyaluronidase on electrocardiographic evidence of necrosis in patients with acute myocardial infarction. *Circulation* 52 (Suppl. II) : 106 (Abstr.) (1975a).

Maroko, P. R., Bernstein, E. F., Libby, P., DeLaria, G. A., Covell, J.W.,Ross, J., Jr., and Braunwald, E.: Effects of intra-aortic balloon counterpulsation on the severity of myocardial ischemic injury following acute coronary occlusion. *Circulation* 45:1150-1159 (1972a).

Maroko, P. R., and Braunwald, E.: Modification of myocardial infarct size after coronary occlusion. *Ann. Intern. Med.* 79:720-733 (1973).

Maroko, P. R., and Braunwald, E.: Effect of metabolic and pharmacologic interventions on myocardial infarct size following coronary occlusion. In *Experimental and Clinical Aspects on Preservation of the Ischemic Myocardium*, A. Hjalmarson and L. Werko, eds. Molndal, Sweden (1976), pp. 125-136.

Maroko, P. R., and Carpenter, C. B.: Reduction in infarct size following acute coronary occlusion by the administration of cobra venom factor. *Clin. Res.* 22:289A (Abstr.) (1974).

Maroko, P. R., Davidson, D. M., Libby, P., Hagan, A. D., and Braunwald, E.: Effects of hyaluronidase administration on myocardial ischemic injury in acute infarction. A preliminary study in 24 patients. *Ann. Intern. Med.* 82:516-520 (1975b).

Maroko, P. R., Kjekshus, J. K., Sobel, B. E., Watanabe, T., Covell, J. W., Ross, J., Jr., and Braunwald, E.: Factors influencing infarct size following experimental coronary artery occlusions. *Circulation* 43:67-82, 1971.

Maroko, P. R., Libby, P., Bloor, C. M., Sobel, B. E., and Braunwald, E.: Reduction by hyaluronidase of myocardial necrosis following coronary artery occlusion. *Circulation* 46:430-437 (1972b).

Maroko, P. R., Libby, P., Covell, J. W., Sobel, B. E., Ross, J., Jr., and Braunwald, E.: Precordial ST segment elevation mapping: An atraumatic method for assessing alterations in the extent of myocardial ischemic injury. The effects of pharmacologic and hemodynamic interventions. *Am. J. Cardiol.* 29:223-230 (1972c).

Maroko, P. R., Libby, P., Ginks, W. R., Bloor, C. M., Shell, W. E., Sobel, B. E., and Ross, J., Jr.: Coronary artery reperfusion I: Early effects on local myocardial function and the extent of myocardial necrosis. *J. Clin. Invest.* 51:2710-2716 (1972d).

Maroko, P. R., Libby, P., Sobel, B. E., Bloor, C. M., Sybers, H. D., Shell, W. E., Covell, J. W., and Braunwald, E.: The effect of glucose-insulin-potassium infusion on myocardial infarction following experimental coronary artery occlusion. *Circulation* 45:1160-1175 (1972e).

Maroko, P. R., Radvany, P., Braunwald, E., and Hale, S. L.: Reduction of infarct size by oxygen inhalation following acute coronary occlusion. *Circulation* 52:360-368 (1975c).

Meyer, K.: Biological significance of hyaluronic acid and hyaluronidase. *Physiol. Rev.* 27:335-359 (1947).

Mueller, H. S., Ayers, S. M., Gregory, J. J., Giannelli, S., Jr., and Grace, W. J.: Hemodynamics, coronary blood flow, and myocardial metabolism in coronary shock: response to l-norepinephrine and isoproterenol. *J. Clin Invest.* 49:1885-1902 (1970).

Mueller, H. S., Ayres, S. M., Religa, A., and Evans, R. G.: Propranolol in the treatment of acute myocardial infarction. *Circulation* 49:1078-1087 (1974).

Muller, J. E., Maroko, P. R., and Braunwald, E.: Evaluation of precordial electrocardiographic mapping as a means of assessing changes in myocardial ischemic injury. *Circulation* 52:16-27 (1975).

Nahum, L. H., Hamilton, W. F., and Heff, H. E.: Injury current in the electrocardiogram. *Am. J. Physiol.* 139:202-207 (1943).

Page, D. L., Caulfield, J. B., Kastor, J. A., DeSanctis, R. W., and Sanders, C. A.: Myocardial changes associated with cardiogenic shock. *N. Engl. J. Med.* 285:133 (1971).

Radvany, P., Davis, M. A., Muller, J. E., and Maroko, P. R.: The effect of minoxidil on regional myocardial blood flow during acute coronary artery occlusion. *Clin. Res.* 23:203A (Abstr.) (1975a).

Radvany, P., Maroko, P. R., and Braunwald, E.: Effects of hypoxemia on the extent of myocardial necrosis after experimental coronary occlusion. *Am. J. Cardiol.* 35:795-800 (1975b).

Redwood, D. R., Smith, E. R., and Epstein, S. E.: Coronary artery occlusion in the conscious dog: Effect of alterations in heart rate and arterial pressure on the degree of myocardial ischemia. *Circulation* 46:323-332 (1972).

Reid, P. R., Taylor, D. R., Kelly, D. T., Weisfeldt, M. L., Humphries, J. O., Ross, R. S., and Pitt, B.: Myocardial-infarct extension detected by precordial ST segment mapping. *N. Engl. J. Med.* 290:123-128 (1974).

Rodbard, S., Williams, C. B., Rodbard, D., and Berglund, E.: Myocardial tension and oxygen uptake. *Circ. Res.* 14:139-149 (1964).

Ross, J., Jr., Sonnenblick, E. H., Kaiser, G. A., Frommer, P. L., and Braunwald, E.: Electroaugmentation of ventricular performance and oxygen consumption by repetitive application of paired electrical stimuli. *Circ. Res.* 16:332-342 (1965).

Russell, R. O., Jr., Rogers, W. J., Mantle, J. A., McDaniel, H. G., and Rackley, C. E.: Glucose-insulin-potassium, free fatty acids, and acute myocardial infarction in man. *Circulation* 53 (Suppl. I) : 207-209 (1976).

Samson, W. E., and Scher, A. M.: Mechanism of ST segment alteration during acute myocardial injury. *Circ. Res.* 8:780-787 (1960).

Sarnoff, S. J., Braunwald, E., Welch, G. H., Jr., Case, R. B., Stainsby, W. N., and Macruz, R.: Hemodynamic determinants of oxygen consumption of the heart with special reference to the tension-time index. *Am. J. Physiol.* 192:148-156 (1958).

Sayen, J. J., Peirce, G., Katcher, A. H., and Sheldon, W. F.: Correlation between epicardial ST segment changes and myocardial metabolism during acute coronary insufficiency. *Circ. Res.* 9:1268-1279, 1961.

Scheuer, J., and Brachfeld, M.: Coronary insufficiency: Relations between hemodynamic, electrical and biochemical parameters. *Circ. Res.* 18:178-189 (1966).

Shaw, CMcK, Jr., Goldman, A., Kennamer, R., Kimura, N., Lindgren, I., Maxwell, M. H., and Prinzmetal, M.: Studies on the mechanism of ventricular activity. VII. The origin of the coronary QR wave. *Am. J. Med.* 16:490 (1954).

Shell, W. E., and Sobel, B. S.: Deleterious effects of increased heart rate on infarct size in the conscious dog. *Am. J. Cardiol.* 31:474-479 (1973).

Sobel, B. E., Bresnahan, G. F., Shell, W. E., and Yoder, R. D.: Estimation of infarct size in man and its relation to prognosis. *Circulation* 46:640-648 (1972).

Somerville, W., and Kevin, S. A.: Angina pectoris and thyrotoxicosis. *Br. Heart J.* 12:245-257 (1950).

Sommers, H. M., and Jennings, R. B.: Ventricular fibrillation and myocardial necrosis after transient ischemia. *Arch. Intern. Med.* 129:780-789 (1972).

Sonnenblick, E. H., Ross, J., Jr., Covell, J. W., Kaiser, G. A., and Braunwald, E.: Velocity of contraction as a determinant of myocardial oxygen consumption. *Am. J. Physiol.* 209:919-927 (1965).

Sybers, H. D., Maroko, P. R., Ashraf, M., Libby, P., and Braunwald, E.: The effect of glucose-insulin-potassium on cardiac ultrastructure following acute experimental coronary occlusion. *Am. J. Pathol.* 70:401-420 (1973).

Szabo, G., and Magyar, S.: Effect of hyaluronidase on capillary permeability, lymph flow and passage of dye-labeled protein from plasma to lymph. *Nature* (Lond.) 182:377-379 (1958).

Watanabe, T., Covell, J. W., Maroko, P. R., Braunwald, E., and Ross, J., Jr.: Effects of increased arterial pressure and positive inotropic agents on the severity of myocardial ischemia in the acutely depressed heart. *Am. J. Cardiol.* 30:371-377 (1972).

Wegria, R., Segers, M., Keating, R. P., and Ward, H. P.: Relationship between the reduction in coronary flow and the appearance of electrocardiographic changes. *Am. Heart J.* 38:90-96 (1949).

Wilson, F. N., MacLeod, A. G., Barker, P. S., Johnston, F. D., and Klostermeyer, L. L.: The electrocardiogram in myocardial infarction with particular reference to the initial deflections of the ventricular complex. *Heart* 16:155-199 (1933).

Wolfson, S., Heinle, R. A., Herman, M. V., et al.: Propranolol and angina pectoris. *Am. J. Cardiol.* 18:345-353 (1966).

Part III

PHYSIOLOGIC MECHANISMS IN MYOCARDIAL ISCHEMIA

Pathophysiology and Therapeutics of Myocardial Ischemia

12

Hemodynamic Alterations in Acute Myocardial Infarction

JOHN K. VYDEN
TERUO TAKANO
TAKESHI OGAWA
HAROLD B. ROSE

INTRODUCTION

In the last decade, significant advances in the management of acute myocardial infarction were made with the advent of the Coronary Care Unit and, in consequence, many deaths from previously fatal cardiac arrhythmias have been avoided. Now, the pulmonary artery balloon flotation catheter provides a new tool for assessing the effects of acute myocardial infarction upon cardiac functions and the modification of disordered function by therapy in physiological terms. As a result, new concepts concerning the disease itself and new treatments have been developed. Two of these new concepts will be discussed in this chapter, namely that: (1) The recognition that the oxygen balance of ischemic myocardium is critical in determining morbidity, at times, even mortality, and (2) the acute myocardial infarction is a collection of sets and subsets of symptoms rather than a homogenous single-disease entity. A third major concept, that is, preservation of the ischemic myocardium, will be dealt with by other authors in this volume.

HEMODYNAMIC PATHOPHYSIOLOGY IN ACUTE
MYOCARDIAL INFARCTION

While size of an acute myocardial infarction is usually the major determinant of the severity of depression of cardiac function, factors other than the infarct size may also induce severe hemodynamic alterations and impairment of cardiac function. Location of the infarct, type and severity of asynergy, hypoxia, acidosis, changes in ventricular compliance, effectiveness of the compensatory mechanisms, and arrhythmias are all important determinants of the hemodynamic effect that will result. For example, a strategically located but small infarct in the intraventricular septum or in the papillary muscle may impose severe hemodynamic burdens by producing a ventricular septal defect or valvular incompetence that may markedly depress cardiac performance, even though the actual size of the infarct may be small. Similarly, contiguous large areas of ischemic, nonfunctioning but viable myocardium may be responsible for severe impairment of left ventricular performance, even when the actual size of the infarct may be relatively smaller at the onset of the clinical syndrome. Changes in compliance in both the infarcted and ischemic segments may also play a significant role in the symptomatology, as well as in the level of depression of left ventricular function.

With a stiffer (less compliant) ventricle, signs and symptoms of pulmonary venous congestion may be present with adequate left ventricular function. Normal left ventricular performance may even be maintained in the face of acute myocardial infarction by effective compensatory mechanisms.

Cardiac output is usually normal in acute myocardial infarction, but occasionally it is increased and a hyperkinetic circulatory state can result. However, when heart failure and "shock" supervene, cardiac output usually falls and a drop of 30-50% is not uncommon (Weil and Shubin, 1969) (Table 1).

Together with a reduction in stroke volume and cardiac output, there is a decrease in the ejection fraction, often with an increase in end-diastolic and end-systolic volumes, a increment in left ventricular diastolic pressure, a decrease in maximal rate of rise of left ventricular pressure (LV max dp/dt) and a diminished peak in mean left ventricular systolic ejection rates.

Since heart rate is often normal or increased in severe acute myocardial infarction, the fall in cardiac output is attributed to re-

Table 1. Hemodynamic analysis of 39 patients with acute myocardial infarction

	Survivors	Non-Survivors	P
Cardiac output L/min	4.4 ± 0.3	3.2 ± 0.7	NS
Heart rate beats/min	88 ± 4	87 ± 6	NS
Mean arterial pressure mmHg	106 ± 3	91 ± 5	<0.005
Pulmonary capillary wedge pressure mmHg	14 ± 2	17 ± 2	NS
Central venous pressure mmHg	8 ± 1	11 ± 2	NS
Stroke volume ml/beat	54 ± 5	36 ± 9	<0.05
Stroke work g-m/beat	88 ± 9	52 ± 15	<0.025
Total systemic vascular resistance 10^3 dynes/sec/cm^{-5}	2.1 ± 1.6	2.6 ± 6.4	NS
Mean tension time index mmHg sec/min	12 ± 0.6	9.9 ± 0.8	<0.005

Hemodynamic measurements were made in a series of 39 patients during the first 24 hr period after acute myocardial infarction.

The data obtained from survivors and non-survivors, including levels of statistical significance between the two groups of data, are shown here.

It is seen that only the values for mean arterial blood pressure (measured intra-arterially), stroke volume, stroke work and mean tension time index are significantly different.

Mean ± SEM

Hypovolemial — a decrease in volume of circulating blood

duced stroke volume. Diminished stroke volume, in turn, be caused by a decrease in cardiac filling pressure, resulting from impaired venous return because of hypovolemia. Hypovolemia is often present without overt evidence of external fluid loss or blood loss. It can be caused by the patient's chronic use of diuretics outside the hospital before infarction, and be due to seepage of fluid volume into vascular spaces and gut; this, in turn, is a consequence of an increased tone of the venous capacitance vessels, resulting from the sympathomimetic discharge that occurs upon infarction. Fluid replacement is now accepted as an essential part of treatment in cases such as these. Diminished stroke volume, on the other hand, may be caused by a decrease in the strength of ventricular contraction. Weakness of ventricular contraction, despite an adequate filling pressure or, in other words, "pump failure," is a source of the hemodynamic maladjustment.

In addition to loss of function of myocardium by infarction or by severe ischemia, and the development of areas of asynergy or dyssynergy (Herman et al., 1967; Langley et al., 1967; Herman and Gorlin, 1969), several other factors contribute to the diminished pumping ability of the heart. These include: (1) a decrease in ventricular performance due to generalized myocardial ischemia and depression secondary to aortic hypertension, with reduced coronary flow; (2) arterial acidosis; (3) hypoxia and the development of ventricular dilatation which further increases myocardial oxygen requirements by Laplace's Law.

In addition, overall cardiac performance may be depressed by the loss of atrial function with atrial fibrillation, or improperly synchronized atrial and ventricular contractions, or by extreme bradycardia or tachycardia.

If a fall in arterial blood pressure occurs, there is a sympatho-adrenal discharge and elevation of blood levels of catecholamines, mediated through the baroreceptor reflexes, which has both beneficial and deleterious effects. The beneficial action of the sympatho-adrenal discharge includes: a positive inotrophic response, redistribution of organ blood flow, and coronary vasodilation (Abboud, 1968). The deleterious consequences involve a prolonged reduction of blood flow to: (a) the kidneys, producing oliguria; (b) the gastrointestinal tract, which may cause mesenteric ischemia; and (c) the musculoskeletal system, resulting in cold, clammy limbs. If the decrease in blood flow to the gastrointestinal tract is severe enough, myocardial depressant factor (MDF) may be released from the ischemic pancreas, causing a further secondary drop in cardiac output. Diminished blood flow in the capillaries leads to venous pooling, systemic acidosis because of lactic acid accumulation resulting from poor tissue perfusion, and the reduction in peripheral blood flow at the microcirculatory levels, which encourages the formation of diffuse intravascular thrombosis.

In addition, some patients—particularly those in acute posterior or inferior myocardial infarction—appear to have a strong vagal discharge which may produce sinus bradycardia, increased atrioventricular block, and depressed atrial and ventricular function. It is, thus, apparent that the effects of a recent myocardial infarction on the performance of the left ventricle cannot be uniform and that several subsets must exist. Therefore, it is important that these subsets be recognized, not only to improve our understanding of the pathophysiology involved, but also to facilitate the rational management of the patient with an acute infarction by the attending physician.

MYOCARDIAL OXYGEN DEMAND

Recent attention has been focused on the oxygen balance of the ischemic myocardium as being a critical factor in determining the morbidity and mortality in the patient with myocardial infarction. Since acute myocardial infarction results from the inability of the coronary arterial system to deliver sufficient oxygen to meet the metabolic demand of the myocardium, it is apparent that there are only two ways to treat this imbalance. One method is to increase oxygen delivery by direct coronary arterial surgery immediately after acute myocardial infarction supervenes, and this procedure is being performed in certain advanced surgical units at the present time. The second method to correct oxygen imbalance is to administer agents that reduce the metabolic activity of the heart and lessen its oxygen demand.

There are four major determinants of myocardial oxygen demand, namely: (1) heart rate, (2) contractility, (3) preload, and (4) afterload (Braunwald, 1969). Thus, interventions that increase myocardial oxygen consumption, such as tachycardia, isoproterenol, digitalis, glucagon and bretylium, in the non-failing heart, are probably contraindicated in the management of acute myocardial infarction (Maroko and Braunwald, 1973). However, other agents, including phentolamine, nitroprusside, beta-adrenergic receptor blockers and corticosteroids, which reduce one or more of these four determinants of myocardial oxygen consumption, will probably assume a far greater role in the future management of acute myocardial infarction.

A number of studies have demonstrated that agents, which reduce systemic vascular resistance, may substantially improve effective cardiac performance in patients with heart failure associated with acute myocardial infarction (Chatterjee et al., 1973a, 1973b; Franciosa et al., 1972; Kelly et al., 1973). Since this improvement is often accompanied by a decrease in several parameters determining myocardial oxygen demand, it has been postulated that ischemic myocardium may also be preserved while hemodynamic function is improving. In the context of severe hypotension, however, most investigators will avoid the use of agents which diminish vascular resistance, fearing that any drop in coronary perfusion pressure will result in unacceptable reductions in myocardial oxygen supply, with consequent increase in the magnitude of ischemia and decrease in cardiac performance. However, recent studies have shown that this is not necessarily the case.

The effectiveness of phentolamine, for instance, in acute myocardial infarction and, particularly, in the management of acute power failure is probably related to its major effect on peripheral arteries and veins rather than to its action on the heart *per se* (Nagasawa et al., 1975). Since this agent dilates the peripheral arterial resistance vessels, the failing heart meets less resistance to ventricular ejection before afterload is reduced. The drug also antagonizes even more effectively constriction of venous capacitance vessels than it does that of the arterial resistance vessels (Abboud et al., 1968). This reduction in peripheral venous return probably contributes to a decrease in (1) ventricular end-diastolic volume, (2) myocardial oxygen need—because of the reduced size of the heart, and (3) alleviation of symptoms of pulmonary congestion (Majid et al., 1971).

Recent studies (Chatterjee et al., 1973a, 1973b; Franciosa et al., 1972; Kelly et al., 1973; Abboud et al., 1968) confirm that upon therapy of acute myocardial infarction, impedance reduction causes an increase in cardiac output and a fall in left ventricular filling pressure, with varying degrees of heart failure. In addition, these investigations indicate that in the presence of cardiogenic shock, the cautious use of drugs, such as phentolamine, can produce increases in cardiac output without a fall in arterial blood pressure.

Modern monitoring equipment which measures capillary wedge pressure and cardiac index demonstrates that at low infusion rates, peripheral vasodilator therapy augments cardiac output and decreases pulmonary wedge pressure, with little change in arterial pressure (Table 2). As the infusion rate is raised, a further increment in cardiac output is frequently observed but arterial blood pressure may begin to diminish. At very high drug infusion rates—comparable to the level of drugs used in treating severe malignant hypertension—pulmonary capillary wedge pressure decreases to low levels, and the cardiac output and arterial blood pressure diminish substantially. Thus, it is possible to "titrate" the desired clinical effect by adjusting the rate of infusion of these drugs. Clinicians

Table 2. Effects of peripheral vasodilator therapy on hemodynamics

Dose	Cardiac Output	Pulmonary Capillary Wedge Pressure	Arterial Pressure
Low	↑	↓	↔
Medium	↑↑	↓	↓
High	↑↑	↓↓	↓↓

At low infusion rates, cardiac output increases and pulmonary capillary wedge pressure falls, with little change in arterial pressure. As infusion rate is augmented, a further rise in cardiac output is frequently observed, but arterial pressure begins to diminish. At very high infusion rates, arterial pressure and pulmonary capillary wedge pressure fall to low levels and cardiac output diminishes substantially.

have, therefore, been liberated at last from cuff blood pressures as a master method of intervention. It appears increasingly important that treatment should be concerned with the determinants of myocardial oxygen demand rather than with arbitrary blood-pressure measurements as has been practiced in the past.

Agents that rapidly reduce afterload and preload present certain problems since they require sophistication in monitoring their effects on myocardial, systemic and peripheral hemodynamics. At the present time, however, this level of sophistication in monitoring is becoming readily available to the internist in many parts of the world. The necessary facilities are thus invaluable not only in large centers but also in more peripheral hospitals.

It is also reasonable to assume that the use of one agent in therapy of acute myocardial infarction does not exclude the concomitant administration of another—to achieve a different beneficial effect. Thus, as more clinical experience is gained, it may be possible to employ one drug specifically to reduce infarct size while another substance, with a more potent effect, may be used to correct some imbalance in systemic hemodynamics by which the equation of the oxygen balance of the heart could be adjusted more effectively.

SUBSETS IN ACUTE MYOCARDIAL INFARCTION

With the advent of bedside hemodynamic monitoring of acute myocardial infarction, it is now apparent that the latter represents a series of hemodynamic sets and subsets rather than a single homogenous disease entity.

It is regrettable that until now, patients with acute myocardial infarction were usually treated with only one therapeutic regime. When hemodynamic measurements were applied to patients with acute myocardial infarction, a number of different groupings of subjects were found that require a particular therapeutic management. Under certain conditions, life and death will depend upon the institution of such therapy. Unfortunately, the therapeutic approach which may be greatly advantageous in one group of patients can, if applied to another group, be equally disastrous. Thus, a beta-adrenergic blocking agent, such as propranoiol, may represent the therapy of choice in a hyperkinetic circulatory state, in acute myocardial infarction but, if given to patients with severely depressed hemodynamic function (e.g., a stroke work index of less than 25 gm-m/m^2 and a left ventricular filling pressure of over 18 mmHg), it could cause total hemodynamic collapse. Thus, it will become essential that the attending physician make more specific choices in the use of therapeutic agents in acute myocardial infarction, and individualize treatment on the basis of the hemodynamic indications particular to each patient.

Of the various methods available for the assessment of left ventricular function, the determination of cardiac index and left ventricular filling pressure is the most simple and the most practical. With the introduction of the balloon-tipped flow-directed catheters, these determinations can now be made at the bedside reliably, repeatedly and safely, without the use of fluoroscopy.

So far, seven groups of patients have been identified, which we shall discuss individually below. However, it is apparent that with further experience, even more subsets of patients may be detected in the future. The groups in question are as follows:

Normal

Some patients with recent myocardial infarction have normal cardiac output and normal left ventricular filling pressures. Approximately 14% of these patients fit these criteria (Chatterjee and Swan, 1973).

Preservation of normal adequate overall pump function in the face of recent myocardial infarction suggests the activity of compensatory mechanisms which are effective in maintaining adequate systemic perfusion. Except for close observation and monitoring for evidence of deterioration of function, these patients will not generally need any specific hemodynamic therapy. However, with the advent of agents which appear to reduce infarct size, consideration should be given to using them in this group in an attempt to preserve ischemic myocardium and, thus, possibly improve long-term prognosis.

Hypovolemia

In hypovolemia, one usually sees a low cardiac index and arterial blood pressure along with the clinical symptomatology of forward failure. In forward failure, the cardiac output is low and the patient exhibits signs of oliguria, cold extremities and obtundation (Table 3). Left ventricular filling pressure is the key to the situation just described. Usually it is very low and can be in the neighborhood of 6 mmHg. Fortunately, a fluid challenge will usually reverse the situation and the patient will improve quickly. Thus, the left ventricular filling pressure should rapidly be brought to a level of 12-14 mmHg. Volume loading will augment cardiac output by the Frank-Starling mechanism in that as the diastolic pressure and volume are raised, the resting fiber length increases as does the stroke volume and the consequent cardiac output. The aim of therapy in this condition is to restore the cardiac index to its normal range, when signs of forward failure will disappear. At no time should symptoms of backward failure, such as dyspnea or crepitations, be present.

The recognition of this subset is vital. If afterload- or preload-reducing agents, such as phentolamine, nitroprusside or corticosteroids, are given, their vasodilating effect could be catastrophic. However, once volume has been restored and the condition of the patient is stable, then the use of such agents as adjunctive therapy in trying to reduce myocardial infarct size could be judiciously undertaken.

Backward Failure without Forward Failure

This subset is diagnosed by the presence of a left ventricular filling pressure exceeding 18 mmHg in the presence of a normal cardiac index. A low cardiac output as manifested by oliguria, obtundation and cold extremities, etc., is absent, but clinical symptomatology of backward failure, such as dyspnea and crepitations in the lungs, will be present.

Table 3. Clinical therapy of acute infarction

Diagnosis	Clinical		Hemodynamic		Therapy	Goal	In-Hospital Mortality Rate
	FF	BF	CI	LVFP			
Normal	0	0	2.2-3.0	<18	Reduction of infarct size	Maintain normal hemodynamics	6%
Hypovolemia	+	0	<2.2	<18	Volume expansion*	LVFP 15-18 CI 2.5-3.5	18%
Backward Failure	0	+	>2.2	>18	Diuretics*	LVFP 15-18	25%
Backward & Forward Failure	+	+	<2.2	>18	Peripheral vasodilator*	LVFP <18 CI >2.5	58%
Shock	++	+	<1.8	>18	Peripheral vasodilator, circulatory assist, consider surgery	LVFP <18 CI >2.5	71%
Shock, Unresponsive to all Therapy	++	++	<1.8	>18	Pressor agents	?Systolic BP 80-90	95%
Hyperdynamic	1st infarct ↑HR ↓BP anxiety		>3.5	<18	Propranolol, sedation*	CI 2.5-3.5	12%

*Together with the correction of the primary hemodynamic problems, an attempt to reduce infarct size (e.g. corticosteroids) should be considered in these subsets.

FF = forward failure (oliguria, cold extremities, obtundation)
BF = backward failure (dyspnea, rales)
CI = cardiac index
LVFP = left ventricular filling pressure

318

The appropriate therapy in this condition is a diuretic agent. This type of drug is easy to administer and effective in reducing left ventricular filling pressure, and it also will not aggravate the imbalance between myocardial oxygen supply and demand. Since central venous pressure (CVP) offers no correlation with radiological evidence of lung failure, further use of CVP monitoring to treat problems of fluid balance in acute myocardial infarction should be discouraged (Forrester et al., 1971). Furosemide is an ideal agent in this situation not only because of its diuretic action, but also because of its marked effect on the peripheral vasculature—it increases venous capacitance and diminishes left ventricular filling pressure before any diuresis is seen (Dikshit et al., 1973). Digitalis appears to be of little use in the management of heart failure in acute myocardial infarction, in contradistinction to its profoundly beneficial effects in congestive heart failure due to chronic heart disease; therefore, it should probably not be used in the situation described above. In this subset, apart from correcting the primary hemodynamic abnormality, in the future, patients should be treated with additional medications in attempts to reduce the size of their infarcts.

Backward and Forward Failure

This subset is diagnosed when a low cardiac index and a high left ventricular filling pressure are found, as manifested by signs of both forward failure (oliguria, cold extremities, obtundation) and backward failure (shortness of breath and crepitation). Diuretics are inadequate in this situation because they do not increase cardiac output and will, therefore, fail to relieve forward failure (Dikshit et al., 1973). Under the circumstances, the probable treatment of choice is a peripheral vasodilator, such as nitroprusside or phentolamine. These agents increase cardiac output and decrease left ventricular filling pressure while simultaneously reducing myocardial oxygen demand. However, even with this advanced form of therapy, the mortality rate is still often over 50% (Table 3).

Cardiogenic Shock

In this subset of patients, oliguria, cold extremities, obtundation—the signs of forward failure become even more pronounced and are coupled with symptoms of backward failure—crepitation and dyspnea. Cardiac index is usually extremely low (beneath 1.8 L/min/m^2).

Usually in this group of patients, one finds that the stroke work index is less than 20 gm-m/m^2 and, if associated with left ventricular filling pressure over 18 mmHg, the mortality rate—in the absence of treatment—is in excess of 95%. These hemodynamic values show that, even in the presence of maximal preloads, measured by left ventricular filling pressure, the performance of the heart is markedly diminished and indicate that the Frank-Starling mechanism has failed. The administration of commonly-used agents, such as norepinephrine, isoproterenol, etc., is probably not beneficial.

Don Michael and his colleagues (1972) have shown that, in this particular group, about half the patients rapidly develop shock. This state of shock is the result of an occlusion of the left main coronary artery or a proximal left anterior descending coronary artery. There arterial occlusion, a major consideration should be emergency coronary artery bypass surgery. While the logistics of such an heroic attempt can sometimes be defeating in this situation, the procedure does appear to improve the patient's chance of survival.

Within the shock group, there is a second subset which includes about 20% of the patients. These subjects usually have mechanical lesions, such as papillary muscle dysfunction and/or mitral regurgitation. In this situation, afterload-reducing agents, such as nitroprusside or phentolamine, can be extremely effective since they decrease myocardial oxygen demand. The patient can usually be maintained on these drugs for a two-week period following the insult of acute myocardial infarction, which allows time for primary healing and scar formation to occur within the heart. Subsequently, elective surgery and replacement of the mitral valve, if necessary, can take place. Other patients in this subset, such as those with acute ventricular septal rupture, may need emergency rather than elective surgery.

A third subset seen in the shock category includes patients with end-stage heart disease. As a rule, this type of patient, with a long history of multiple myocardial infarctions, is maintained outside the hospital on high doses of digitalis and diuretics. It is apparent that any further insults will quickly put the patient into shock and near death. Until artificial hearts become available, the only reasonable form of therapy, at present, again involves the use of impedance-reducing agents. Upon *post mortem* examination, these patients are found to have an enlarged heart of which often 50 to 80% consists of scar tissue resulting from previous infarcts.

When vasodilator therapy is used in these patients, it may produce substantial improvement in hemodynamics, and the side effects of lowering coronary diastolic perfusion pressure can be reduced by concomitant use of mechanical circulatory assistance. Considerable decrease in hospital mortality can be achieved by such therapy.

Chatterjee and coworkers (1976) have recently shown that with aggressive therapy in all forms of shock, the mortality rate in hospital can be cut from 100% to 44%. However, the long-term prognosis is none the best since in the two following years, many of these patients succumb to their disease and—as a result—the survival rate is about 27%.

Unresponsive Shock

In this group of patients where surgery cannot be undertaken, or vasodilator therapy has been unsuccessful or systolic arterial blood pressure falls beneath 70 to 80 mmHg, the physician may turn to pressure agents, such as dopamine or, possibly, norepinephrine. However, the usual in-hospital mortality rate in this situation is in excess of 95%.

Hyperdynamic Group

In a small subset of patients with acute myocardial infarction, there exists a hyperdynamic group in which the arterial blood pressure and the cardiac index are often very high (Table 3). This syndrome is frequently found in anxious young men with their first infarct. Pulmonary capillary wedge pressure in these subjects is in the low normal range. Apart from sedation, the usual treatment consists of beta-adrenergic receptor blockade with an agent, such as propranolol, in order to try and normalize the cardiac index and arterial blood pressure. Once more, the effect of propranolol in this situation is to promptly reduce myocardial oxygen requirements and, possibly, infarct size.

The diagnosis of the hyperdynamic circulatory state is imperative since the use of a negative inotropic agent, e.g., propranolol, in some of the other subsets of patients may have catastrophic effects since it could precipitate total hemodynamic collapse.

Preservation of Ischemic Myocardium

Research on methods for preserving myocardium rendered ischemic by acute myocardial infarction constitutes one of the most exciting areas in cardiology today. Potential benefits could be enormous both for the critically-ill patient, where they could mean the difference between life and death, and in cases of uncomplicated infarction where limiting the infarct size could result in a smaller scar and improved long-term prognosis. Different interventions agents preserve ischemic myocardium by different mechanisms. These include agents, such as corticosteroids, nitrites, glucose-insulin-potassium, hyaluronidase, beta-blocking drugs, oxygen, and certain forms of circulatory assistance (Maroko and Braunwald, 1973). Early clinical trials indicate that, corticosteroids and propranolol seems effective if used in a carefully-monitored dose range (Morrison et al., 1976; DeMello et al., 1976).

A full discussion of agents which apparently reduce infarct size can be found elsewhere in this monograph.

CONCLUSION

Many aspects of the etiological factors involved in the pathogenesis of acute myocardial infarction still remain an enigma. However, in recent years, significant advances have been made in our understanding of the hemodynamic derangements it causes and new therapeutic approaches to dealing with this life-threatening condition are being vigorously pursued. The underlying cause of the disease—nodular arteriosclerosis—has not yet yielded many of its secrets to research and its treatment is still highly problematical. The practicing cardiologist must concern himself mainly with the sequelae of a heart attack. He has come to recognize that the hemodynamic disturbance is profound and can feed upon itself by activating neurohumoral and vascular mechanisms which—if not properly treated—can carry the patient into more treacherous waters.

The concept of a balance between myocardial oxygen demand and supply being crucial for cardiac function, now allows the use of new therapeutic modalities which, even five years ago, would have been thought impossible because of a mistaken concern and fixation by the attending physician to keep the patient's arterial blood pressure high at all costs. Much greater attention is now being paid to the venous bed and its contribution to the preload of the infarcted heart, an aspect which was almost totally ignored in the past.

Careful examination of the hemodynamic disarrangement makes it possible, at present, to differentiate among diverse hemodynamic patterns which may result in acute myocardial infarction, and institute specific forms of treatment appropriate for each particular subset. Thus, the hyperkinetic patient can now be distinguished from the hypodynamic one. Different types and degrees of heart failure are found to involve different pathogenic mechanisms, and conditions which are clinically mimicked by hypovolemia can be distinguished from them.

Thus, the practicing physician, supported by his colleagues in experimental and clinical research, can move forward in the management of acute myocardial infarction with the confidence that his attempts to stem the tide of death from the nation's number one killer will be increasingly successful.

ACKNOWLEDGMENT

The authors wish to thank for the excellent secretarial assistance of Maricathryn Evans and Betty Garrigues in preparing this manuscript.

REFERENCES

Abboud, F. M.: The sympathetic nervous system and alpha adrenergic blocking agents in shock. *Med. Clin North Am.* 52:1049-1060 (1968).

Abboud, F. M., Schmid, P. C., and Eckstein, J. W.: Vascular responses after alpha-adrenergic receptor blockade. I. Responses of capacitance and resistance vessels to norepinephrine in man. *J. Clin. Invest.* 47:1-9 (1968).

Braunwald, E.: Bowditch Lecture. The determinants of myocardial oxygen consumption. *Physiologist* 12:65-93 (1969).

Chatterjee, K., Parmley, W. W., Ganz, W., Forrester, J. S., Walinsky, P., Crexells, C., and Swan, H. J. C.: Hemodynamic and metabolic responses to vasodilator therapy in acute myocardial infarction. *Circulation* 48:1183-1193 (1973a).

Chatterjee, K., Parmley, W. W., Swan, H. J. C., Berman, G., Forrester, J. S., and Marcus, H. S.: Beneficial effects of vasodilator agents in severe mitral regurgitation due to dysfunction of subvalvar apparatus. *Circulation* 48:684-690 (1973b).

Chatterjee, K., and Swan, H. J. C.: Hemodynamic profile of acute myocardial infarction. In *Myocardial Infarction*, E. Corday and H. J. C. Swan, eds. Williams and Wilkins Company, Baltimore (1973), pp. 51-61.

Chatterjee, K., Swan, H. J. C., Kaushik, V. S., Jobin, G., Magnusson, P., and Forrester, J. S.: Effects of vasodilator therapy for severe pump failure in acute myocardial infarction on short-term and late prognosis. *Circulation* 53:797-802 (1976).

DeMello, V. R., Roberts, R., and Sobel, B. E.: Deleterious effects of methylprednisolone in patients with evolving myocardial infarction. *Circulation* 53 (Suppl. 1): 204-206 (1976).

Dikshit, K., Vyden, J. K., Forrester, J. S., Chatterjee, K., Prakash, R., and

Swan, H. J. C.: Renal and extrarenal effects of furosemide in congestive heart failure after acute myocardial infarction. *N. Engl. J. Med.* 288: 1087-1090 (1973).

Don Michael, T. A., Forrester, J. S., Allen, H. N., and Swan, H. J. C.: Identification of clinical subsets in cardiogenic shock. *Am. J. Cardiol.* 29:280 (Abstr.) (1972).

Forrester, J. S., Diamond, G., McHugh, T. J., and Swan, H. J. C.: Filling pressures in the right and left sides of the heart in acute myocardial infarction. *N. Engl. J. Med.* 285:190-193 (1971).

Franciosa, J. A., Guina, N. H., Limas, C. J., Rodriguera, E., and Cohn, J. N.: Improved left ventricular function during nitroprusside infusion in acute infarction. *Lancet* 1:650-654 (1972).

Herman, M. V., and Gorlin, R.: Implications of left ventricular asynergy. *Am. J. Cardiol.* 23:538-547 (1969).

Herman, M. V., Henile, R. A., Klein, M. D., and Gorlin, R.: Localized disorders in myocardial contractions: Asynergy and its role in congestive heart failure. *N. Engl. J. Med.* 277:222-226 (1967).

Kelly, D. T., Delgado, C. E., Taylor, D. R., Pitt, B., and Ross, R. S.: Use of phentolamine in acute myocardial infarction associated with hypertension and left ventricular failure. *Circulation* 47:729-735 (1973).

Langley, J. O., Martinez, A., Fakhro, A., Duvoisin, P., and Harrison, T. R.: Paradoxical precordial motion and wasted left ventricular work: The concept of cardiac dysnergy. *Am. Heart J.* 73:349-361 (1967).

Majid, P. A., Sharma, B., and Taylor, S. H.: Phentolamine for vasodilator treatment of severe heart failure. *Lancet* 2:719-723 (1971).

Maroko, P., and Braunwald, E.: Modification of myocardial infarction size after coronary occlusion. *Ann. Inter. Med.* 79:720-733 (1973).

Morrison, J., Reduto, L., Pizzarello, R., Geller, K., Maley, T., and Gullota, S.: Brief communication: Modification of myocardial injury in man by corticosteroid administration. *Circulaton* 53 (Suppl. I): 200-203 (1976).

Nagasawa, K., Vyden, J. K., Forrester, J. S., Groseth-Dittrich, M. F., Corday, E., and Swan, H. J. C.: Effect of phentolamine on cardiac performance and energetics in acute myocardial infarction. *Circ. Shock* 2:5-11 (1975).

Weil, M. H., and Shubin, H.: Cardiogenic shock. Pathogenesis and rationale of therapy. *Cor. Heart Dis.* 1 (Suppl. II): 165-178 (1969).

Pathophysiology and Therapeutics of Myocardial Ischemia

13

Enzymatic Estimation
of Infarct Size

ROBERT ROBERTS
BURTON E. SOBEL

INTRODUCTION

Enzymatic estimation of infarct size, based on serial changes in plasma creatine kinase (CK) activity, was initially evaluated in experimental animals. Studies in rabbits showed that after coronary occlusion, the weight of infarct in the left ventricle was linearly related to the amount of CK activity depleted from myocardium (Kjekshus and Sobel, 1970). Other studies in dogs demonstrated that myocardial CK depletion 24 hr after coronary occlusion correlated directly with infarct size estimated morphologically (Maroko et al., 1972). The regional distribution of myocardial CK depletion was found to correlate with reduced blood flow (Kjekshus and Sobel, 1970), ST-segment elevation (Kjekshus et al., 1972), and histologically demonstrable necrosis (Maroko et al., 1971; Ruegsegger et al., 1959).

To estimate infarct size *in vivo*, a model was developed utilizing serial changes in plasma CK activity. These studies, performed in conscious dogs, demonstrated that the amount of CK activity released into blood was a relatively constant function (15%) of total

325

CK depleted from myocardium (CK_d) and that both were directly related to the extent of myocardial damage (r = .96, n = 22) (Shell et al., 1971). The amount of CK lost in a gram of homogenous infarct was determined experimentally. Thus, based on an estimate of CK activity released into the circulation, infarct size could be estimated in terms of CK gram equivalents (CK-g-eq) (Shell et al., 1971).

APPLICATIONS TO PATIENTS

Infarct size was calculated in an analogous fashion from serial changes in plasma CK—activity in patients with acute myocardial infarction, and was found to correlate closely with early mortality and morbidity (Sobel et al., 1972), depression of left ventricular ejection fraction (Kostuk et al., 1973), decreased compliance, and impaired hemodynamics (Mathey et al., 1974). Recently, infarct size was found to correlate with the incidence of early ventricular dysrhythmia associated with acute myocardial infarction (Roberts et al., 1975d). Bleifeld et al. (1974) demonstrated that enzymatically estimated infarct size correlated closely with morphological estimates in patients who succumbed early after infarction (r = .98). These findings suggest that the ratio of CK released into blood to CK depleted from myocardium remains relatively constant in patients, as is the case in experimental animals.

Recently, accurate assessment of infarct size has become increasingly important, particularly in studies concerned with evaluation of selected interventions. Enzymatic estimates of infarct size in patients have been employed in several centers (Mathey et al., 1974; Norris et al., 1975; Sobel et al., 1976), and shown to be useful in assessing selected pharmacological and physiological interventions designed to protect ischemic myocardium.

EVALUATION OF PARAMETERS

Despite some clinical utility of enzymatic estimations of infarct size in its current state of development, refinements and improvements in the approach are required (Roberts et al., 1975d). Estimates of infarct size based on CK time-activity curves depend on several parameters, one of which is the assumed fractional disappearance rate of CK activity from the circulation (k_d). Since marked hemodynamic alterations may occur in association with acute myo-

Table 1. CPK disappearance determined repetitively*

Dog Number	Day			
	First	Second	Third	Mean
1	4.3	4.1	4.4	4.1
2	5.6	5.2	5.0	5.3
3	6.2	5.7	6.3	6.3
4	4.9	5.4	5.6	5.3
5	3.8	4.2	3.9	4.0

*Results expressed are fractional disappearance rates (min^{-1}) x 10^3. Note: CPK and CK are used interchangeably in this chapter.

cardial infarction, it was necessary to determine their influence, if any, on k_d.

Our early studies utilized changes in total plasma CK activity, which restricted estimation of infarct size to patients without severe complications. Patients with shock, hypotension, or intramuscular injections were excluded to avoid the influence of CK released from non-cardiac sources. Subsequently, a quantitative assay for CK isoenzymes was developed (Roberts et al., 1974). The MB CK isoenzyme was found in man to be a virtually specific marker of myocardium, and thus to provide a more specific index for use in estimating infarct size (Roberts et al., 1975c).

CK DISAPPEARANCE

To assess the disappearance rate of CK, partially purified canine heart CK was injected intravenously in conscious dogs (Roberts et al., 1975a; Roberts et al., 1973). The disappearance of CK activity approximated a mono-exponential function. As we have noted previously, the disappearance rate varied markedly from animal to animal (.004-.007 min^{-1}) (Shell et al., 1971; Roberts et al., 1975c). To determine whether the disappearance rate remained constant within the same animal from day to day, repeated determinations of k_d were performed daily in 5 animals for 3 consecutive days. As shown in Table 1, there was $<10\%$ variation of k_d within each animal.

To determine whether k_d was influenced by hemodynamic derangements simulating those seen in patients with acute myocardial infarction, interventions were performed in conscious dogs (Roberts and Sobel, 1975a). One week prior to each intervention, the dogs were instrumented with monitoring devices. In one group of animals, at the same time inflatable cuffs were placed around the inferior vena cava, for subsequent use in decreasing cardiac output. Flow probes were placed around the aorta for measurement of cardiac output. In other animals, cuffs were placed around the renal, hepatic, or celiac arteries for subsequent use in decreasing renal, or hepatic celiac flow. Again, flow probes were placed distally. All these devices were exteriorized. When the animals had completely recovered from the operation, partially purified canine myocardial CK was injected intravenously, and k_d was determined during a 3-4-hr interval prior to each intervention and for 3-4-hr after the onset of each, so that each animal could serve as its own control. Reduction of cardiac output by 67% did not affect k_d. When renal flow was decreased bilaterally by 80% (n = 5), celiac flow cut down by 70% (n = 5), or hepatic flow completely interrupted (n = 5), no significant alteration of k_d occurred (Fig. 1).

[14]C-CK was injected intravenously and used to determine k_d before, during and after infarction, in conscious dogs, produced by occlusion of the left anterior descending coronary artery. Under those conditions, tracer disappearance is independent of release of endogenous enzyme. In each experiment, k_d before, during and after infarction in the same animal was virtually identical (n = 5) (Roberts and Sobel, 1975b).

Results of these experiments indicate that although k_d varied from animal to animal, it is remarkably constant within the same subject and insensitive to marked hemodynamic alterations, similar to those associated with massive myocardial infarction and to infarctions *per se*.

These studies emphasize the importance of using the individualized estimates of k_d in experimental as well as clinical studies (Norris et al., 1975).

Panels A, B, C, and D illustrate the lack of effect of decreased cardiac output, decreased celiac, renal and hepatic flow, respectively, on plasma CPK disappearance rate performed in conscious dogs. Purified CPK was injected at zero time and, following a control period, the intervention was performed as indicated by the dotted line. There was slight slowing, initially, after constriction of hepatic artery (D) but, in spite of sustained occlusion, k_d returned to that of control.

1

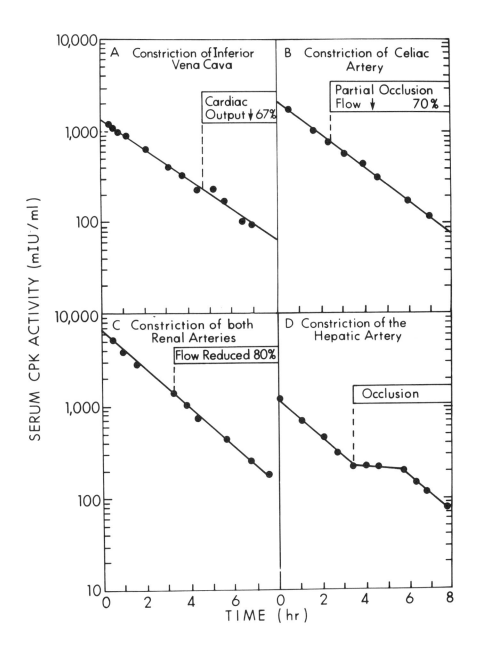

ESTIMATION OF INFARCT SIZE BASED ON PLASMA MB CK

To evaluate the specificity of MB CK as a marker of myocardial injury, we performed studies using a new quantitative, fluorometric kinetic assay (Roberts et al., 1975b). Tissue samples obtained from patients during surgery performed for diagnostic and therapeutic purposes were assayed fresh for CK isoenzymes. Only skeletal muscle, heart, brain and gut contained significant CK and, as shown in Fig. 2, MB CK is found virtually exclusively in human myocardium where it constitutes approximately 15% of total CK (Roberts et al., 1975b). Other studies were performed in patients undergoing a variety of non-cardiac surgical procedures, all of whom exhibited marked elevation in total plasma CK activity but no increase in plasma MB CK (Roberts and Sobel, 1976). Similar results were obtained in patients given intramuscular injections (Roberts et al., 1974), and in others undergoing cardiac catheterization (Roberts et al., 1975b). A comparison of plasma total and MB CK time-activity curves after myocardial infarction is illustrated in Figs. 3 and 4. Fig. 3 shows results obtained in a patient with uncomplicated myocardial infarction versus one complicated with intramuscular injections in Fig. 4. From such curves, parameters were developed for calculation of infarct size based on changes in plasma MB CK (Roberts et al., 1975a). Utilization of changes in MB CK facilitates extension of the method to patients with hypotension, cardiogenic shock, or intramuscular injections (Gutovitz et al., 1976).

SUMMARY

Our initial formulation for estimation of infarct size has been employed in studies designed to clarify prognosis and to assess interventions. The method has been improved by elucidation of factors affecting creatine kinase (CK) disappearance rates, and utilizations of changes in MB CK rather than CK, to extend the approach to patients with infarction complicated by release of non-cardiac CK.

ACKNOWLEDGMENTS

This work was supported, in part, by Washington University School of Medicine, U. S. Public Health Service SCOR in Ischemic Heart Disease 1 P17 HL 17646-01.

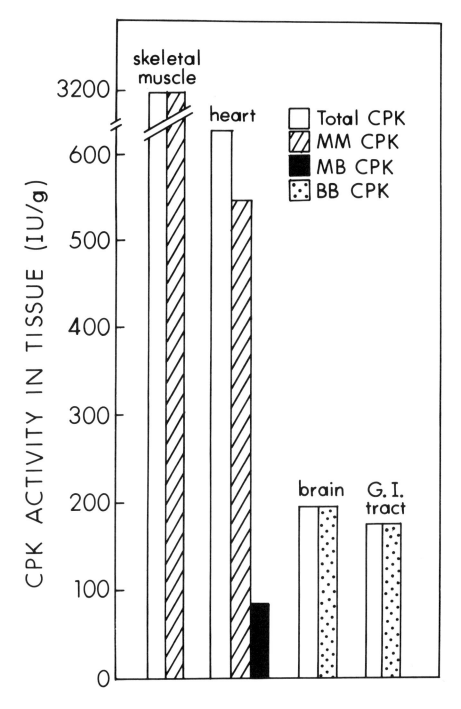

2

This illustrates the creatine phosphokinase (CPK) isoenzyme composition of human tissues analyzed fresh.

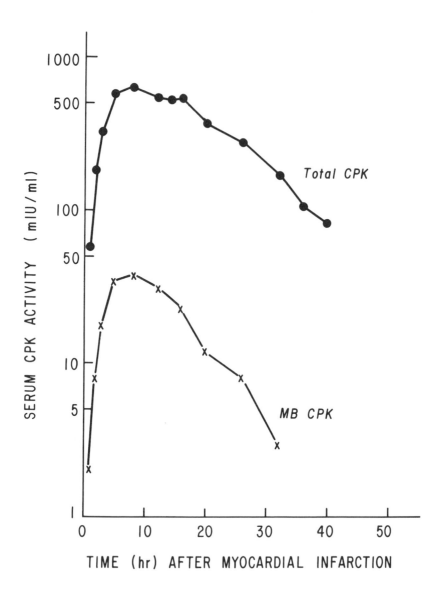

3 This illustrates the similarity between plasma time-activity curves of total CPK and MB CPK in a patient with uncomplicated infarction.

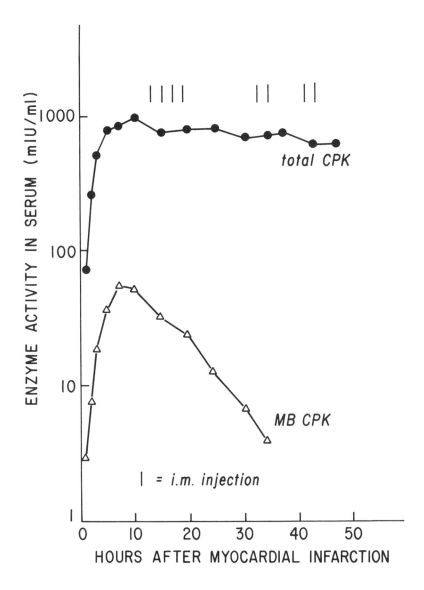

4

This illustrates the lack of similarity between plasma time-activity curves of total CPK and MB CPK in a patient with infarction and i.m. injection. Release of MM CPK from skeletal muscles keeps the total CPK level elevated, the return of MB CPK to normal being unaffected since release of MB CPK from skeletal muscles did not occur.

We gratefully acknowledge Ms Linda Wilson and Carole Goodell for the preparation of this manuscript.

REFERENCES

Bleifeld, W., Mathey, D., and Hanrath, P.: Serial studies of serum creatine phosphokinase for intravital estimation of infarction size. In *Proceedings, 7th World Congress of Cardiology* (1974), p. 123.

Gutovitz, A. L., Roberts, R., and Sobel, B. E.: Progressive necrosis: A common denominator of cardiogenic shock. *Circulation* 54:724-733, 1976.

Kjekshus, J. K., Maroko, P. R., and Sobel, B. E.: Distribution of myocardial injury and its relation to epicardial ST-segment changes after coronary artery occlusion in the dog. *Cardiovasc. Res.* 490-499 (1972).

Kjekshus, J. K., and Sobel, B. E.: Depressed myocardial creatine phosphokinase activity following experimental myocardial infarction in rabbit. *Circ. Res.* 27:403-414 (1970).

Kostuk, W. J., Ehsani, A. A., Karliner, J. S., Ashburn, K. L., Ross, J. Jr., and Sobel, B. E.: Left ventricular performance after myocardial infarction assessed by radioisotope angiocardiography. *Circulation* 47:242-249 (1973).

Maroko, P.R., Kjekshus, J. K., Sobel, B. E., Watanabe, T., Covell, J. W., Ross, J. Jr., and Braunwald, E., Factors influencing infarct size following experimental coronary artery occlusion. *Circulation* 43:67-82 (1971).

Maroko, P. R., Libby,, P., Ginks, W. R., Bloor, C. M. Shell, W. E., Sobel, B. E., and Ross, J. Jr.: Coronary artery reperfusion: 1. Early effects in local myocardial function and the extent of myocardial necrosis. *J. Clin. Invest.* 51:2710-2716 (1972).

Mathey, D., Bleifeld, W., Hanrath, P., and Effert, S.: Attempt to quantitate relation between cardiac function and infarct size in acute myocardial infarction. *Br. Heart J.* 36:271-279 (1974).

Norris, R. M., Whitlock, R. M. L., Barratt-Boyes, C., and Small, C. W.: Clinical measurement of myocardial infarct size: Modification of a method for the estimation of total creatine phosphokinase release after myocardial infarction. *Circulation* 51:614-620 (1975).

Roberts, R., Ambos, H. D., Carlson, E. M., and Sobel, B. E.: Improved quantification of myocardial infarction based on analysis of serum CPK isoenzymes. *Am. J. Cardiol.* 35:166 (1975a).

Roberts, R., Gowda, K. S., Ludbrook, P. A., and Sobel, B. E.: The specificity of elevated serum MB CPK activity in the diagnosis of acute myocardial infarction. *Am. J. Cardiol.* 36:433-437 (1975b).

Roberts, R., Henry, P. D., Shell, W. E., and Sobel, B. E.: The effect of hemodynamic changes on disappearance of serum CPK activity. *Clin. Res.* 21: 197 (1973).

Roberts, R., Henry, P. D., and Sobel, B. E.: An improved basis for enzymatic estimation of infarct size. *Circulation* 52:743-754 (1975c).

Roberts, R., Henry, P. D., Witteveen, S. A. G. J., and Sobel, B. E.: Quantifications of serum creatine phosphokinase (CPK) isoenzyme activity. *Am. J. Cardiol.* 33:650-654 (1974).

Roberts, R., Husain, A., Ambos, H. D., Oliver, G. C., Cox, J. Jr., and Sobel,

B. E.: Relation between infarct size and ventricular arrhythmia. *Br. Heart J.* 37:1169-1175 (1975d).

Roberts, R., and Sobel, B. E.: Factors affecting disappearance of creatine phosphokinase (CPK) from the circulation. *Clin. Res.* 23:205A (1975a).

Roberts, R., and Sobel, B. E.: The effect of experimental myocardial infarction on CPK disappearance. *Circulation* (Suppl. II) 51 and 52:232. (1975b).

Roberts, R., and Sobel, B. E.: Elevated plasma MB creatine phosphokinase activity. *Arch. Intern. Med.* 136:421-424 (1976).

Ruegsegger, R. B., Nydick, I., Frieman, A., and LaDue, J. S.: Serum activity patterns of glutamic oxaloacetic transaminase, glutamic pyruvic transminase and lactic dehydrogenase following graded myocardial infarction in dogs. *Circ. Res.* 7:4-10 (1959).

Shell, W. E., Kjekshus, J. K., and Sobel, B. E.: Quantitative assessment of the extent of myocardial infarction in the conscious dog by means of analysis of serial changes in serum creatine phosphokinase (CPK) activity. *J. Clin. Invest.* 50:2614-2625 (1971).

Sobel, B. E., Bresnahan, G. F., Shell, W. E., and Yoder, R. D.: Estimation of infarct size in man and its relation to prognosis. *Circulation* 46:640-648 (1972).

Sobel, B. E., Roberts, R., and Larson, K. B.: Estimation of infarct size from serum MB creatine phosphokinase activity. Applications and limitations. *Am. J. Cardiol.* 37:474-485 (1976).

14

Cardiac Lymph Studies in Acute Myocardial Ischemia

MARIO FEOLA

INTRODUCTION

Until now, scant attention has been paid to interstitial fluid dynamics in acute myocardial infarction. It is generally assumed that myocardial cell injury results from an inadequate supply of oxygen and nutrients, and sight is lost of the fact that it is the interstitial fluid that ultimately carries these substances, while also rinsing the cells of their waste products and any toxic compound resulting from altered conditions.

Access to the interstitial fluid of the heart can be gained by way of the cardiac lymphatic system. Ranvier (1889) stated: "The mammalian heart is a lymph sponge, as much as the frog's heart is a blood sponge." The 'intramyocardial lymphatic plexus' of the left ventricle drains into a 'subepicardiac plexus,' whence into an 'anterior interventricular trunk' which follows the course of the left anterior descending coronary artery, a 'marginal trunk' which follows the obtuse marginal artery and a 'posterior interventricular trunk' which follows the posterior descending branch of the circumflex artery (Patek, 1939). These trunks converge into one 'main supracardiac lymph channel' which runs behind the pulmonary artery toward a 'cardiac lymph node' situated in the space between the superior vena cava and the brachiocephalic artery. This channel can be cannulated and most of the lymph of the left ventricle can be collected (Drinker et al., 1940). Studies in normal dogs have revealed that lymph flow of the left ventricle amounts to an average 4-5 ml/hr (Drinker et al., 1940; Miller et al., 1964; Ullal et al., 1972; Feola and Glick, 1975). It has been shown that this flow obeys Starling's Law on interstitial fluid formation. Thus, an increase in hydrostatic capillary pressure from venous congestion (Leeds et al., 1970), or a reduction of colloid osmotic pressure from large infusions of cristalloid solutions (Wasserman and Mayerson, 1952), or altered capillary permeability from anoxia (Maurer, 1940) increase cardiac lymph flow. It has also been shown that lymph drainage can be enhanced by the administration of sympathomimetic drugs through the increase in the force of contraction of the left ventricle (Drinker et al., 1940).

On the basis of these studies, it appeared possible to investigate the changes in interstitial fluid, taking place during ischemia, by means of the cardiac lymph. It also seemed possible to gain a measure of interstitial fluid dynamics by injecting a vital dye into the myocardium, and studying the times of its appearance and clearance at various levels of the lymphatic system.

EXPERIMENTAL STUDIES

Experiments were conducted in mongrel dogs, 25-30 kg in body weight, with hematocrit values of $45 \pm 5\%$ and plasma protein concentration of 4 ± 0.5 gm %. The animals were anesthetized with sodium pentobarbital (30 mg/kg, i.v.) and ventilated with room air via an endotracheal tube, using a Harvard respirator. Adjustments were made to keep arterial blood pH between 7.35 and 7.45, PO_2 above 80 mm Hg, and pCO_2 between 35 and 45 mm Hg. Hemodynamic monitoring included heart rate, obtained from a standard ECG, arterial and central venous pressures, determined by means of catheters inserted into the aorta and the superior vena cava, and connected to P23db Statham pressure transducers.

The heart was exposed through the left fourth intercostal space and suspended in a pericardial cradle. The cardiac lymphatic system was visualized by the intramyocardial injection of 0.2 ml of Evans blue dye.

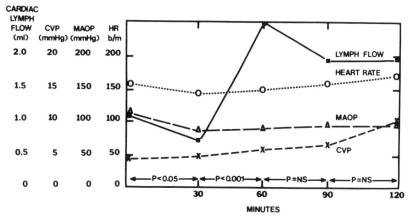

**CARDIAC LYMPH FLOW, CENTRAL VENOUS PRESSURE,
MEAN AORTIC PRESSURE, HEART RATE IN ACUTE MYOCARDIAL ISCHEMIA**

1 Diagram of changes in lymph volume in relation to hemodynamic changes. Lymph flow dropped from 1.09 ± 0.03 ml (30 min of base-line condition) to 0.74 ± 0.03 ml during the first 30 min of ischemia, to rise to 1.79 ± 0.08 ml during the following 30 min of ischemia. Thereafter, it remained elevated with respect to base-line. P-values in the figure refer to these changes. Heart rate did not change significantly. Mean aortic pressure (MAOP) dropped during the first 30 min of ischemia from 108 ± 5 to 85 ± 4 mm Hg ($p < 0.05$); subsequent changes were not statistically significant. Central venous pressure (CVP) increased progressively from 4.4 ± 0.4 to 13 ± 0.5 mm Hg ($p < 0.005$).

In one group of experiments, the supracardiac lymph channel was cannulated and cardiac lymph was collected for 2 hr before and 2 hr after occlusion of the circumflex artery (Feola and Glick, 1975). Fig. 1 shows the changes in lymph flow in relation to the hemodynamic alterations.

The changes in lymph composition are summarized in Table 1. Ischemic injury of the blood capillaries was reflected in significant increases in lymph total protein content (up an average 67%) and red-blood-cell concentration (up an average 400%). Ischemic myocardial-cell injury was reflected in significant increases in K-ion

Table 1. Changes in cardiac lymph flow and composition during
acute myocardial ischemia

	2 hr control		2 hr ischemia	
	Lymph	Serum	Lymph	Serum
Volume flow (ml)	4.3 ± 0.32		6.6 ± 0.52*	
pH	7.55 ± 0.016	7.45 ± 0.01	7.31 ± 0.015*	7.45 ± 0.01
Potassium (mEq/L)	3.7 ± 0.24	4.0 ± 0.15	4.3 ± 0.27*	3.8 ± 0.12
CPK (units)	241.0 ± 14.4	36.4 ± 2	381.0 ± 45.4*	39.2 ± 2.4
Acid P-ase (units)	2.2 ± 0.22	0.9 ± 0.08	2.88 ± 0.30*	0.83 ± 0.14
Protein content (g)	0.18 ± 0.019		0.24 ± 0.020*	
Red blood cells (x10^6)	0.150 ± 0.010		0.790 ± 0.075*	
Lactate (mg%)	14.0 ± 1.3	15.4 ± 1.6	33.0 ± 5.5*	14.4 ± 2

Numbers represent mean values ± standard error.
* = p < 0.05 relative to preceding interval.

concentration and in creatine phosphokinase (CPK) and acid P-ase enzyme activities. The shift to anaerobic metabolism produced higher levels of lactate and H-ions.

In a second group of experiments, the supracardiac lymph channel was not cannulated and the natural conditions of lymph drainage were not disturbed. In 9 dogs (sham group), the circumflex artery was isolated but not occluded. Evans blue dye (0.2 ml) was injected into the posterior-lateral wall of the left ventricle and the times of dye appearance and clearance were studied at four levels: the subepicardiac plexus, the supracardiac lymph channel, the cardiac lymph node, and the right lymphatic duct. Two injections were made, one after completion of the surgical preparation (T_1) and one 2 hr later (T_2). In 9 other dogs, the appearance and clearance time were studied at baseline (T_1) and 2 hr after occlusion of the circumflex artery (T_2).

In the sham group, the times of appearance and clearance were the same after the two injections. In the ischemic group, the appearance time at the subepicardiac plexus level was the same before and after coronary occlusion, but the appearance time at the other levels was prolonged during ischemia. All clearance times were greatly extended during ischemia. These data are presented in Fig. 2.

The hemodynamic changes upon occlusion of the circumflex artery were characterized by an early decline of the mean aortic

APPEARANCE – CLEARANCE TIMES OF EVANS BLUE DYE

	CONTROL (T₁)		ISCHEMIA (T₂)	
	APPEARANCE	CLEARANCE	APPEARANCE	CLEARANCE
RIGHT LYMPHATIC DUCT	10 ± 2	20 ± 5	30 ± 5	> 120
CARDIAC LYMPH NODE	10 ± 2	20 ± 5	30 ± 5	> 120
SUPRA CARDIAC COLLECTOR	5 ± 2	20 ± 5	15 ± 5	60 ± 10
SUBEPICARDIAC PLEXUS	< 1	10 ± 2	< 1	30 ± 5
MYOCARDIAL SPOT				

2 Diagram of changes in lymph drainage. These data refer to the group of experiments in which the circumflex artery was ligated. Numbers represent mean values in minutes ± standard error.

pressure, followed by partial recovery and a progressive rise in central venous pressure (changes similar to those obtained in the first group of experiments).

Tissue blocks of the anterior and lateral walls of the left ventricle were taken at the end of the experiment and water content was measured by wet/dry weight differential. In the sham group, myocardial water content was the same in the two areas sampled, measuring $76 \pm 1.1\%$. In the ischemic group, the water content of the ischemic myocardium increased to $80 \pm 1\%$. This increase was statistically significant ($p < 0.005$).

Tissue sections of ischemic myocardium clearly confirmed the development of interstitial edema (Fig. 3).

In one dog, a lymphogram of the ischemic area plus the entire draining system was obtained by the method of Celis et al. (1968). This is shown in Fig. 4.

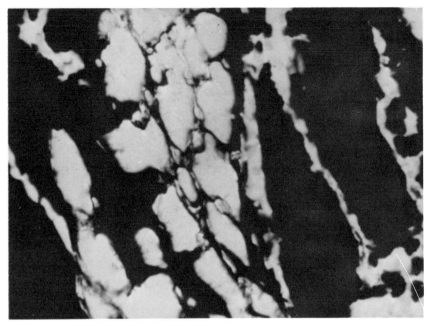

3 Photomicrograph of section of ischemic myocardium. India ink (0.2 ml) was injected into the ischemic myocardium 5 min before excision of the heart. (Hematoxylin and Eosin: original magnification × 650). Large interstitial spaces are seen filled with stained fluid.

CONCLUSIONS

The conclusions derived from these experiments are the following.

Increases in Lymph Production during Myocardial Ishemia

Except for an immediate period after coronary occlusion, lymph flow was greater during ischemia than under baseline conditions. This finding has recently been confirmed by other investigators (Uhley et al., 1976). The increase can be explained on the basis of a rise in blood capillary permeability, evidenced by the significantly augmented lymph protein content and red-blood-cell concentration.

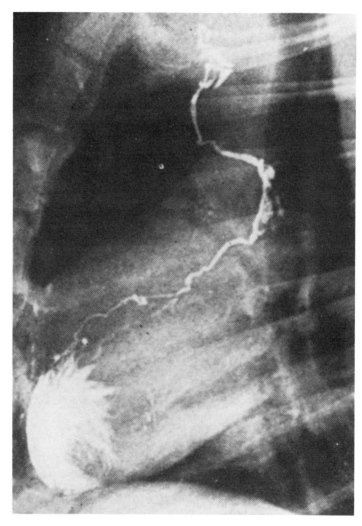

4 Roentgenogram of dog heart showing the lymph draining system of the left ventricle. Contrast medium (an emulsion of lipoidol F-glycerol-soy bean lecithin-glucose) was injected into the apical portion of the lateral wall of the left ventricle 2 hr after ligation of the circumflex artery. After 15 min, the heart arrested in ventricular fibrillation. A roentgenogram was immediately obtained. The supracardiac and terminal lymph channels appear markedly dilated.

Impairment of Lymph Drainage during Myocardial Ischemia

The appearance-clearance times of vital dye injected into the ischemic myocardium were greatly prolonged, compared to those of dye injected into normal myocardium. A pooling of lymph in dilated channels was evident in the lymphogram.

Lymph in any single tissue is moved by a combination of at least three factors: an active lymphatic pump, represented by active contractions of the lymphatic channels; a tissue pump, represented in the heart by its rhythmic contractions; and an arterial pump which is the force generated by arterial pulsations (Taylor et al., 1973). During acute myocardial ischemia, it is readily seen how these mechanisms fail: the suppression of the arterial pump, consequent to coronary occlusion; the impairment of the tissue pump, due to hypokinesis of the ischemic portion of the left ventricle; and the ischemic injury to the lymphatic vessels. Furthermore, it has been suggested (Wegria, 1964) that the increase in central venous pressure represents an obstruction to lymph efflux at its venous terminal. The fact that lymph flow was increased when the main lymphatic channel was cannulated, while lymph drainage was impaired when that channel was left intact, tends to attribute a great deal of importance to the obstructive mechanism.

Development of Interstitial Edema from Increased Lmyph Production + Impaired Lymph Drainage

On the basis of the experimental findings presented above and other reported observations, the following hypothesis (Fig. 5) has been formulated, concerning the role of the cardiac lymphatic system in the pathophysiology of myocardial infarction.

The importance of this role remains to be ascertained. It can be speculated, at this time, that the interstitial stagnation of a fluid rich in proteins, H-ions, lactic acid, lysosomal enzymes and, possibly, other substances, such as prostaglandins and kinins, cannot have but a harmful effect on the injured cells.

This hypothesis is supported by some observations showing an aggravation of ischemic myocardial injury in dogs subjected to lymph obstruction (Kline et al., 1964). Conversely, preliminary experiments (Feola et al., 1973) have shown a reduction of ischemic injury in animals in which the main lymphatic channel was cannulated and the lymph drained.

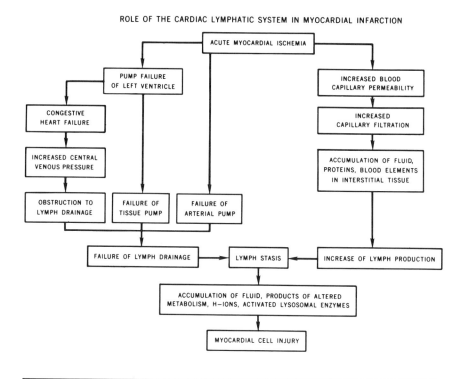

ROLE OF THE CARDIAC LYMPHATIC SYSTEM IN MYOCARDIAL INFARCTION

5   Diagram of an hypothesis. Close relationship exists between the cardiac lymph and myocardial ischemic injury, as indicated by our studies and reports of other investigators.

ACKNOWLEDGMENT

This work was supported by the Southeastern Pennsylvania Chapter of the American Heart Association.

REFERENCES

Celis, A., Del Castillo, H., Marquez, H., Alcantara, R., and Mijangos, D.: Radiologic demonstration of the lymphatic circulation of the heart. *Acta Radiol.* 4:48-489, 1966.

Drinker, C. K., Warren, M. D., Maurer, F. W., and McCarrell, J. D.: Flow, pressure and composition of cardiac lymph. *Am. J. Physiol.* 131:43-55 (1940).

Feola, M., and Glick, G.: Cardiac lymph flow and composition in acute myocardial ischemia in dogs. *Am. J. Physiol.* 229(1):44-48 (1975).

Feola, M., Glick, G., and Pick, R.: Interrelations between cardiac lymph and experimental infarction in dogs. *Clin. Res.* 21:418 (1973).

Kline, I. K., Miller, A. J., Pick, R., and Katz, L. N.: Effects of chronic impairment of cardiac lymph flow on myocardial reactions after coronary artery ligation in dogs. *Am. Heart J.* 68:515-523 (1964).

Leeds, S. E., Uhley, H. N., Sampson, J. J., and Friedman, M.: The cardiac lymphatics after ligation of the coronary sinus. *Proc. Soc. Exp. Biol. Med.* 135:59-62, (1970).

Maurer, F. W.: The effects of decreased blood oxygen and increased blood carbon dioxide on the flow and composition of cervical and cardiac lymph. *Am. J. Physiol.* 131:331-348 (1940).

Miller, A. J., Ellis, A., and Katz, L. N.: Cardiac lymph: flow rates and composition in dogs. *Am. J. Physiol.* 206:63-66 (1964).

Patek, P. R.: The morphology of the lymphatics of the mammalian heart. *Am. J. Anat.* 64:203-250 (1939).

Ranvier, L.: *Traité technique d'histologie*, 2nd ed. F. Savy, Paris (1889), p. 275.

Taylor, A. E., Gibson, W. H., Granger, H. J., and Guyton, A. C.: Interaction between intracapillary and tissue forces in the overall regulation of interstitial fluid volume. *Lymphology* 6:192-208 (1973).

Uhley, H. N., Leeds, S. E., and Elevitch, F. R.: Canine cardiac lymph potassium, pH and flow after experimental myocardial infarction. *Proc. Soc. Exp. Biol. Med.* 151:146-148 (1976).

Ullal, S. R., Kluge, T. H., Kerth, W. J., and Gerbode, F.: Flow and composition of cardiac lymph in dogs. *Ann. Surg.* 175:299-304 (1972).

Wasserman, K., and Mayerson, H. S.: Mechanisms of plasma protein changes following saline infusion. *Am. J. Physiol.* 170:1-10 (1952).

Wegria, R., Zeker, H., and Entrup, R. W.: Effect of an increase in systemic venous pressure on the formation and evacuation of lymph. *Acta Cardiol.* (Brux.) 19:193-216 (1964).

Discussion

Vyden, Roberts and Feola

DR. PETER R. MAROKO (*Harvard Medical School*): Dr. Feola, I measured pH in cardiac lymph and it was about 8 in my experiments. I attributed this high pH to the fact that it took so long to collect the lymph that the CO_2 was lost. Does that sound like a reasonable explanation?

DR. MARIO FEOLA (*Jefferson Medical College*): Perhaps, but I collected the lymph under a layer of mineral oil. We still found the pH to be on the alkaline side.

DR. ALLAN M. LEFER (*Jefferson Medical College*): Dr. Roberts, in the experiments you described, zymosan, which is a well-known reticulo-endothelial (RE) system blocking agent, prevented clearance of CPK. However, I am mystified by your experiment in which you did a total hepatectomy and did not find any change in the clearance rate; I believe that most RE investigators would agree that 90% of the active phagocytic cells of the RE system are located in the liver. How do you reconcile these two experiments?

DR. ROBERT ROBERTS (*Washington University School of Medicine*):   I cannot really offer a reconciliation. However, we are now looking at this problem in little more detail for another reason. Perhaps, zymosan does not block the RE system. This agent may, in fact, be more tied up with complement and this may be an immunological mechanism. If that is the case, then perhaps we can get around the apparent contradiction by some other means.

DR. STANLEY GLAUSER (*Temple University School of Medicine*):   Dr. Vyden, you indicated that oxygen decreases infarct size. Our analysis indicates that hyperbaric oxygen does not significantly decrease infarct size; and I was wondering if you wanted to elaborate on what you meant by an "oxygen effect."

DR. JOHN K. VYDEN (*UCLA School of Medicine*):   Dr. Braunwald, in his presentation, showed that, when oxygen was increased to 40% from the average room air value of 20%, a diminution in infarct size occurred.

DR. MAROKO: The only point that I was making was that non-hyperbaric oxygen is useful, but I have no data on hyperbaric oxygenation.

DR. GERALD WEISSMAN (*NYU School of Medicine*):   I would like to ask Dr. Roberts if he has studied CPK-disappearance time in whole blood in which polymorphonuclear leukocytes and platelets are present when zymosan is added, because not only does this drug mobilize the alternative pathway of complement activation, and by virtue of feedback—the Hageman factor, but it also causes substantial release of proteases from the white cells present in whole blood; therefore I shall be curious to see whether you have simply added zymosan to whole blood containing formed elements to determine if CPK disappeared.

DR. ROBERTS: Yes, if CPK is incubated in whole blood, just at 37°, the half-life for dog CPK is about 8 hr, whereas *in vivo* it is about 2 hr. However, if you add zymosan, the CPK half-life is much longer and goes up to about 14 hr.

DR. WEISSMANN: Was the zymosan added after or before the CPK?

DR. ROBERTS: It was added after CPK.

DR. JOHN MORRISON (*North Shore University Hospital, Man-hassett, N. Y.*):   Just a comment on Dr. Vyden's presentation. I would caution against the sweeping condemnation of digitalis in acute myocardial infarction in man. In the dog model where artificial congestive heart failure is induced, the ST segment mapping system seems to improve somewhat with ouabain. We have looked at digoxin in the setting of Killip class III acute myocardial infarction in man. Here, the CPK loss appears to diminish, although there are no hemodynamic changes.

In a similar group of patients, where furosemide (i.v.) was given, the hemodynamics improved, but there was no change in CPK loss. I think we have to be very careful in such situations, because hemodynamic changes that appear to show a betterment do not always agree with changes in infarct size.

DR. VYDEN: I take note of Dr. Morrison's comments. Obviously, as time goes on, we are going to reveal more and more of these anomalies. I think the one which strikes me the most is the fact that phentolamine, which has been a mainstay of treatment by the Harvard group, has been replaced by nitroprusside, largely due to the high cost of phentolamine. Dr. Maroko has observed that there may have been some situations in which ST segment elevation occurred with nitroprusside, which would tend to render us more cautious in employing this agent and, possibly, reconsider the use of phentolamine, or perhaps administer other agents, such as isosorbide and nitroglycerine, which are also very useful.

Concerning digitalis, Dr. William Shell is now working with us and according to his data, this drug usually enhances myocardial CPK efflux. However, I do not have any specific data on the subset of patients in heart failure. Therefore we shall take note of your comments and most certainly consider them in future studies.

DR. MAROKO: In the experimental animal, digitalis may either increase or decrease ischemic injury, depending on the hemo-dynamic state of the subject. If there is no heart failure and myocardial oxygen consumption rises due to the positive ino-tropic effect, we find an increase in ischemic injury; whereas, when digitalis is given in the presence of cardiac failure, it decreases myocardial oxygen utilization by decreasing the size of the heart. This would reduce ischemic injury. Probably, something similar happens in patients.

DR. GLAUSER: I would like to ask Dr. Feola this question. Does cardiac lymph clot, and if so, is there any change in clotting after inducing prolonged ischemia?

DR. FEOLA: We did not heparinize our dogs, but we filled the lymph catheter with a weak heparin solution, 5 to 10 units/ml, therefore we have not seen lymph clot. I did not look for platelets in cardiac lymph but a few red blood cells appear after collecting it. However, we centrifuge the lymph to eliminate any blood cells.

15

Myocardial Cell-Volume Control in Ischemic Injury

ROBERT B. JENNINGS
HAL K. HAWKINS
MARY L. HILL

INTRODUCTION

After sudden occlusion of a major branch of coronary artery in the normal dog, the least collateral arterial flow is found in the inner myocardium. Flows in this region routinely are depressed to 5-15% of those found prior to occlusion (Kloner et al., 1975; 1976). This condition is termed "severe" or "low-flow" ischemia (Jennings et al., 1975). On the other hand, collateral arterial flow in the subepicardial myocardium is greater than that in the subendocardial and may reach 50% of the flow noted prior to occlusion. Ischemia with high flow differs from severe ischemia in the sense that metabolite exchange in the ischemic cells is facilitated by the greater collateral flow. Regions of intermediate depression in arterial flow (moderate ischemia) also exist within the ischemic region. These generally are located in the outer one-half of the free ventricular wall. Thus, the acutely ischemic myocardium of the dog contains an ischemic gradient which ranges from low-flow ischemia in the subendocardial region to intermediate and high-flow ischemia in the subepicardial myocardium.

351

Our work has been aimed at learning what event or series of events leads ischemic injury to become irreversible. What change or changes occurring within the cell dictate that it will die even if the cause of the injury is removed by reperfusing the tissue with arterial blood? Most of our studies on this question have been carried out on open-chest anesthetized dogs, utilizing the large area of ischemia produced by high occlusion of the circumflex branch of the left coronary artery. The posterior papillary muscle is included in the ischemic area and serves as a source of severely ischemic tissue for study of the structural, functional and biochemical events occurring *in vivo* as a consequence of ischemia. The anterior wall of the heart, which is supplied by the anterior descending artery, serves as control nonischemic tissue.

Temporary occlusion studies have shown that 50-60% of the cells of the posterior papillary muscle have passed the point of no return after 40 min, and that almost all of the cells of this muscle are irreversibly injured by 60 min of ischemia (Jennings and Reimer, 1974). This change to irreversibility is heralded, at 60 min, by the tissue changing from a deep red to pink-gray (see Fig. 3 in Jennings and Ganote, 1974, for an illustration of this phenomenon). Thus, by concentrating on the grossly abnormal tissue, it is possible to take samples which include large quantities of irreversibly injured cells contaminated to only a small extent with reversibly injured tissue.

Previously, we have shown that striking and characteristic ultrastructural changes occur in the irreversibly injured cells (Jennings and Ganote, 1974), and that mitochondria isolated from such cells show defective function (Jennings and Ganote, 1976). Also, the irreversibly injured cells react to reperfusion of arterial blood by swelling explosively, by developing striking contraction bands, and by accumulating large quantities of calcium phosphate within the mitochondria (Shen and Jennings, 1972; Whalen, et al., 1974; Kloner et al., 1974b). Finally, the swollen cells show defects in the plasma membrane of the sarcolemma (Jennings, 1975; Ganote et al., 1976). The membrane defects, and failure of the irreversibly injured cells to exclude Ca^{2+} and maintain their volume after reperfusion have led to the studies of cell-volume control in normal and injured tissue *in vitro*, which are described below.

TEST SYSTEM FOR CELL-VOLUME REGULATION

The heart is excised quickly and cooled to about 4°C in a large volume of ice-cold isotonic KCl. The papillary muscles are removed

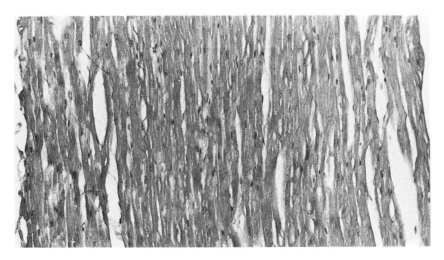

1 This micrograph shows the thickest portion of a freehand slice of posterior papillary muscle after 60 min incubation at 37°C. Note the increase in the interstitial space. The tissue is less compact because of the release of tissue tension, secondary to the slicing procedure. Hematoxylin and eosin. Mag. × 100.

and placed *en bloc* in ice-cold Krebs-Ringers-Phosphate (KRP) buffered to pH 7.4. After trimming the papillary muscle into small blocks, the tissue is sliced free hand, parallel to the long axis of the muscle and the cells of the muscle. The slices are about 8 × 8 mm and 0.1 to 0.7 mm thick. The thickest portion of the slice is about 40 and the thinnest about 18 cells thick (Fig. 1) (Grochowski et al., 1976).

These free-hand slices, incubated with KRP at 37°C in an O_2 atmosphere, will maintain a constant tissue H_2O, Na^+, K^+, and Mg^{2+} for as long as 3 hr. The inulin-diffusable space of the tissue is about 30% of the tissue water. Each slice is surrounded by six sides of cut cells. Inside the slice are normal uncrushed cells supported by diffusion of oxygen. A vascular system is not required for sustaining metabolism, and ion or H_2O exchange. Presumably, endogenous glycogen, fatty acids or amino acids serve as substrates. The regulation of volume is a function of the uncrushed inner cells of the slice.

The ultrastructure of the internal cells of the slice during incubation remains intact and indistinguishable from control myocardium. However, the cut cells on the periphery show signs of dam-

Table 1. Comparison of H_2O and electrolytes in control
unincubates vs incubated slices[†]

H_2O	Na	K	Mg
	Ml or mmol/100 g dry tissue		
	Unincubated		
337.6	17.2	39.6	4.9
± 4.48	± 1.71	± 1.49	±0.18
	Incubated 60 min at 37°C		
377.3	31.5	32.1	4.3
± 6.02**	± 3.67*	± 3.62	±0.27
	Cooled 30 min at 0°C		
432.0	63.1	13.2	4.3

[†]Four dogs were used. Values are means ± S.E. mean. The unincubated slices were weighed directly for analysis of water and electrolytes. The incubated slices were shaken in 15 ml of KRP, at 37°C, with continuous gassing with hydrated O_2 for 60 min. The slices were removed, blotted, and dried to constant weight at 105°C. Electrolytes were extracted with 0.75 ml HNO_3 and determined by flame absorption spectrophotometry (Jennings et al., 1970).

* $p < 0.05$; ** $p < 0.01$ by a two-tailed paired t test.

age, including mitochondrial Ca^{2+} accumulation and contraction bands (Grochowski et al., 1976; Ganote et al., 1976).

The data in Table 1 compares H_2O and electrolytes of control and incubated slices. Incubation of slices for an hour at 37°C results in a significant, small increase in total tissue water (TTW) and Na^+, and a decrease in K^+ and Mg^{2+}. This rise in H_2O content probably is partially an artifactual underestimation of TTW of control slices because of the drying that occurs when the tiny unincubated slices are weighed. However, swelling of the cut cells on the edge of the slice during incubation also contributes to the increased TTW. The Na of the incubated tissue also augments significantly, presumably because of increase in the interstitial space due to a loosening of the tissue during the process of cutting, plus Na^+ entering the cut cells of the edge of the slice. The drop in K^+ is invariably present and appears to be a function of the presence of cut cells on the slice periphery.

The adenosine triphosphate (ATP), creatine phosphate (CP), and glucose-6-phosphate (G-6-P) of various types of control and sliced tissue are shown in Table 2. Tissue frozen *in situ* with liquid

Table 2. Metabolites of control LV, unincubated and incubated slices*

TISSUE	TREATMENT	ATP	CP	G-6-P
		μmol/g wet wt		
LV	Freezing *in situ*	5.8 ± 0.16	8.0 ± 0.70	
PP slices	Cooled	5.7 ± 0.35	2.3 ± 0.5	3.1 ± 2.1
PP slices	Warm 60 min	2.5 ± 1.1	6.1 ± 0.1	0.29 ± 0.15

*The frozen *in situ* left ventricle (LV) data is from Brasch et al., (1968). The results are from 3 dogs and are means ± SE mean. Control papillary muscle quickly cooled en bloc prior to slicing is labelled PP cooled. These slices were weighed and placed directly into 3.6% PCA for extraction. The PP slices which were incubated for 60 min in warm KRP also were weighed and placed directly into 3.6% PCA. The metabolites were determined by the methods of Lamprecht et al., (1974), and Lamprecht and Trautschold, (1974).

nitrogen shows a high ATP and CP, and low G-6-P and lactate (Brasch et al., 1968; Wollenberger and Krause, 1968). If the heart is excised and cooled prior to preparing free-hand slices, tissue ATP remains unchanged from control. However, CP is reduced greatly as a consequence of the brief period of anaerobic metabolism which occurs while the tissue is being cooled (Brasch et al., 1968). Incubation of the slices, under conditions which maintained volume, resulted in tripling of tissue CP and in halving of tissue ATP. The G-6-P, which had accumulated because of anaerobic glycolysis occurring while the tissue was being cooled, was reduced in the incubated tissue. Thus, active metabolism maintained significant net high-energy phosphate in functioning control tissue.

MYOCARDIAL SWELLING INDUCED BY COLD INCUBATION

The effect of metabolic inhibition by cold on slice volume is shown in Table 1. Incubation of normal slices at 0-1°C results in massive cell swelling. Sodium increases markedly and much of the K+ of the cells of the slice is lost to the medium. Presumably the medium containing Na and Cl enters the cells of the slice, down the

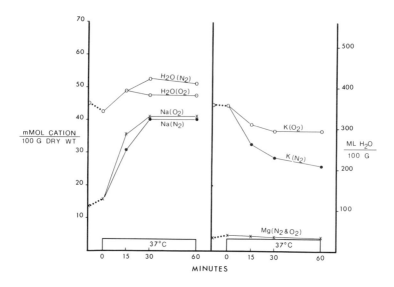

2 Cation and water content of slices incubated at 37°C in nitrogenated and oxygenated media. Each value is the mean of a duplicate or triplicate analysis by techniques described in detail in Grochowski et al. (1976).

concentration gradient from the media to cell water, while K^+ diffuses in the opposite direction. Tissue Mg^{2+} remains unchanged during the period of cold-induced respiratory arrest, probably because most intracellular Mg^{2+} is bound to adenine nucleotides (Page and Polimeni, 1972). The inulin-diffusable space is unchanged by swelling of the slice in the cold (Grochowski et al., 1976). Inulin is excluded by the cell membrane and, therefore, remains unaffected by the cell swelling.

Resumption of metabolism, by rewarming the cold slices to 37°C, is followed by a return of the water and Na content toward levels noted in incubated control tissue. Moreover, much of the K^+ lost during the period of arrested metabolism is reaccumulated. Both the accumulation of K^+ and the extrusion of Na occur against a significant concentration gradient. The capacity of tissue injured *in vitro* or *in vivo* to maintain volume, either with or without being swollen in the cold, is a measure of the integrity of the cells. We

Table 3. Capacity of anoxic LV tissue to control volume

	GAS	H_2O	Na	K	Mg
		Ml or mmol/100 gm dry tissue			
Incubated tissue	O_2	380.	41.6	36.2	3.9
30 min cold	O_2	432.	63.1	13.2	4.3
30 min cold 60 min warm	O_2	388.	44.9	21.5	3.8
30 min cold 60 min warm	N_2	422.	54.9	13.8	3.3

**Results are from a single experiment (Dog 2344). Incubated tissue refers to slices in KRP for 60 min at $37°C$. Each value is the mean of three slices. Measurements were made by methods described in footnote to Table 1. The N_2 medium was saturated with N_2 prior to use. In addition, the flasks were continuously gassed with hydrated N_2 during incubation.

shall show, subsequently, that cells damaged by ischemia *in vivo* eventually lose their capacity to maintain their volume.

EFFECT OF ANOXIA ON MYOCARDIAL CELL VOLUME REGULATION

The effect of anoxia, induced by saturation of the media with N_2, on cell-volume control was studied in slices of healthy left ventricular papillary muscle tissue. Slices were placed directly in warm nitrogenated or oxygenated media for various time intervals, and were then analyzed for H_2O and electrolytes. Results of a representative experiment are plotted in Fig. 2. Those in oxygenated media showed good volume control and exhibited no significant changes in H_2O content; the K^+ and Mg^{2+} remained constant at about 60-70% or more of the level observed in control unincubated tissue; the Na content doubled. The anoxic slices in this experiment were similar to the oxygenated ones, except for a slight increase in H_2O and significantly less K^+ per 100 g of dry tissue. The results show that anaerobic glycolysis provided enough energy to support significant volume regulation for 60 min.

The effect of anoxia on the capacity of slices swollen in the cold to restore volume and K^+ to control levels is shown in Table 3. Ar-

Table 4. Myocardial electrolytes and water after permanent
ischemia *in vivo* *

TISSUE	TIME (in min)	H$_2$O	Na	K	Mg	Ca	Cl
		Ml	or	m mol/100 g dry weight			
LV	Control	355.9 ± 32.0	19.1 ± 1.0	41.5 ± 2.1	5.0 ± 0.16	0.4 ± 0.2	13.8 ± 2.0
PP	40	358.7 ± 19.0	21.2 ± 1.6	40.1 ± 1.1	5.0 ± 0.19	0.5 ± 0.4	14.7 ± 0.9

*Data from Whalen et al. (1974). Results are mean ± standard error of the mean.
LV = left ventricle
PP = papillary muscle

rest of metabolism by cold for 30 min resulted in a 52-ml or 14% increase in TTW, and a 52% drop in K$^+$; resumption of metabolism in an oxygenated environment at 37°C resulted in a return of TTW to control levels. Much Na was pumped out of the cell with the H$_2$O and much of the K$^+$ was regained. Conversely, the anoxic tissue (N$_2$) could not support any reaccumulation of K$^+$, even though a small quantity of H$_2$O and Na was lost during the 60 min of anaerobic glycolysis. Thus, energy from anaerobic glycolysis is insufficient to support cell-volume regulation if the tissue is swollen and has lost K$^+$ prior to the onset of anaerobic metabolism.

Healthy tissue, suddenly made severely ischemic *in vivo*, functions primarily by anaerobic glycolysis as do anoxic heart slices *in vitro* (Fig. 2, Table 3) (Jennings et al., 1975). If the results of the *in vitro* experiments, plotted in Fig. 2, are applicable to *in vivo* conditions, it seems likely that severely ischemic myocardium would exhibit no marked swelling for the first 30-60 min of ischemia, even if sufficient plasma was available to support swelling. The TTW and electrolyte findings *in vivo*, after 40 min of severe ischemia (Whalen et al., 1974), are consistent with this assumption in that no changes are noted in posterior papillary muscle (PP) and left ventricle (LV) (Table 4). This result suggests strongly that cell volume is maintained by anaerobic glycolysis for at least the first 40 min of ischemia. The alternate hypothesis, i.e., that arterial flow is so low that insufficient plasma water is provided to support swelling, seems improbable (Jennings et al., 1975; Kloner et al., 1976).

It appears unlikely that cell swelling accentuates the severity of ischemic injury in areas of severe ischemia until after the cells have passed the point of no return. The failure to demonstrate changes in arterial collateral flow, as a function of persistent ischemia, further supports this conclusion. No data are currently available about the role cell swelling may play in regions of moderate to high-flow ischemia. Although cell swelling of sufficient degree to prevent reflow of arterial blood does not occur acutely in severely ischemic myocardium, the "no reflow" phenomenon does take place eventually in some parts of the injured tissue. Kloner et al. (1974a), have shown that ischemic vascular damage is probably the reason for its occurrence. The thrombosis and hemorrhage they observed in areas of no reflow presumably prevent the latter and create the "no reflow" phenomenon.

CELL VOLUME REGULATION IN IRREVERSIBLE ISCHEMIC INJURY IN VIVO

While cell volume changes cannot be detected *in vivo* after 60 min of ischemic injury, there is excellent biological evidence, from ultrastructural and reflow studies, that these cells are irreversibly injured (Fig. 3) (Grochowski et al., 1976; Jennings and Ganote, 1974). Because there is enormous swelling and Ca^{2+} entry in such cells after reflow of arterial blood (Whalen et al., 1974; Shen and Jennings, 1972), it seemed likely that the irreversibly injured cells would exhibit defective volume regulation in the *in vitro* freehand slice volume-test system.

In fact, slices of PP injured by 60 and 120 min of severe ischemia *in vivo* cannot maintain cell volume and electrolytes (Ganote et al., 1976). These data are shown in Table 5. There was a 45-ml increase in tissue water, associated with a massive rise in Na and a very marked decrease in K^+ and Mg^{2+}. Of note is the fact that cold-induced swelling of normal tissue produces similar findings (Table 3), except that the Na is not as high and Mg^{2+} remains unchanged.

The inulin-diffusable space (IDS) of tissue irreversibly injured by 60 min of ischemia is increased by 55 ml (Table 5). These data indicate that some tissue water, in a compartment not previously penetrated by inulin, e.g., intracellular H_2O, has been penetrated by a molecule with a molecular weight of 5000. This observation suggests that cell-membrane permeability to this molecule is altered in the irreversibly injured cells or that the membrane of these cells

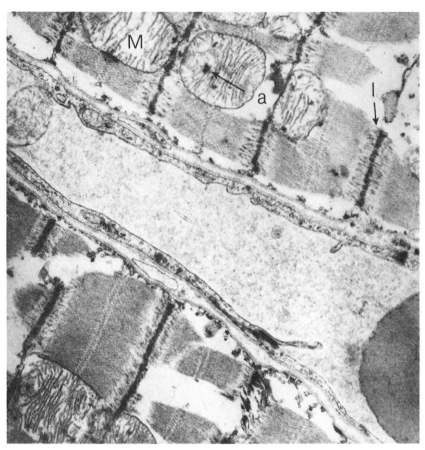

3   PP after 60 min of ischemic injury **in vivo**. Parts of two cells and a capillary are shown. The myofibrils are relaxed. I bands are prominent. Mitochondria (M) are enlarged due to an increase in matrix space. Amorphous matrix densities (a) are prominent in most mitochondrial profiles. At this magnification, the sarcolemma appears intact. The capillary endothelium shows no abnormalities aside from a decrease in pinocytotic vesicles. Osmium fixation stained with uranyl acetate and lead citrate (Mag. × 12,700). [Reproduced from Ganote et al. (1976), with permission of the Editor of the **Journal of Molecular and Cellular Cardiology**.]

Table 5. Water and electrolytes in control and injured myocardium after
in vitro incubation at 37°C†

	H_2O	IDS	Na	K	Mg
	ml	or		m mol/100 g 60 min ischemia	
LV	371.5 ± 11.0	141. ± 11.	61.9 ± 3.0	29.9 ± 1.98	4.2 ± 0.24
PP	426.0** ± 10.0	196.** ± 20.	90.8** ± 2.92	11.3** ± 1.72	2.6** ± 0.17

†LV and PP are anterior and posterior papillary muscles slices, respectively. IDS is the inulin diffusable space in ml/100 g dry tissue. The probability that the difference between LV and PP (damaged) tissue is statistically significant by a two-tailed paired t test is **p < 0.01. The medium is oxygenated KRP buffered to pH 7.4. Six dogs were used in this experiment. The higher Na values in this table are due to a constant artifact not present in more recent experiments (see Tables 1 and 3). These data were abstracted from Ganote et al. (1976).

contains defects large enough to allow inulin to enter.

The IDS can be used to estimate the intracellular H_2O of the tissue: TTW-IDS = intracellular cell water/100 g dry tissue. The results of this calculation, in the injured tissue system presented in Table 5, suggest that the cell water of the irreversibly injured cells is not altered. After 60 min of ischemia, cell water is 230.5 ml in LV and 230 ml in PP (Table 5). Thus, if one accepts the assumption that the inulin molecules remain extracellular, the augmented IDS indicates that the PP edema is caused by an increase in interstitial fluid. Since ultrastructural study shows that cell swelling is present in the PP, it seems likely that parts of the intracellular space have been penetrated by inulin and have become a part of the extracellular space, without a concomitant loss in the total mass of the tissue (Jennings, 1975). This leads to the TTW being lower than it would have been if the cell were intact, swollen and capable of excluding inulin.

Associated with the failure of cell-volume regulation are striking changes in the ultrastructure of the plasma membrane of the sarcolemma of the ischemic cells. These are best detected in cold swollen PP tissue. If one places slices of normal LV and damaged

PP in cold KRP, both tissues will swell markedly. However, the PP shows pronounced subsarcolemmal bleb formation as well as mito-chondrial swelling (Fig. 3). In addition, plasma membrane in the region of the subsarcolemmal blebs disappears or persists only as circular profiles, leaving residual glycocalyx to mark the site of the sarcolemma (Fig. 4). The resulting defects in the sarcolemma are large enough to allow both inulin and Ca^{2+} to enter the intracellular water. Whether these defects are the primary cause of the influx of inulin and Ca^{2+} is not established.

Incubation of PP slices from irreversibly damaged PP, at 37°C, is associated with contraction of most of the myofibrils. This pre-sumably is due to Ca^{2+} in the intracellular H_2O; Ca^{2+} entry can be documented by electron microscopy, since it is accumulated as elec-tron-dense granules in the mitochondria of some of the cells. No Ca^{2+} entry is seen in nonischemic control tissue.

Since the addition of an exogenous substrate, such as succinate, has no beneficial effect on volume control of the irreversibly injured cells, it seems unlikely that the observed defect is due to substrate deficiency. However, preliminary data shows that the irreversibly injured tissue does contain less than 5% of the ATP and CP found in control tissue. These results suggest that irreversible injury is associated with exhaustion of a component necessary for the opera-tion of the Na-K pump. Further work is required on this point.

The results of these experiments provide objective evidence that cell-volume control is deficient in cells which have just entered a state of irreversible injury. Associated with the failure of cell-volume control are defects in the structure of the plasma membrane of these cells. It seems likely that cell-membrane integrity was al-tered during the period of ischemia *in vivo* in such a way that the *in vitro* test system employed allowed detection of the sarcolemmal defect. In any event, our observations establish that defective cell-volume regulation is a very early event in irreversible injury of the myocardium.

SUMMARY

The effects of anoxia *in vitro* or ischemia *in vivo* on cell volume regulation were investigated, using free-hand slices of dog papillary muscles incubated in Krebs-Ringers-Phosphate media. Anoxia *in vitro* did not result in loss of myocardial cell-volume control, unless the cells were swollen prior to the onset of anoxia. Myocardial cells

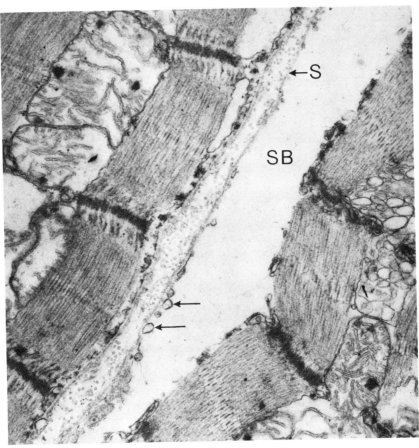

4   Slice of PP shown in Fig. 4 after 60 min incubation at 0-1°C. TTW
was increased by more than 50%. The swelling included formation
of a subsarcolemmal bleb (SB) which is of interest because the
plasma membrane of the sarcolemma is incomplete over the bleb.
The irregular circular profiles are believed to be remnants of the
plasma membrane (arrows). The basement membrane of the
sarcolemma appears intact (S). The myofibrils have remained
relaxed. The mitochondria appear swollen and contain no densities
aside from the amorphous matrix densities which were present prior
to incubation (Max × 25,200). [Reproduced from Ganote et al.
(1976), with permission of the Editor of the **Journal of Molecular
and Cellular Cardiology**.]

irreversibly injured by a brief episode of severe ischemia *in vivo* swelled when incubated *in vitro*. In addition, they had no capacity to maintain cation concentrations and had an increased inulin-diffusable space. This loss of cell-volume control was associated with striking defects in the plasma membrane of the irreversibly injured cells. Defective sarcolemmal structure or permeability appears to be an early characteristic feature of irreversible ischemic injury.

ACKNOWLEDGMENTS

This work was in part supported by NIH Grant 7-RO1-HL 18833 and Contract NO1-HV 52999.

Some of the experiments reported in this lecture were performed at Northwestern University in association with Charles E. Ganote, M.D. and Eugene C. Grochowski, M.D., Ph.D. The details of these experiments are given in Ganote et al. (1976), and Grochowski et al. (1976). Jonathan Worstall provided excellent technical assistance in the experiment shown in Fig. 2.

REFERENCES

Brasch, W., Gudbjarnason, S., Puri, P. S., Ravens, K. G., and Bing, R. J.: Early changes in energy metabolism in the myocardium following acute coronary artery occlusion in anesthetized dogs. *Circ. Res.* 23:429-438 (1968).

Ganote, C. E., Jennings, R. B., Hill, M. L., and Grochowski, E. C.: Experimental myocardial ischemic injury. II. Effect of *in vivo* ischemia on dog heart slice function *in vitro*. *J. Mol. Cell Cardiol.* 8:189-204 (1976).

Grochowski, E. C., Ganote, C. E., Hill, M. L., and Jennings, R. B.: Experimental myocardial ischemic injury. I. A comparison of Stadie-Riggs and free-hand slicing techniques on tissue ultrastructure, water and electrolytes during *in vitro* incubation. *J. Mol. Cell Cardiol.* 8:173-187 (1976).

Jennings, R. B.: Cell volume regulation in acute myocardial ischemic injury. *Acta Med. Scand.* (Suppl. 587): 83-92 (1975).

Jennings, R. B., and Ganote, C. E.: Structural changes in myocardium during acute ischemia. *Circ. Res.* (Suppl. III) 35:156-172 (1974).

Jennings, R. B., and Ganote, C. E.: Mitochondrial structure and function in acute myocardial ischemic injury. *Circ. Res.* (Suppl. I) 38:80-91 (1976).

Jennings, R. B., Ganote, C. E., and Reimer, K. A.: Ischemic tissue injury. *Am. J. Pathol.* 81:179-198 (1975).

Jennings, R. B., Moore, C. B., Shen, A. C., and Herdson, P. B.: Electrolytes of damaged myocardial mitochondria.. *Proc. Soc. Exp. Biol. Med.* 135:515-522 (1970).

Jennings, R. B., and Reimer, K. A.: Salvage of ischemic myocardium. *Mod. Concepts Cardiovasc. Dis.* 43:125-130 (1974).

Kloner, R. A., Ganote, C. E., and Jennings, R. B.: The "no-reflow" phenomenon after temporary coronary occlusion in the dog. *J. Clin. Invest.* 54·1496-1508 (1974a).

Kloner, R. A., Ganote, C. E., Reimer, K. A., and Jennings, R. B.: Distribution of coronary arterial flow in acute myocardial ischemia. *Arch. Pathol.* 99: 86-94 (1975).

Kloner, R. A., Ganote, C. E., Whalen, D., and Jennings, R. B.: Effect of a transient period of ischemia on myocardial cells. II. Fine structure during the first few minutes of reflow. *Am. J. Pathol.* 74:399-422 (1974b).

Kloner, R. A., Reimer, K. A., and Jennings, R. B.: Distribution of collateral flow in acute myocardial ischemic injury—Effect of propranolol therapy. *Cardiovasc. Res.* 10:81-90 (1976).

Lamprecht, W., Stein, P., Heinz, F., and Weisser, H.: Creatine phosphate. In *Methods of Enzymatic Analysis*, H. U. Bergmeyer, ed. Academic Press, New York (1974), pp. 1777-1781.

Lamprecht, W., and Trautschold, I.: Determination of ATP with hexokinase and glucose-6-phosphate dehydrogenase. In *Methods of Enzymatic Analysis*. H. U. Bergmeyer, ed. Academic Press, New York (1974), pp. 2101-2110.

Page, E., and Polimeni, P. I.: Magnesium exchange in rat ventricle. *J. Physiol.* (Lond.) 224:121-139 (1972).

Shen, A. C., and Jennings, R. B.: Myocardial calcium and magnesium in acute ischemic injury. *Am. J. Pathol.* 67:417-440 (1972).

Whalen, D. A., Jr., Hamilton, D. G., Ganote, C. E., and Jennings, R. B.: Effect of a transient period of ischemia on myocardial cells. I. Effects on cell volume regulation. *Am. J. Pathol.* 74:381-398 (1974).

Wollenberger, A., and Krause, E.: Metabolic control characteristics of the acutely ischemic myocardium. *Am. J. Cardiol.* 22:349-359 (1968).

16

Lysosomes in Ischemic Myocardium, with Observations on the Effects of Methylprednisolone

GERALD WEISSMANN
SYLVIA HOFFSTEIN
DORIS GENNARO
ARTHUR C. FOX

INTRODUCTION

The objectives of our studies to date were to delineate the sequential morphological, cytochemical and biochemical changes that occurred in the course of regional myocardial ischemia, and to seek pharmacological means to minimize these changes. Since lysosomes contain a variety of hydrolytic enzymes (Hirschhorn, 1974) capable of causing some of the morphological sequelae of ischemic injury, and since ischemia induces a degree of acidosis (Effros et al., 1975) which approaches the pH optima of these enzymes, we began with a study of the distribution of lysosomal enzymes in normal and ischemic canine myocardial tissue. We have now documented the ubiquitous distribution of two marker lysosomal enzymes in the sarcoplasmic reticulum of normal myocardial cells. During ischemic injury, these lysosomal hydrolases are solubilized and disappear from their characteristic, membrane-bound locations. This redistribution of lysosomal hydrolases from membrane-bound organelles to the cytosol correlated with ultrastructural indications of cell injury (Hoffstein et al., 1975b) and with subcellular fractionation studies, which showed an increase in soluble, unsedimentable lysosomal enzymes in extracts from infarcted myocardium (Hoffstein et al., 1976). In addition, we have shown that loss of sarcolemmal integrity is also an early event in ischemic injury and can occur in cells with otherwise intact organelles (Hoffstein et al., 1975a).

LYSOSOMAL INVOLVEMENT IN CELL INJURY

Ultrastructural Evidence

Ischemia and its consequent intracellular acidosis are known to disrupt lysosomes in various cell types (de Duve and Beaufay, 1958; Holtzer and Van Lancker, 1958; Nelson, 1966), permitting acid hydrolases to gain access to the cytosol. Such intracellular release of lysosomal enzyme may be one of the mechanisms by which myocardial ischemia leads to cell injury and death, since enzymes normally contained within lysosomes have been shown to be capable of degrading many biologically significant intracellular and extracellular macromolecules. Ultrastructural studies of irreversibly injured, ischemic myocardial cells show a variety of morphological changes, many of which could be caused by the intracellular release of hydrolytic enzymes. Normal myocardial cells contain considerable amounts of glycogen, a moderately densely staining ground cytoplasm, and mitochondria with dense matrices. Cells irreversibly injured by ischemia contain no visible glycogen, have electron-lucent areas where the ground cytoplasm should be, mitochondria which are devoid of matrix, and I bands with a characteristic moth-eaten appearance (Jennings et al., 1965; 1969; Heggtveit, 1971/72; Herdson et al., 1965; Kloner et al., 1974; Korb and Totovic, 1969; Hoffstein et al., 1975a, 1975b).

All of these changes could be caused if lysosomal hydrolases were no longer membrane-bound but released into the cytosol to digest cytoplasmic constituents. The importance of the release of hydrolases from myocardial lysosomes in the pathogenesis of ischemic injury has been questioned, since some studies have shown that myocardial cells contain few lysosomes (Abraham et al., 1967; Buchanan and Schwartz, 1967; Topping and Travis, 1974). Most of the lysosomal enzyme activity, localized by conventional cytochemical procedures, was found in residual or lipofuscin bodies in the perinuclear region (Abraham et al., 1967). Only a few lysosomes could be located in the distal regions of the cell (Topping and Travis, 1974). Furthermore, earlier electron-microscopic observation of irreversibly injured ischemic myocardial cells seemed to show no alteration in residual bodies, and their limiting membranes appeared intact (Kloner et al., 1974). The redistribution of acid hydrolases from the particulate to the soluble subcellular fraction after ischemia might, therefore, only reflect changes in lysosomes from endothelial and interstitial cells and not from cardiac cells. However, fractionation (Holtzer and Van Lancker, 1958; Nelson, 1966; Romeo et al., 1966; Canonico and Bird, 1970; Gottwick et al., 1974; Rugh et al., 1974; Stauber and Bird, 1974) and cytochemical (Topping and Travis, 1974; Stauber and Bird, 1974; Pearce, 1965a, 1965b; Hudgson and Pearce, 1969) studies of skeletal and myocardial tissue suggested the possibility that acid hydrolases might be located in the sarcoplasmic reticulum of muscle cells as well as in classical primary and secondary lysosomes and Golgi bodies. We have shown by means of ultrastructural cytochemistry (Hoffstein, 1975b) that the sarcoplasmic reticulum of myocardial cells does indeed contain acid hydrolases and that these hydrolases are released during early ischemic injury. Furthermore, Brunk and Ericsson (1972b) have shown that lysosomal hydrolases may leak through what appear to be morphologically intact lysosomal membranes.

Cytochemical Evidence

We have localized cytochemically (Hoffstein et al., 1975a; 1975b) the lysosomal marker enzymes, acid phosphatase and aryl sulphatase, in lateral sacs associated with the sarcolemma, in tubules, and in the longitudinal sarcoplasmic reticulum elements between myofibrils, and adjacent to mitochondria. The distribution of sarcoplasmic reticulum in myocardial cells is so widespread and the presence of acid phosphatase and aryl sulphatase activity within the sarcoplasmic reticulum so ubiquitous that membrane-bound reaction product can be seen in orderly arrays throughout normal cells. Ischemically injured myocardial cells from 3½-hr and 24-hr infarctions show cytoplasmic damage that correlates with a reduction in the acid hydrolase positive elements of the sarcoplasmic reticulum. Thus, severely injured cells showed little reaction product but that which was present was found within lateral sacs or vesiculated elements of the sarcoplasmic reticulum. Moderately damaged cells showed less reduction in these acid hydrolase-positive vesicles than did severely injured cells. The latter are completely devoid of glycogen but moderately injured cells from the marginal zone of $3\frac{1}{2}$-hr infarcts may show focal depletion of glycogen in a few areas of cytoplasm. Those areas contained fewer acid phosphatase reactive sarcoplasmic reticulum elements than did adjacent areas of the same cell. These data, in addition to our other work (Hoffstein et al., 1975a; 1975b; 1976) showing that such lytic injury to the cytoplasm can occur in the presence of an intact sarcolemma, suggested that at least some of the pathology found in ischemic myocardial cells may result from the intracellular release of lysosomal hydrolases from the sarcoplasmic reticulum (SR).

The cytochemical localization of acid hydrolases in the SR of rat cardiac (Topping and Travis, 1974) and skeletal muscle (Pearce, 1965a, 1965b; Hudgson and Pearce, 1969) has previously been reported by other investigators. However, relatively few reaction-positive SR profiles were demonstrated. The essential difference between their methods and ours was that we have employed DMSO to increase the rate of deposition and amount of reaction product (Brunk and Ericsson, 1972b) so that small amounts of enzyme activity could be localized within restrictive limiting membranes (Romeo et al., 1966). DMSO presumably acts by increasing the accessibility of the substrate to the fixed enzyme without altering its specific localization (Brunk and Ericsson, 1972a; Bainton and Farquhar, 1968).

Biochemical Evidence

The basis for the concept that release of lysosomal hydrolases occurs in ischemic myocardium as a result of lysosomal rupture, and that this may produce tissue autolysis, has been reviewed recently by Brachfeld (1969) and by Sobel (1972). Lysosomal acid hydrolases were demonstrated in beef heart by Romeo and coworkers (1966), who noted that heart lysosomes seemed less fragile than those in liver. Brachfeld and Gemba (1965) reported that lysosomal cathepsin was released into myocardium rapidly after ligation of the anterior descending coronary artery, and that rat hearts rendered toxic with digitalis released lysosomal enzymes into the bathing medium (Oran and Brachfeld, 1970). Ricciutti et al. (1968) demonstrated an increase in acid phosphatase in infarcted canine myocardium, suggesting a decrease in lysosome stability. Fractionation studies of ischemic cardiac (Sobel, 1972; Leighty et al., 1967; Raven and Gudbjarnason, 1969; Ricciutti, 1972a, 1972b) and skeletal muscle (Arcangeli et al., 1973) support this hypothesis by showing that lysosomal marker enzymes shift from the particulate to the soluble fraction within the first few hours of ischemia.

Cell Fractionation Evidence

The unusual localization of acid hydrolases in myocardial tissue meant that fractionation techniques, suitable for the isolation of lysosomes in other tissues, might not suffice to produce adequately high yields of granule-associated lysosomal enzymes in normal canine myocardium. Ordinary homogenization and differential sedimentation (de Duve and Beaufay, 1958) in 0.25 or 0.34 molar sucrose, using a Teflon homogenizer (conditions sufficient to obtain good lysosomal preparation from liver, kidney, leukocytes, etc.), were inadequate to demonstrate sufficient sedimentable lysomes in homogenized normal myocardium. Instead, it was necessary to devise special fractionation techniques to demonstrate lysosomes sedimenting as a post-nuclear pellet at $120,000 \times g$ for 2 hr in sucrose homogenates (0.25-0.34 molar sucrose). The size and density of the demonstrable lysosomes, isolated biophysically, seem compatible with the structures seen in the electron microscope. The special maneuver employed was to permit the shear-fractured vesicles to "reseal" on standing (60 min) in sucrose (Hoffstein et al., 1976). With the new fractionation procedures, it became possible to obtain lysosomal preparations from dog myocardium of better stability than any previously reported in the literature (Ricciutti, 1972a, 1972b; Arcangeli et al., 1973; Spath et al., 1974). This method provides a relatively high yield of granule-associated or "latent" enzyme activity from normal myocardial tissue, an important prerequisite for testing various therapeutic maneuvers designed to stabilize lysosomal membranes during ischemia. A high yield of sedimentable lysosomal enzyme activity in normal tissue permits one to demonstrate differences with statistical significance in experiments involving treatment effects.

Biochemically, the lysosomal preparations obtained in this fashion showed that lysosomes can be secured from the endocardium in a more reproducible and less "fragile" state than can those from the epicardium, in transmural biopsies of the ventricular wall dissected into endo- and epicardial halves. After establishing a reliable fractionation procedure for normal endocardium—which left better than 50% of the lysosomal enzymes, acid phosphatase and beta-glucuronidase in the pelletable post-nuclear fraction—we were able to show a significant redistribution of these enzymes from the pelletable to the soluble fraction 2 hr post infarction in ischemic endocardium (Hoffstein et al., 1976). Redistribution of lysosomal enzymes in the overlying ischemic epicardium was not significantly different from the random labilization that we found in normal epicardium. At this early period, cells in the epicardium are known to be ischemic but not irreversibly injured (Kloner et al., 1974, 1975). Thus, the fractionation data for redistribution correlates with the cytochemical and physiological data.

EVIDENCE FOR EARLY IMPAIRMENT OF CELL MEMBRANE INTEGRITY

Loss of sarcolemma integrity is another early event in ischemic injury. Several histological studies of ischemic myocardium (Shnitka and Nachlas, 1973; Kent, 1966, 1967; Dusek et al., 1971) have shown that irreversibly-injured cells are characterized by loss of glycogen and the acquisition of diastase-resistant periodic acid Shiff-staining (PAS) properties. Kent (1966, 1967) has shown that this PAS-positive staining is due to plasma glycoproteins which penetrate the injured sarcolemma. Albumin and IgG diffuse into dog myocardial cells within an hour after ischemia is induced. Fibrinogen has been identified in the center of human myocardial infarcts but only albumin and IgG are found at the periphery of infarcts at 3 to 4 hr. Studies in our laboratory, using colloidal lanthanum to detect alterations in sarcolemmae permeability at the ultrastructural level, have shown that the sarcolemma loses its integrity very early (within 1 hr) in the center of the infarcted area (Abraham et al., 1967).

The use of lanthanum as a tracer has shown that these two morphological consequences of ischemia, loss of glycogen and altered sarcolemmae permeability, do not necessarily coincide in marginally injured cells although they do so in obviously necrotic cells. In the marginal area of early infarctions, we found a correlation between permeability to lanthanum and contractility in the presence of intact organelles and glycogen stores. Cells with strong contraction bands showed these features in regions with those bands although a greater degree of damage to organelles can sometimes be seen in other parts of the same cell.

Our data suggest that cell injury in the marginally ischemic area and, perhaps, in the center of the infarct may occur by at least two mechanisms involving loss of membrane integrity. In one, an early event is the loss of sarcolemmal integrity, leading to uncontrolled entry of ions and macromolecules into the cells and concomitant loss of soluble cytoplasmic constituents. The second pathway appears to involve early intracellular release of substances (possibly from lysosomes) which exert glycogenolytic and proteolytic effects. In the presence of an intact sarcolemma these processes may lead to an increase in osmotic pressure and consequent intracellular edema. Indeed, lack of synchrony in these two mechanisms of cell injury may account for some of the morphological heterogeneity characteristic of ischemic lesions. Further lanthanum and other tracer studies of short-term occlusions in which the injury is known to be reversible should help clarify the problem.

PHARMACOLOGICAL INTERVENTION: MEMBRANE STABILIZERS

Since so much accumulated information suggested that ischemic injury to myocardial cells involved an impairment of membrane function, the obvious move was to see whether steroids, which apparently can act upon biomembranes in general to increase their stability (Weissmann, 1973), were capable of reducing the size of the necrotic lesion, or reducing the extent of the solubilization of lysosomal enzymes, or both. After establishing a reliable fractionation procedure, we were able to show that, in dogs given 50 mg/kg of methylprednisolone one-half hour after induction of myocardial infarction, there was significant inhibition of lysosomal redistribution into the supernatant fraction of infarcted endocardium at 2 hr post infarction. No such changes were seen in epicardium (Figs. 1, 2). In addition, ultrastructural evaluation of myocardial tissue injury, in random samples of ischemic myocardium from treated and untreated animals, showed a significant difference in the number of tissue samples with morphological signs of irreversible cell injury, indicating a possible reduction in infarct size by the steroid (Hoffstein et al., 1976).

POSSIBLE ROLES FOR LYSOSOMES IN EXPANSION OF NECROTIC LESION

In the final stages of ischemically-induced myocardial cell death, it is clear that loss of integrity is observed of both lysosomal

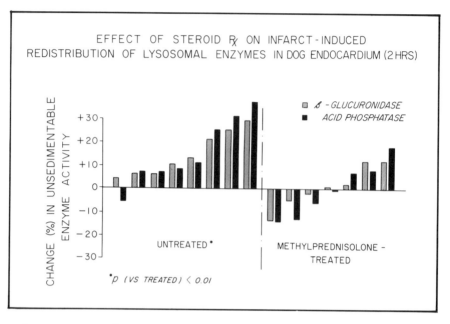

1   Change in unsedimentable (100,000 × g, 15 min) enzyme activity in ischemic dog endocardium 2 hr after ligation of left anterior descending coronary artery. Differences recorded between percentage of β-glucuronidase and acid phosphatase, rendered unsedimentable in ischemic and remote (uninjured) tissue. Methylprednisolone (50 mg/kg) given 30 min after ischemia.

membranes and the sarcolemmae. A mechanism, therefore, exists that permits lysosomal hydrolases to escape to the extracellular milieu. Furthermore, this leakage of hydrolytic enzymes begins early in ischemia and progresses as the necrotic lesion enlarges. Lysosomes are known to contain proteases capable of degrading macromolecules to biologically active peptides which may be significant in causing inflammation and, perhaps, in spreading the necrotic lesion. Thus, a lysosomal location has been found for an enzyme capable of converting plasminogen to plasmin and a similar location has been reported for a tissue-kininogen activator. In addition, a neutral protease has been identified in myocardial tissue extracts, which cleaves the serum protein C_3 into chemotactively-active products (Hirschhorn, 1974). One of the products of C_3 cleavage is C_3b which can activate an amplification loop in the complement

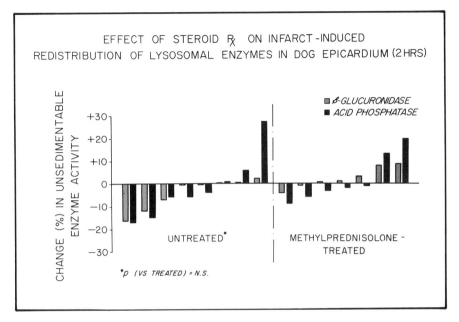

2 Change in unsedimentable (100,000 × g, 15 min) enzyme activity in ischemic dog epicardium 2 hr after ligation of left anterior descending coronary artery. Differences recorded between percentage of β-glucuronidase and acid phosphatase rendered unsedimentable in ischemic and remote (uninjured) tissue. Methylprednisolone (50 mg/kg) given 30 min after ischemia.

pathway, leading to the activation of the terminal complement sequence. The latter components of the activated complement sequence are capable of injuring outer membranes of bystander cells, with the resultant loss of the usual homeostatic control of ion flux (Ruddy, 1974). Thus activation of complement, by products released from cells early in ischemia, may be one of the mechanisms by which the necrotic lesion enlarges.

SUMMARY

These studies thus far cannot be taken as proving or disproving a primary role for lysosomal enzymes in provoking the tissue injury of myocardial infarctions. It is entirely possible that primary changes, involving the plasma membrane, myofibrillar elements or mitochondria, are responsible for the loss of tissue integrity during ischemia. Nevertheless, they provide clear evidence that lysosomes are among the organelles injured early in the course of myocardial infarction. They also show that it is not only possible to demonstrate early lysosomal rupture during myocardial infarction, but also that glucocorticoid—given after the acute insult—can regularly inhibit the redistribution of lysosomal enzyme from a sedimentable into a non-sedimentable fraction of ischemic canine myocardial homogenates. These results correlate with the findings of Libby et al. (1973), who have demonstrated reduction of infarct size with steroid administration at 6 hr after infarction, and with those of Maroko et al. (1972), who showed that ischemic tissue can be rescued hours after the initial insult.

ACKNOWLEDGMENTS

This work was aided by grants from the National Institutes of Health (AM-11949 and HL-19072), the New York Heart Association and the Whitehall Foundation.

REFERENCES

Abraham, R., Morris, M., and Smith, J.: Histochemistry of lysosomes in rat heart muscle. *J. Histochem. Cytochem.* 15:596-599 (1967).

Arcangeil, P., Del Soldata, P., Digiesi, V., and Melani, F.: Changes in the activities of lysosomal enzymes in striated muscle following ischemia. *Life Sci.* 12:13-23 (1973).

Bainton, D. F., and Farquhar, M. G.: Differences in enzyme content of azurophil and specific granule of polymorphonuclear leukocytes. II Cytochemistry and electron microscopy of bone marrow cells. *J. Cell Biol.* 39: 229-317 (1968).

Brachfeld, N.: Research on acute myocardial infarction. *Circulation* 39, 40 (Supp. IV): 202-215 (1969).

Brachfeld, N., and Gemba, T.: Mechanisms of cell death: Release of lysosomal hydrolases after ischemia. *Clin. Res.* 13:524 (1965).

Brunk, U. T., and Ericsson, J. L. E.: Demonstration of acid phosphatase in *in vitro* cultured cells. Significance of fixation, tonicity and permeability factors. *Histochem. J.* 4:349-363 (1972a).

Brunk, U. T., and Ericsson, J. L. E.: Cytochemical evidence for the leakage of acid phosphate through ultrastructurally intact lysosomal membranes. *Histochem. J.* 4:479-491 (1972b).

Buchanan, W. E., and Schwartz, J. B.: Lysosomal enzyme activity in heart and skeletal muscle of cortisone treated rats. *Am. J. Physiol.* 212:732-737 (1967).

Canonico, P. G., and Bird, J. W. G: Lysosomes in skeletal muscle tissue, Zonal centrifugation evidence for multiple cellular sources. *J. Cell. Biol.* 45:321-333 (1970).

de Duve, C., and Beaufay, H.: Tissue fractionation studies 10. Influence of ischemia on the state of some bound enzymes in rat liver. *Biochem. J.* 73: 610-616 (1958).

Dusek, J., Rana, G., and Kahn, D. S.: Healing process in the marginal zone of an experimental myocardial infarct. Findings in the surviving cardiac muscle cells. *Am. J. Pathol.* 62:321-340 (1971).

Effros, R. M., Haider, B., Ettinger, P. O., Ahmed, S. S., Oldewortel, H. A., Marold K., and Reagan, T. J.: *in vivo* myocardial cell pH in the dog: response to ischemia and infusion of alkal. *J. Clin. Invest.* 55:1100-1110 (1975).

Gottwik, M. G., Kirk, E. S., and Weglicki, W. B.: Myocardial lysosomal hydrolases 1 hour following coronary occlusion: Effect of collateral blood flow. *Circulation* 50:176, (Abst.) (1974).

Heggtveit, H. A.: Morphological alterations in the ischemic heart. *Cardiology* 56:284-290 (1971-72).

Herdson, P. B., Sommers, H. M., and Jennings, R. B.: A comparative study of the fine structure of normal and ischemic dog myocardium with special reference to early changes following temporary occlusion of a coronary artery. *Am. J. Pathol.* 46:367-386 (1965).

Hirschhorn, R.: Lysosomes in inflammation. In *The Inflammatory Process,,* Vol. 1, B. W. Zweifach, L. Grant and R. McCluskey, eds. Academic Press, New York and London (1974), p. 259.

Hoffstein, S. T., Gennaro, D. E., Fox, A. C., Hirsch, J., Streuli, F., and Weissmann, G.: Colloidal lanthanum as a marker for impaired plasma membrane permeability in ischemic dog myocardium. *Am J. Pathol.* 79:206-217 (1975a).

Hoffstein, S., Gennaro, D., Weissmann, G., Hirsch, J., Streuli, F., and Fox, A. C.: Cytochemical localization of lysosomal enzyme activity in normal and ischemic dog myocardium. *Am J. Pathol.* 79:193-206 (1975b).

Hoffstein, S., Weissmann, G., and Fox, A. C.: Lysosomes in myocardial infarction: Studies by means of cytochemistry and subcellular fractionation, with observations on the effects of methylprednisolone. *Circulation* 53 (Suppl.) I:34-39 (1976).

Holtzer, B. S., and Van Lancker, J.: The release of acid phosphatase and beta-glucuronidase from cytoplasmic granules in the early course of autolysis. *Am. J. Pathol.* 35:563-573 (1958).

Hudgson, P., and Pearce, G. W.: In *Disorders of Voluntary Muscle*, 2nd ed., L. Walton, ed. Little Brown, Boston (1976), pp. 277-294.

Jennings, R. B., Baum, J. H., and Herdson, P. B.: Fine structural changes in myocardial ischemic injury. *Arch. Pathol.*, 79:135-143 (1965).

Jennings, R. B., Sommers, H. M., Herdson, P. B., and Kaltenbach, J. P.: Ischemic injury of the myocardium, *Ann. N.Y. Acad. Sci.* 156:61-78 (1969).

Kent, S. P.: Intracellular plasma protein: A manifestation of cell injury in myocardial ischemia. *Nature* (Lond.) 210:1279-1281 (1966).

Kent, S. P.: Diffusion of plasma proteins into cells: A manifestation of cell injury in human myocardial ischemia. *Am. J. Pathol.* 50:623-637 (1967).

Kloner, R. A., Ganote, C. E., and Jennings, R. B.: The "no-flow" phenomenon after temporary coronary occlusion in the dog. *J. Clin. Invest.* 54:1496-1508 (1974).

Kloner, R. A., Ganote, C. E., Reimer, K. A., and Jennings, R. B.: Distribution of coronary arterial flow in acute myocardial ischemia. *Arch. Pathol.* 99: 86-94 (1975).

Kloner, R. H., Ganote, C. E., Whalen, D. A., and Jennings, R. B.: Effect of a transient period of ischemia on myocardial cells. II. Fine structure during the first few minutes of reflow. *Am. J. Pathol.* 74:399-413 (1974).

Korb, G., and Totovic, V.: Electron microscopic studies on experimental ischemic lesions of the heart. *Ann. N. Y. Acad. Sci.* 156:48-60 (1969).

Leighty, E. G., Stoner, C. D., Ressallat, M. M., Tasananti, G. T., and Sirak, H. D.: Effects of acute asphyxia and deep hypothermia on the state of binding of lysosomal acid hydrolases in canine cardiac muscle. *Circ. Res.* 21:59-67 (1967).

Libby, P., Maroko, P. R., Bloor, C. M., Sobel, B. E., and Braunwald, E: Reduction of experimental myocardial infarction size by corticosteroid administration. *J. Clin. Invest.* 52:599-607 (1973).

Maroko, P. R., Libby, P., Ginks, W. R., Bloor, C. M., Shell, W. E., Sobel, B. E., and Ross, J. Jr.: Coronary artery reperfusion. I. Early effects on local myocardial function and the extent of myocardial necrosis. *J. Clin. Invest.* 51:2710-2716 (1972).

Nelson, D.: Hepatic lysosome and serum enzyme alterations in rats exposed to high altitude. *Amer J. Physiol.* 211:651-655 (1966).

Oran, E., and Brachfeld, N.: Myocardial metabolism and lysosomal expression of digitalis toxicity. *Circulation* 42 (Suppl. III): 7007 (1970).

Pearce, G. W.: Electron microscopy in the study of muscle disease. *Ann. N. Y. Acad. Sci.* 138:138-150 (1965a).

Pearce, G. W.: Research in muscular dystrophy. *Proceedings 3rd Symposium.* J. B. Lippincott Co., Philadelphia (1965b) pp. 146-173.

Ravens, K. G., and Gudbjarnason, S.: Changes in the activities of lysosomes in infarcted canine heart muscle. *Circ. Res.* 24:851-857 (1969).

Ricciutti, M. A.: Myocardial lysosome stability in the early stages of acute ischemic injury. *Am. J. Cardiol.* 30:492-497 (1972a).

Ricciutti, M. A.: Lysosomes and myocardial cellular injury. *Am. J. Cardiol.* 30: 498-502 (1972b).

Ricciutti, M., Scherlag, B., Stein, E., and Damato, A.: Lysosome stability and coronary artery occlusion. *Clin. Res.* 16:245 (1968).

Romeo, D., Stagni, N., Sottacasa, G. L., Pugliarello, M. C., DeBernard, B., and Vittur, F.: Lysosomes in heart tissue. *Biochim. Biophys. Acta.* 130:4-80 (1966).

Ruddy, S.: The complement and properdin systems. In *Madiators if Inflammation,* G. Weissmann, ed. Plenum Press, New York, (1974), pp. 113-140.

Rugh, R. C., Gottwik, M. G., Owens, K., McNamara, D. B., and Weglicki, W. B.: Subcellular localization of acid hydrolases in normal and dystrophic muscle. *Fed. Proc.* 34:257 (Abstr.) (1974).

Shnitka, T. K., and Nachlas, M. M.: Histochemical alterations in ischemic heart muscle and early myocardial infarctions. *Am. J. Pathol.* 42:507-527 (1973).

Sobel, B. E.: Biochemical and morphologic changes in infarcting myocardium. *Hosp. Pract.* Vol. 53:59-71 (1972).

Spath, J. A., Lane, D. L., and Lefer, A. M.: Protective action of methylprednisolone on the myocardium during experimental myocardial ischemia in the cat. *Circ. Res.* 35:44-51 (1974).

Stauber, W. T., and Bird J. W. C.: Zonal fractionation studies of rat skeletal muscle lysosome-rich fractions. *Biochem. Biophys.* Acta. 338: 234-245 (1974).

Topping, T .M., and Travis, D. F.: An electron cytochemical study of mechanisms of lysosomal activity in the rat left ventricular mural myocardium. *J. Ultrastruct. Res.* 46:1-22 (1974).

Weissmann, G.: Effects of corticosteroids on the stability and fusion of biomembranes. In *Asthma*, L. Lichtenstein and K. F. Austen, eds. Academic Press, New York and London (1973), pp. 221-223.

17

Metabolic Cellular Interrelationships during Myocardial Ischemia

NORMAN BRACHFELD

INTRODUCTION

A discussion of subcellular biochemical interrelationships during normal function and under conditions of myocardial ischemia might best be introduced by contrasting the two major components of myocardial cellular energy utilization. The myocardial cell performs as an isothermal engine that converts the potential chemical energy of metabolic fuel into an easily utilizable storage form, the pool of high-energy phosphate compounds. These molecules are subsequently utilized to meet two distinct types of demand, each expressed during one of the major divisions of the cardiac cycle. Energy consumption must, therefore, be considered as applicable to quite different but related cellular functions. When the supply of energy is limited, as occurs during severe ischemia, the response of each energy-dependent compartment which differs significantly, is expressed as hemodynamic and metabolic malfunction and has important implications for the maintenance of cellular viability. Table 1 outlines these requirements.

Table 1. Energy-requiring process of the myocardial cell

External Work (Systolic) + Internal Work (Diastolic)
= Total Energy Utilization

A. EXTERNAL WORK - SYSTOLIC ENERGY UTILIZATION

   1. Intramyocardial Tension (Stress)

      a. Ventricular pressure
      b. Intraventricular volume
      c. Myocardial mass

   2. Contractile State of the Heart

      a. Force velocity relation
      b. Maximal velocity of myocardial contraction (V Max)

   3. Heart Rate

B. WORK OF INTERNAL MAINTENANCE - DIASTOLIC ENERGY UTILIZATION

   1. Maintenance of Internal Cellular Milieu

      a. Substrate transport
      b. Intracellular oxidative phosphorylation
      c. RNA, protein, carbohydrate, lipid synthesis (macromolecules)

   2. Active Ion Transport (Na^+, Ca^{++})

      a. May consume 20-45% of total energy utilized by cell
      b. Thermogenesis

         i. Thyroid hormone
         ii. Catecholamines
         iii. Ion transport
         iv. Energy derived from hydrolysis of ATP and not utilized is expressed as heat or "entropy"

   3. Coronary Perfusion Pressure

      a. MVO_2 may relate to flow and oxygen availability under normoxemic conditions. Hetero-homogeneous perfusion may determine recruitment of contractile elements.

   4. Mechano-Chemical Transduction - Heat Production

      a. Internal work — 12-18% of total heat production
      b. Heat production is linearly related to peak developed tension
      c. Includes degraded work plus work of re-establishing internal biochemical conditions

   5. Cardiac Resting Heat

      a. About 2.5 ml O_2/100 g tissue
      b. Increases as resting tension rises
      c. Increases with an increase in calcium permeability

   6. Active Heat Production

      a. Heat in excess of resting heat
      b. Includes initial and recovery heat

   7. Tension-Independent Heat

      a. Increases with rate of stimulation
      b. May depend upon ion-pump mechanisms

THE ENERGY REQUIREMENTS OF MYOCARDIAL CONTRACTILITY

Systolic Energy Utilization

The greatest demand on cellular energy production, estimated as 80-90% of the total, is made during the performance of systolic, external pressure and flow work. Such activity is expressed thermodynamically as an increase in the entropy of the cell as it approaches an equilibrium state. When nutritional flow is compromised, there is an almost immediate reduction in the ability of the contractile components of the cell to perform normally. External work declines. Indeed, this may be viewed as a homeostatic attempt to match work performance to the availability of fuel. The possibility of making adjustments in this supply and demand relationship is utilized clinically when pharmacological agents are introduced to reduce myocardial oxygen requirements.

Preoperative ventriculographic evidence of akinesia or dyskinesia, with restoration to normal contractile activity after administration of inotropic agents or vasodilators, or following successful coronary artery bypass surgery, often provides dramatic clinical evidence to support the theoretical consideration that the non-contractile cell may retain the potential for recovery. It provides the framework for medical and surgical efforts to protect the ischemic myocardium and reduce infarct size.

The Work of Internal Maintenance - Diastolic Energy Utilization

The remaining 10-20% of the energy produced by the cell is quantitatively smaller but meets an equally important cellular requirement. It is utilized for the performance of internal cellular work—the work of internal maintenance. Since it is consumed during diastole, the so-called "resting state," it cannot be measured by orthodox hemodynamic parameters and is quantitated in terms of oxygen consumption or heat production. It may be defined as that energy necessary to maintain the cell in a state that is remote from its environment. Although we have traditionally expressed myocardial function in mechanistic terms, it must be remembered that the cell retains the synthetic and biological potential required of all living tissue, and must perform all the "work" necessary to maintain an appropriate internal cellular environment. During the "resting"phase of contraction, the cell consumes negentropy from its environment and utilizes it to reduce the increase in entropy induced by contraction, thus preparing for the ensuing systole. These "housekeeping" tasks include the support of ion and molecular transport, repair or replacement of subcellular particles, synthesis of molecules utilized for enzymatic or structural purposes, metabolic degradation of substrate, additional energy production and storage as well as other essential tasks. Thus, each cardiac cycle recapitulates the life of the organism as a whole.

When energy availability is reduced by inadequate perfusion, the degree of flexibility expressed by a decrement of mechanical performance is not matched by a reduction in diastolic requirements. The energy required for internal cellular maintenance is relatively fixed. As oxygen consumption falls, the work required to maintain an appropriate cellular environment consumes a proportionately greater percentage of that which is available. The cell ceases to contract normally and eventually becomes asystolic. It, nevertheless, maintains viability, damage is potentially reversible and normal function may be restored. What little oxygen and substrate is available is directed toward the maintenance of a homeostatic state as close to normal as possible. All internal mechanisms are mobilized to retain viability.

Utilization of marginal supplies of oxygen has widespread biological ramifications and obviously represents an extraordinarily unstable state. When flow falls below this irreducible minimum requirement for even brief periods of time, the life of the cell is threatened and irreversible damage may occur.

Disruption of the energy-producing or consuming pathway is reflected by measurable distortions of virtually all metabolic processes as well as by evidence of mechanical and electrical malfunction. Such changes are the cause of the clinical abnormalities we observe when we evaluate patients with ischemic heart disease.

"ISCHEMIC HEART DISEASE" - A MISNOMER

Coronary artery disease leads to a unique type of metabolic cardiac abnormality that interferes with the chemical transformation of potential energy in sufficient amounts to support contractility and, ultimately, threatens cellular viability. The term "ischemic heart disease" is actually a misnomer. It does not involve the heart as a whole. The vascular process is most often segmental and may affect one or more vessels, with varying degrees of severity. Nutritional insufficiency is rarely fixed and occurs only during the most extreme reductions in flow or increases in demand. It usually terminates in cell death. Most frequently, the ischemic state oscillates in severity determined by many factors, including non-uniform distribution of collateral flow and metabolic demands which, in turn, are regulated by the contractile state, heart rate, perfusion pressure, wall stress or tension as a function of blood pressure and cardiac volume, and both humoral and pharmacological influences. It is thus an intermittent cellular disease of regional distribution, never a global phenomenon.

Metabolism implies living tissue, and the processes of ischemic metabolism are dynamic phenomena in a constant state of flux and demonstrating an extreme degree of instability. The margin between myocardial cell life and death is often difficult to accurately define. There is rarely a sharp line of demarcation between reversible and irreversible damage.

Not too long ago, we naively assumed that myocardial infarction was an all-or-none type of injury which consisted of a central zone of homogeneously necrotic tissue, surrounded by a slim periphery of ischemic myocardium. This is certainly not the case. The "infarct" is rarely discrete but most often consists of multiple borderzones with cell populations that present (at least initially) as a heterogenous mixture of constantly changing proportions. Such cells have widely different metabolic and hemodynamic expressions, and provide evidence of normal, mild, moderate and severe ischemic metabolism and contractile ability. We may find essentially normal cells consuming energy at normal or supernormal rates, and utilizing it to perform normal internal and external work, lying adjacent to cells that are contracting poorly or not at all, and whose total or near-total energy consumption is devoted to the maintenance of viability. In the surviving organ, this state of scattered segments of "diseased" tissue most frequently comprises less than 20% of total myocardial mass.

The unique nature of the ischemic heart-disease process bears emphasis. The great majority of its victims demonstrate intermittent symptomatic expression which may be precipitated by many known and unknown factors. Others may be symptom free, yet show "ischemic" ST-segment changes during normal daily activities (Kennedy et al., 1976). A diverse spectrum of responses may be produced in different patients who suffer from the same degree of coronary luminal narrowing. Indeed, those with severe angina pectoris and those with severe chronic congestive heart failure may be considered to represent opposite ends of the clinical spectrum (Roberts et al., 1974). Patients with angina alone and no evidence of previous myocardial infarction may demonstrate normal myocardium or, at most, patchy subendocardial scarring. In those with congestive heart failure, ventricular aneurysm formation and transmural scarring are often present. In the former, ischemic heart disease is expressed as recurrent pain; in the latter—as dyspnea. The pathological studies reported by Roberts and coworkers (1974) stress that the explanation does not reside in the coronary arteries (Roberts et al., 1974). One may speculate that, in the former group of patients, energy demands intermittently exceed nutritional flow to a degree that is sufficient to precipitate a pain and/or hemodynamic response (or electrocardiographic changes in the absence of pain) but not great enough to exceed the requirements for internal maintenance. With reduction in demand or return of flow, normal function resumes. In the latter group, nutritional flow has proven inadequate to maintain viability and necrosis ensues. Disparate responses of this type have long troubled those interested in the gross pathology of coronary artery disease and suggest that the "supply and demand" concept, which we use to describe the balance upon which coronary vascular reserve is based, may be overly simplistic and ignore many as yet unknown but significant factors.

PROTECTION OF THE ISCHEMIC MYOCARDIUM

It is barely 15 years since the first units specifically dedicated to the care of patients with myocardial infarction were inaugurated in this country. Continuous electrocardiographic monitoring and use of antidysrhythmic drugs, and electrical cardioversion and defibrillation have substantially reduced mortality from previously lethal dysrhythmias. Unfortunately, mortality related entirely to the quantitative amount of ischemic or necrotic myocardium remains alarmingly high.

The recent interest in the development of techniques designed to protect the ischemic myocardium and reduce infarct size is an attempt to move off this therapeutic plateau, and indicates a potentially new era in our approach to ischemic heart disease. We have seen a progression from monitoring and treating dysrhythmias as they occurred, to the aggressive use of antidysrhythmic drugs and, more recently, to the application of interventions developed to support ischemic, but viable tissue.

The experimental techniques described by several centers have not long ago been reviewed by Braunwald and Maroko (1974) ; in general, these methods attempt to increase myocardial oxygen supply, reduce myocardial oxygen demand or increase metabolic support. Although many have proven successful under laboratory conditions, none have as yet been applied as routine therapy. They are outlined in Table 2. The potential efficacy of such therapeutic interventions, whether medical or surgical, is directed toward improving *relative* nutritional flow to multiple, small areas whose loss of viability often leads to loss of the entire organ. Success or failure undoubtedly relates to the quantitative mass of tissue involved, its location and the degree of pre-existing disease.

MEASUREMENT OF INFARCT SIZE

Evaluation of the success of an intervention requires an adequate animal model for experimental study and an accurate, objective, easily utilizable method for the measurement of the mass of ischemic or infarcted myocardium, or for the prediction of ultimate infarct size. Regrettably, these requirements have so far not been met.

The most frequently utilized techniques at the present time include precordial ST-segment mapping, enzyme measurements and myocardial imaging. Unfortunately, all remain in the developmental stage and require further refinement. The first two have proven to be less valuable as a routine tool than initial reports had indicated. They undoubtedly provide evidence of deterioration of cell-membrane polarization and enzymatic proof of cell damage. However, at the current state of the art, they are of greater qualitative than quantitative value. Furthermore, these techniques are not only cumbersome but often also imprecise, time consuming, not easily reproduceable in less experienced hands and subject to a variety of non-controllable variables.

Epicardial ST-Segment Mapping

Epicardial ST-segment mapping has, in general, shown a good correlation with subsequent pathological study. Unfortunately, extrapolation to precordial mapping has proven less than satisfactory. Its use as a quantitative tool is challenged by our ignorance of the true causes of such distortions of membrane polarization. ST-segment changes certainly demonstrate deterioration of repolarization

Table 2. Interventions which aid the preservation of the ischemic myocardium
(After Braunwald and Maroko, 1974)

A. DECREASING MYOCARDIAL OXYGEN DEMAND

   1. Beta Blockade, Propranolol
   2. Glycosides in Congestive Heart Failure
   3. Counterpulsation

      a. Intra-aortic balloon
      b. External counterpulsation

   4. Nitroglycerin
   5. Decrease in Preload

      a. Ethacrynic acid
      b. Furosamide

   6. Decrease in Afterload with Hypertension

      a. Arfonad
      b. Nitroprusside

   7. Inhibition of Lipolysis

      a. Beta-pyridyl-carbinol

B. INCREASING MYOCARDIAL OXYGEN SUPPLY

   1. Directly

      a. Coronary artery reperfusion
      b. Elevation of arterial PO_2
      c. Thrombolytic agents

   2. Through Collateral Vessels

      a. Elevation of perfusion pressure with: methoxamine, phenylephrine, norepinephrine
      b. Internal and external counterpulsation

   3. Increasing Plasma Osmolality

      a. Mannitol, dextran, sucrose, glucose

   4. Increasing coronary flow

      a. Methylprednisolone?

C. AUGMENTING ANAEROBIC METABOLISM (PRESUMED)

   1. Glucose-Insulin-Potassium
   2. Hyptertonic Glucose
   3. Reversal of Electron Flow

      a. Glucose-malate-glutamate
      b. Glucose-oxaloacetate-a-oxoglutarate

   4. Increasing Cardiac Glycogen Stores

      a. Propranolol
      b. Reserpine
      c. Physical training
      d. Increased utilization of FFA

Table 2. Interventions which aid the preservation of the ischemic
myocardium *(continued)*

D. ENHANCING TRANSPORT OF SUBSTRATE TO THE ISCHEMIC ZONE (PRESUMED)

   a. Hyaluronidase

E. PROTECTING AGAINST HETEROLYTIC AND AUTOLYTIC PROCESSES

   1. Hydrocortisone, Methylprednisolone
   2. Cobra Venom Factor

F. REVERSAL OF ABNORMAL MITOCHONDRIAL OXIDATIVE PHOSPHORYLATION
BY CALCIUM ION DURING ISCHEMIA (EXPERIMENTAL)

   1. Chelation - EDTA
   2. Ca^{++} Antagonists - Verapamil

G. MISCELLANEOUS

   1. Maintenance of Body Pool of Purine Bases

     a. Allopurinol

   2. Reversal of Inhibition of Adenine Nucleotide Translocase by Long-Chain Acyl CoA
esters L-Carnitine

   3. Kallikrein Antagonists

---

but are non specific reflections of disturbances in ion transport, energy metabolism or unknown cause. They may be seen in such nonischemic processes as those associated with cardiomyopathies, body position, hyperventilation, ventricular hypertrophy, left bundle-branch block (LBBB), the Wolf-Parkinson-White syndrome, "Prinzmetal angina" without intrinsic coronary artery disease, increased sympathetic tone, early depolarization, left ventricular aneurysm, pericarditis and other unknown factors that may be responsible for the false-positive ST-segment depressions noted during treadmill tests in subjects with normal coronary arteries.

Serum CPK

Quantitation of infarct size by serial determination of creatine-phosphokinase (CPK) activity necessitates a delay prior to administration of a planned intervention, is less accurate than was initially suggested, requires multiple biochemical determinations and availability of computer time for curve-fitting techniques that permit comparison of projected CPK values to serial changes actually observed. Such determinations are made by analysis of a highly complex biological system. The main difficulties encountered relate to the many factors that affect the fractional disappearance rate of CPK, and include pharmacological interventions following admission to hospital and hemodynamic alterations in cardiac output. Such changes are said to be capable of producing an error of as much as $\pm 15\%$ from the mean calculated mass (Roe and Starmer, 1975). Variations in myocardial depletion rate, extracellular, intravascular and lymphatic distribution space, and the proportion of the enzyme that appears in each space are all capable of introducing significant errors in less than expert hands. A number of technical problems encountered in the assay methodology itself has further complicated its use. Finally, there is a rapid temperature-related and sometimes unpredictable breakdown of CPK within tissue and a high activation energy. A rise in body temperature of one degree, which may occur during acute myocardial infarction, can increase the error of the determination by as much as 20%. The method and assay technology have been subject to intensive current investigation and have been considerably improved. The addition of CPK isoenzyme determinations also promises to further refine the accuracy of the CPK technique.

Radioisotope Myocardial Imaging

Efforts to improve the definition of myocardial imaging by accumulation of radioisotope in the area of ischemia or surrounding normal myocardium holds promise for the future and appears to be especially well suited for evaluation of those interventions that might improve nutritional flow.

Clinical Implications

There is currently no consistently effective simple means for measuring myocardial infarct size in man. The clinical applications of many of the interventions described have been extrapolated from animal studies. However promising they may appear, cardiologists have been unable to utilize them adequately *in vivo* and provide objective evidence of ability to protect the ischemic myocardium or reduce infarct size. Encouraging results must be interpreted by less than satisfactory prospective epidemiological data evaluation.

Despite these *caveats*, it must be acknowledged that animal models have provided encouraging findings to support the potential efficacy of many of the therapeutic approaches outlined above. Furthermore, early clinical applications have also been encouraging. It would not be unduly optimistic to expect that most hospital units will have an acceptable technique for the quantification of infarct size, a measure of the potential extent of injury, its degree of reversibility and a means for determining and evaluating optimal therapy in the not too distant future.

PATHOGENESIS OF ISCHEMIC TISSUE INJURY

Cellular ischemia may be said to exist when reduction in arterial flow proves insufficient to meet oxygen demand (Jennings, 1970). Adequate perfusion may be prevented by a decrease in perfusion pressure and flow, induced by large-vessel insufficiency as well as by a *temporary* increase in peripheral myocardial vascular resistance, secondary to arteriolar vasoconstriction, an increase in intra-myocardial pressure, a reduction in capillary perfusion due to endothelial cell swelling or to a rate-related decrease in diastolic perfusion time. Furthermore, there is suggestive evidence that, under rare circumstances, coronary vasospasm may play a role in decreasing perfusion.

Histologic Evidence of Ischemia

The series of studies reported by Jennings et al. (1975) has established an optical and electron-microscopic basis for tissue response to a decrease in flow. The use of nuclide-labeled microspheres, to yield sequential instantaneous estimates of local flow, has confirmed that it is possible to quantitate regional differences in depressed flow and, thus, of severity of ischemia within the same zone. Both vasoactivity and the anatomic location of collateral-flow channels, supplied by arteriolar and larger anastomosis, determines the supply of potential nutritional flow. This non-uniformity of ischemic injury—necrotic cells being mixed with normal, mildly, moderately and severely ischemic cells—is further complicated by existence of a transmural flow gradient. Oxygen tension (PO_2) is more markedly reduced in the subendocardium than in the subepicardium. There are also lateral gradients which insure that the center of the ischemic zone receives less flow than does the periphery (Jennings et al., 1975). These anatomic gradients are accompanied by metabolic transmural tissue gradients for glycogen, lactate, high-energy phosphate and other metabolites (Karlsson et al., 1973; Griggs et al., 1972).

Reversible and Irreversible Ischemic Tissue Injury

There is rarely a sharp line of demarcation between reversible and irreversible ischemic damage. Necrosis may be evident as early as 20 min after cessation of primary vessel flow and be progressive, with more and more cells succumbing over a period of 24 hr (Jennings et al., 1960; Jennings and Reimer, 1974). In some experimental studies, histological evidence of irreversibility, that is, necrosis or scarring did not occur until 1-7 days after reflow (Jennings et al., 1960). These studies and those of Alonso and coworkers (1973) indicate that myocardial infarction is not a completed process upon early admission to hospital despite demonstration of diagnostic ECG and enzyme changes. They suggest a continuum of changes, with probable progression of necrosis and extension of the initial area of infarction for hours or days after these patients come under observation. The possibility of therapeutic intervention is, thus, a very real challenge for the future.

ANGINA PECTORIS AND CORONARY INSUFFICIENCY, THE PRE-INFARCTION STATE OF ISCHEMIC HEART DISEASE

The foregoing analysis suggests that there is value in our ability to identify a significant reduction in coronary reserve capacity with some degree of precision prior to a coronary event.

In many cases, we need do little more than review a patient's history and complete a physical examination. Further diagnostic refinement, though not truly quantitative, is provided by the use of graded exercise electrocardiography. Coronary angiography is *not* an acceptable tool for the functional evaluation of coronary reserve. It should not be utilized for this purpose and when so misapplied may lead to inappropriate diagnostic conclusions and therapeutic intervention. Carefully performed ventriculographic studies that include evaluation of hemodynamic parameters, pressure-volume analysis, ejection-fraction calculation, etc., and visualization of ventricular-wall motion are proving to be of increasing value. They contribute, as do echocardiographic studies, to our understanding of the functional meaning of insufficient nutritional flow. Right-heart catheterization at the time of coronary angiography and ventriculography permits atrial pacing and coronary sinus blood sampling. Such stress studies are of particular value since they offer an opportunity for combining coronary anatomic definition, determination of ventricular function, electrocardiographic response to stress and biochemical quantitation of evidence of ischemic metabolism. This technique not only offers many diagnostic advantages but establishes a true baseline against which response to subsequent therapy may be measured.

Regional Myocardial Metabolism

The introduction of surgical and medical techniques for improving relative or absolute nutritional flow to ischemic cells makes it of more than academic interest for us to determine, with some degree of precision, the severity of myocardial ischemia and its anatomic location. The biochemical characterization of ischemic myocardium has as its major focus the identification of ischemic, yet viable and potentially salvageable myocardium which, without successful intervention, is almost certainly destined to be transformed into infarcted tissue. Once this has occurred, restoration of coronary blood flow can do little to improve function and has been implicated in hemorrhagic infarction. Continuous refinement of techniques, improvement in assay sensitivity and careful selection of metabolic parameters may make it possible to quantify and predict the extent of injury, determine its degree of reversibility and help provide a guideline for evaluating optimal intervention.

Graded atrial pacing during cardiac catheterization has proven to be an effective, sensitive and objective means for challenging coronary vascular reserve. The pacing stimulus is increased until a target rate has been reached, severe chest pain is induced or diagnostic ischemic changes are noted during a continuously monitored electrocardiogram.

Ischemic Myocardial Metabolism

In 1947, Bing et al. reported catheterization of the coronary sinus and middle cardiac vein in man and soon exploited this technique to describe the normal myocardial patterns of substrate utilization. The development of techniques to measure coronary flow *in vivo* and the application of sophisticated biochemical-assay methodology permitted the evaluation of pathways utilized in the cellular metabolism of the major substrate classes under normal and abnormal conditions. The heart was shown to demonstrate wide substrate adaptability and to be capable of utilizing most nutritional substances. It normally extracted glucose, pyruvate, lactate and free fatty acids but was capable of consuming acetate, ketone bodies and amino acid under appropriate circumstances. Extraction patterns were influenced by many factors, including absolute and relative arterial concentrations, and the permeability of the plasma membrane which sets transport thresholds. Oxidative metabolism was shown to be markedly flow dependent since oxygen extraction was near maximal at rest. An increase in demand for available free energy, most often induced by an increase in work, showed a near linear correlation with enhancement of coronary flow.

CLINICAL APPLICATION OF METABOLIC STUDIES

Wollenberger (1949) and Olson (1959) suggested that a defect in myocardial energetics may be induced by an insufficient production of energy, a defective storage of energy, or an inability to utilize energy efficiently. They suggested an approach by which biochemical data that had previously been of essentially academic interest could be utilized in a clinical setting. It soon became apparent that this information was more applicable in the experimental animal and during steady-state performance in man. It was subject to all of the limitations imposed by intact biological systems and often failed to detect subtle changes in metabolic balance. It also assumed homogeneous myocardial perfusion. Substrate storage and dilutional problems caused by metabolic pools made it difficult to equate consumption of substrate with its utilization without isotopic substrate labeling. Explanations for the infrequent but puzzling lack of reproduceability, when metabolic pacing-stress studies were performed in patients with coronary artery disease, have only lately become apparent and recent modifications of this technique have enhanced its diagnostic value.

VARIABILITY OF PERFUSION TO THE ISCHEMIC ZONE

The absence of biochemical evidence of ischemia after pacing in patients with known coronary disease often occurs as a result of mixing problems or non-uniform distribution of perfusion. Drainage from ischemic zones may be diluted by effluent flow from normal areas of the ventricle. Mixing of effluent from tissues with different metabolic rates may induce a variety of errors in interpretation. Furthermore, if the coronary effluent from the ischemic area drains into the coronary sinus proximal to the position of the tip of the catheter, it cannot be sampled. The introduction of multiple-site sampling of myocardial venous drainage by Herman et al. (1967) has improved our ability to detect and localize regional abnormalities. This clinical study was confirmed by evaluation of regional metabolic changes in the myocardium following ligation of the anterior descending coronary artery of the dog. Samples of venous effluent drawn from a position deep in the great cardiac vein were compared to those taken from the ostia of the coronary sinus (Obeid et al., 1972). Confirmation was also obtained by Owen et al. (1970) in experiments that compared metabolic changes in local venous and coronary sinus blood after acute coronary arterial occlusion. Corday and coworkers (1974) have emphasized that the metabolic consequences of coronary arterial insufficiency must be studied by assay of samples draining the zone of ischemia. When the left circumflex artery is experimentally occluded, drainage from the great cardiac vein represents the venous return from the non-ischemic area perfused by the left anterior descending coronary artery. An intra-coronary balloon catheter has been designed to separate the venous blood which originates from ischemic and non-ischemic myocardium; it permits localization and assessment of regional myocardial oxygen and substrate metabolism (Corday et al., 1974).

DIAGNOSTIC IMPLICATIONS OF ISCHEMIC METABOLIC CHANGES

Hoffstein et al. (1975) have utilized colloidal lanthanum to demonstrate that injury to the plasma membrane is an early event in the pathogenesis of ischemic cellular damage. Increased permeability to ions and macromolecules is noted before overt structural changes appear. Although virtually all metabolic pathways are affected by a critical reduction in flow, our ability to demonstrate abnormal arteriovenous differences for specific compounds at rest, post myocardial infarction or after a pacing-induced stress is determined by many factors. These include membrane binding and permeability, the severity of ischemia, the sensitivity of our assays, sampling sites and times, the nutritional state of the patient and other variables. Although apparently paradoxical, it is evident that with total cessation of flow tissue metabolism becomes completely anaerobic and soon ceases. While abnormal metabolic intermediates will accumulate within the cell, the absence of washout will preclude appearance of such substances in venous drainage. As one progresses to areas of moderate to mild ischemia, flow insures that substrate will reach the injured cells and energy production can proceed via a mixture of aerobic and anaerobic metabolism. Washout can occur and venous sampling will provide evidence of abnormal metabolism. Mildly ischemic tissue probably provides the greatest amount of these by-products (Jennings et al., 1975; Opie, 1975).

Pacing-Induced Ischemia

Venous sampling after pacing-induced ischemia has proven particularly useful in the evaluation of patients with atypical chest pain, normal resting and exercise electrocardiograms, and angiograms compatible with moderate coronary artery disease. Such patients often pose difficult diagnostic and therapeutic problems which may be resolved by metabolic studies. This approach is equally applicable for determination of the effectiveness of surgical or pharmacological intervention for coronary artery disease. If proper precautions are taken in the interpretation of data, atrial pacing and coronary sinus sampling may offer an objective method for the biochemical demonstration of myocardial ischemia (Brachfeld, 1974).

Pacing-induced stress in man is accompanied by measurable changes in all major substrate classes. Fig. 1 illustrates the changes in carbohydrate metabolism that have proven to be of diagnostic value. Group I, control patients, are compared to patients with angina pectoris of variable severity. In both groups, fractional glucose extraction was augmented in response to pacing and was unrelated to arterial concentration (Most et al., 1972). Enhanced anaerobic carbohydrate metabolism was noted in patients with coronary insufficiency, however, and was demonstrated by marked differences in lactate metabolism. At rest, lactate extraction in the control group exceeded that in group II patients by 33%. In both, lactate extraction fell during pacing. In control patients, this decrease was compatible with the enhanced glucose extraction and glycogenolysis associated with an increase in myocardial work. Mean fractional extraction was 13%, well within the normal range. In patients who were unable to meet the demands of an increase in heart rate, glycolysis "overloaded" oxidative pathways and the pattern of lactate metabolism were reversed from extraction to "production." There was a net *negative* anteriovenous balance of 34%.

Free fatty acid (FFA) metabolism is also quite sensitive to alterations in oxygen availablity. Fig. 2 compares sodium palmitate

METABOLIC STUDIES IN ANGINA PECTORIS

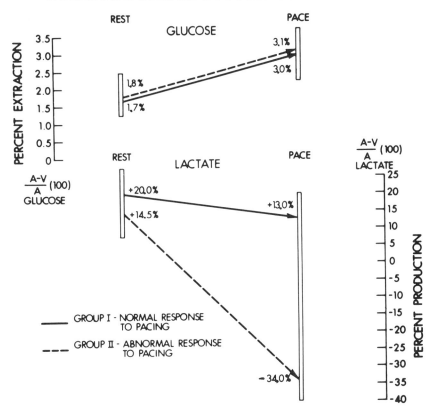

1   Metabolic cellular interrelationships during myocardial ischemia.

metabolism, evaluated by both chemical and radionuclide methodology. Patients with normal nutritional flow demonstrated an enhancement of myocardial fractional extraction of this FFA, which exceeded the resting state by 15.6%. In those with pacing-induced ischemia, the normal pattern was reversed and extraction fell 37%. It is of further interest that, despite this decrease in extraction, the oxidation of FFA which was transported into the cell increased significantly (Brachfeld et al., 1971).

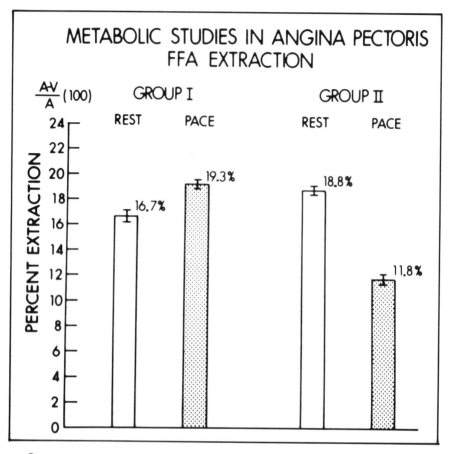

2   Metabolic cellular interrelationships during myocardial ischemia.

Estimation of Myocardial Ischemia Based upon Pacing-Induced Venous Lactate Data

The general availability, accuracy and ease of methods for assay of serum lactate concentration has established its popularity for diagnostic and investigative evidence of enhanced anaerobic glycolytic activity. Authors of preceding chapters in this volume have commented on the metabolic pathways responsible for this "production" of lactate by ischemic myocardium.

Table 3. Significant factors in evaluating myocardial lactate data

1. Nutritional Status of the Patient
   a. Infusion of glucose, pyruvate or lactate. There is a positive correlation between lactate extraction and arterial lactate concentration
   b. Arterial lactate is elevated with shock, hypoxia
   c. Diabetes
   d. Elevated serum FFA concentration may suppress extraction of carbohydrate and induce pyruvate efflux
2. Alkalosis, Hyperventilation, Bicarbonate Infusion
3. Catheter Placement, Inadequate Sampling, Segmental Disease
   a. Sampling site may be proximal to vein draining ischemic area
   b. Drainage from ischemic area may be meager or absent
   c. Dilution of ischemic drainage by normal venous efflux

The validity of this estimation requires that the muscle-cell membrane be freely permeable to lactate and pyruvate, and that there be an equilibrium between cytoplasmic and mitochondrial NADH concentration—assumptions that are not entirely justified. If the clinician is aware of potential pitfalls, misinterpretation may be avoided and this extrapolation considered valid for all practical purposes (Opie et al., 1973; Gorlin, 1972). Table 3 lists some of the factors of importance in evaluating myocardial venous lactate data. Although patients with myocardial ischemia may show evidence of enhanced glycolysis when coronary reserve is challenged, myocardial glycolysis is accelerated by many factors in the absence of coronary artery disease. Despite adequate oxygenation if the capacity of the hydrogen shuttle is exceeded, lactate may be formed from pyruvate.

Potential Pitfalls in Evaluation of Myocardial Venous Lactate Data

Pacing studies should not be performed unless the subject is in a steady (basal) nutritional, metabolic and hormonal state. Sampling, after an overnight fast which induces a period of active metabolism of elevated FFA, is accompanied by suppression of circulating glucose, lactate and pyruvate concentration, as well as inhibition of pyruvate dehydrogenase activity, so that an increased amount of pyruvate is converted to lactate. Glycolysis is also depressed by citrate-induced inhibition of phosphofructokinase (PFK) activity, extraction of carbohydrate is reduced, and myocardial arteriovenous differences are difficult to determine accurately. Starved rats show a decrease in their myocardial L/P ratio. Conversely, hyperglycemia caused by glucose infusion will enhance its extraction and the formation of both pyruvate and lactate, prevent steady-state determinations, and produce a transit time artifact (Gorlin, 1972). Exercise-stress tests, popular for evaluation of coronary insufficiency, cannot be utilized for estimation of myocardial glycolysis, because of the accompanying increase in arterial lactate concentration, and have been replaced by pacing-induced stress. Shock and generalized hypoxia, from whatever cause, are also associated with marked elevations in arterial lactate concentration and constitute a contraindication for coronary sinus studies.

Henderson et al. (1969) have postulated compartmentation of tissue lactate, and demonstrated differing transmembrane concentration gradients for lactate and pyruvate. The rate of pyruvate efflux from the isolated heart was shown to exceed that of lactate by 10-fold. Many investigators have, therefore, abandoned pyruvate determinations and L/P ratios in favor of a lactate assay alone, recognizing that the loss in sensitivity is compensated for by increased reliability.

The relative inhibition of membrane transport of glucose in diabetes mellitus reduces glycolytic flux, and is associated with a decrease in L/P ratio and with pyruvate accumulation. In studies performed with the isolated diabetic heart, the addition of insulin enhanced glycolytic flow, but pyruvate accumulation persisted. Further, the elevation in circulating FFA and ketone bodies, noted in poorly controlled diabetes, leads to citrate-induced inhibition of PFK activity and further depresses glycolysis. Both FFA and ketone bodies are extracted from the arterial blood in preference to lactate and, when present in significant concentrations, will distort the L/P ratios of the coronary venous samples and cause a misleading drop in the calculated percentage of lactate extraction. Enhanced insulin resistance or latent diabetes, frequently noted in the post-coronary state, must also be considered when such studies are performed.

Other hormones and drugs (growth hormone, cortisol, heparin) modulate glycolytic flux by mobilization of FFA. Perhaps, the most common mechanism for the mobilizaton of FFA from adipose depots is that stimulated by an increase in catecholamine secretion. Patients undergoing diagnostic pacing studies often demonstrate anxiety symptoms and elevated blood-catecholamine levels, especially when paced to the onset of angina. Finally, it must be noted that glucagon has been shown to accelerate conversion of phosphorylase "b" to "a," thus enhancing glycogenolysis and increasing the output of lactate.

Scheuer and Berry (1967) reported that alkalosis increased myocardial lactate production as well as exogenous glucose and endogenous glycogen utilization during normal oxygenation. These effects were noted irrespective of whether pH changes occurred as a result of lowering PCO_2 or by increasing the bicarbonate content. The mechanism involved appears to be a stimulation of PFK activity. The Pasteur effect is disrupted by alkalosis since PFK activity is relieved from ATP inhibition by an elevation of pH.

During hypoxia, metabolic alkalosis is associated with improved ventricular pressure and rate of pressure rise, neither oxygen consumption nor lactate production is increased, and L/P ratios are lower than in controls. Huckabee (1958) also reported lactate production in hyperventilating human subjects. Thus, alkalosis alone may double lactate production.

It is evident that evaluation of lactate data may be inconclusive without simultaneous determination of pH, bicarbonate concentration and arteriovenous glucose levels.

Hexokinase and PFK activity may be accelerated in the isolated heart preparation by an acute increase in work (Neely et al., 1972). Glucose and glycogen consumption rises, as does output of lactate and pyruvate. Lactate production is similarly doubled when contractility is enhanced by raising the calcium concentration of perfusate solutions (Kuhn and Pachinger, 1972). Other more exotic causes of lactate production in the face of normal oxygenation include cardiac transplantation, uncoupling or interruption of the respiratory chain by cyanide, a variety of idiopathic cardiomyopathies, phenformin-induced and idiopathic lactic acidosis, and alcohol ingestion. The latter agent taken in excessive quantities increases cytoplasmic hydrogen-ion content at a rate greater than that at which it can be shuttled to the mitochondrion for oxidation.

Despite great care, one may still fail to obtain evidence of ischemia by relying on evidence of anaerobic glycolysis alone. It would, therefore, seem wise to simultaneously evaluate several parameters during pacing studies. Table 4 outlines ischemia-induced metabolic abnormalities that may be recognized by coronary venous sampling and analysis.

Table 4. Metabolic abnormalities induced by cardiac pacing

1. Increased glucose extraction
2. Decrease in lactate extraction, lactate production
3. FFA extraction decreased, oxidation increased
4. Negative potassium balance
5. Adenosine release into coronary venous blood
6. Prostaglandin F (PGF) release into venous blood
7. Bradykinin release into venous blood
8. Alanine release into venous blood
9. Fall in venous pH, oxygen desaturation

ADDITIONAL DIAGNOSTIC METABOLIC ABNORMALITIES ASSOCIATED WITH PACING-INDUCED ISCHEMIA

A negative potassium balance induced by pacing was reported by Parker and coworkers (1970) and demonstrated experimentally by Opie et al. (1972) in hearts whose ischemic zone comprised more than 15% of total heart volume. Opie also reported an increase in coronary venous inorganic phosphate that exceeded arterial concentration by more than 15-20% and was felt to reflect the intracellular breakdown of high-energy phosphate compounds (Opie et al., 1972). Fox and his group (1974) reported the release of adenosine into coronary sinus blood of patients paced to the onset of angina and found such release to be a valuable supplementary index of the early effects of ischemia on myocardial metabolism. Berger et al. (1976) recently described release of prostaglandin F (PGF) in 11 of 12 patients paced to the onset of angina. Although the precise site of PGF release was not known, its correlation with regional myocardial ischemia suggested that this potent substance may also play a physiological role in the cellular response to ischemia. Bradykinin, another physiological vasoactive substance, has been identified in the coronary venous effluent of patients with significant coronary-artery disease by Pitt and coworkers (1969). Alterations in amino-acid metabolism, during ischemia, leading to release of alanine both at rest and after pacing was reported by Mills et al. (1975). Finally, a fall in venous pH and oxygen desaturation of venous samples often, although not invariably, accompanies pacing-induced angina.

CONCLUSIONS AND SOME UNSOLVED PROBLEMS

The initial impact of the coronary-care concept on mortality from myocardial infarction has been realized. Recent experimental reports indicate that we are entering into a new phase in the treatment of coronary insufficiency and myocardial ischemia. The contemporary approach stresses cellular support for the threatened myocardium rather than accepting infarction as an inevitable and essentially untreatable pathological event. I have attempted to outline current biochemical methods for characterization of the ischemic process by regional metabolism since it appears evident that such definition will prove of both diagnostic and prognostic value.

Unfortunately, as old problems are solved, new ones continue to appear. We remain baffled by the high incidence of myocardial infarction occurring at rest in previously asymptomatic patients and in some few patients with "normal" coronary arteries. The pathogenesis of the so-called "Prinzmetal angina" is still an enigma as is the true relationship between angina pectoris and myocardial infarction. Are these two separate diseases or different limbs of the same tree? The existence of coronary vasospasm and its potential for inducing myocardial ischemia was speculated upon over 50 years ago but has long been thought of as an anatomic impossibility. Nevertheless, reports are appearing with increasing frequency that offer convincing angiographic evidence that coronary vasospasm may be implicated as a cause of myocardial ischemia in man (Maseri et al., 1975). Finally, many of us continue to wonder if an adaptation to a state of chronic ischemia is possible or, indeed, if ischemia can exist on a chronic basis without ultimately evolving into myocardial infarction.

ACKNOWLEDGMENTS

This work was supported by the New York Cardiac Center, the Lincoln National Life Insurance Company, the Massachusetts Mutual Life Insurance Company, the North American Reassurance Company, the Manhattan Life Insurance Company, the Home Life Insurance Company, the Estelle Ferkauf Foundation, and the Hearst Foundation.

REFERENCES

Alonso, D. R., Scheidt, S., Post, M., and Killip, T.: Pathophysiology of cardiogenic shock. *Circulation* 48:588-596 (1973).

Berger, H. J., Zaret, B. L., Speroff, L., Cohen, L. S., and Wolfson, S.: Cardiac prostaglandin release during myocardial ischemia induced by atrial pacing in patients with coronary artery disease. *Cir. Res.* 38:566-571 (1976).

Bing, R. J., Vandam, L. D., Gregoir, F., Hansdelman, C., Goodale, W. T., and Eckenhoff, J. E.: Catheterization of coronary sinus and middle cardiac vein in man. *Proc. Soc. Exp. Biol. Med.* 66:239-240 (1947).

Brachfeld, N.: Ischemic myocardial metabolism and cell necrosis. *Bull. N. Y. Acad. Med.* 50:261-293 (1974).

Brachfeld, N., Keller, N,. Tarjan, E., Klein, S. A., and Apstein, C.: Myocardial metabolism following pacing induced stress. *Circulation* (Suppl.) 44:145 (1971).

Braunwald, E., and Maroko, P. R.: The reduction of infarct size - An idea whose time (for testing) has come. *Circulation* 50:206-209 (1974).

Corday E. Lang, T., Meerbaum, S., Gold, H., Hirose, S., Rubins, S., and Dalcastro, M.:Closed chest model of intracoronary occlusion for study of regional cardiac function. *Am. J. Cardiol.* 33:49-59 (1974).

Fox, A. C., Reed, G. E., Glassman, E., Kaltman, A. J., and Silj, B. B.: Release of adenosine from human hearts during angina induced by rapid atrial pacing. *J. Clin. Invest.* 53:1447-1457 (1974).

Gorlin, R.: Assessment of hypoxia in the human heart. *Cardiology* 57:24-34 (1972).

Griggs, D. M., Tchokoev, V. V., and Chen, C. C.: Transmural differences in ventricular tissue substrate levels due to coronary constriction. *Am. J. Physiol.* 222:705-709 (1972).

Henderson, A. H., Craig, R. J.: Gorlin, R., and Sonnenblick, E. H.: Lactate and pyruvate kinetics in isolated perfused rat hearts. *Am. J. Physiol.* 217: 1752-1756 (1969).

Herman, M. V., Elliott, W. C., and Gorlin, R.: An electrocardiographic, anatomic metabolic study of zonal myocardial ischemia in coronary heart disease. *Circulation* 35:834-846 (1967).

Hoffstein, S., Gennaro, D. E., Fox, A. C., Hirsh, J., Streuli, F., and Weissmann, G.: Colloidal lanthanum as a marker for impaired plasma membrane permeability in ischemic dog myocardium. *Am. J. Pathol.* 79:207-218. (1975).

Huckabee, W. E.: Relationship of pyruvate and lactate during anaerobic metabolism. *J. Clin. Invest.* 37:244-263 (1958).

Jennings, R. B.: Myocardial ischemia observations, definitions and speculations (Editorial) *J. Mol. Cell. Cardiol.* 1:345-349 (1970).

Jennings, R. B., Ganote, C. E., and Reimer, K. A.: Ischemic tissue injury. *Am. J. Pathol.* 81:179-198 (1975).

Jennings, R. B., and Reimer, K. A.: Salvage of ischemic myocardium. *Mod. Concepts Cardiovasc. Dis.* 43:125-130 (1974).

Jennings, R. B., Sommers, H. M., Smyth, G. A., Flack, H. A. and Linn, H.: Myocardial necrosis induced by temporary occlusion of a coronary artery in the dog. *Arch. Pathol.* 70:68-78 (1960).

Karlsson, J., Templeton, G. H., and Willerson, J. T.: Relationship between epicardial S-T segment changes and myocardial metabolism during acute coronary insufficiency. *Circ. Res.* 32:725-730 (1973).

Kennedy, H. L., Underhill, S. J., Caralis, D. G., Kahn, A. M. and Poblete, P. F.: Detection of non-anginal or "silent" ischemia ST segment depression in patients with ischemic heart disease. *Am. J. Cardiol.* 37:147 (1976).

Kuhn, P., and Pachinger, O.: The effect of calcium on myocardial lactate production under aerobic conditions. *J. Mol. Cell. Cardiol.* 4:171-174 (1972).

Maseri, A., Mimmo, P., Chierchia, S., Mavchesi, C., Pesola, A., and L'Aggate,, A.: Coronary artery spasm as a cause of myocardial ischemia in man. *Chest* 68:625-633 (1975).

Mills, R. M., Mudge, G. H., Taegtmeyer, H., Gorlin, R., and Lesch, M.: Alterations of myocardial amino acid metabolism in coronary artery disease. *Circulation* 51, 52 (Suppl. II): 11-90 (1975).

Most, A. S., Gorlin, R., and Soeldner, J. S.: Glucose extraction by the human myocardium during pacing stress. *Circulation* 45:92-96 (1972).

Neely, J. R., Denton, R. M., England, P. J., and Randle, P. J., The effects of increased heart work on the tricarboxylic acid cycle and its interactions with gylcolysis in the perfused rat heart. *Biochem. J.* 128:147-159 (1972).

Obeid, A., Smylvan, H., Gilbert, R., and Eich, R. H.: Regional metabolic changes in the myocardium following coronary artery ligation in dogs. *Am. Heart J.* 83:189-196 (1972).

Olson, R. E.: Myocardial metabolism in congestive heart failure. *J. Chron. Dis.* 9:442-464 (1959).

Opie, L.: Metabolism of free fatty acids, glucose and catecholamines in acute myocardial infarction. *Am. J. Cardiol.* 36:938-953 (1975).

Opie, L., Owen, P., Thomas, M., and Samsoh, R.: Coronary sinus lactate measurements in assessment of myocardial ischemia. *Am. J. Cardiol* 32:295-305 (1973).

Opie, L. H., Thomas, M., Owen, P., and Shulman, G.: Increased coronary venous inorganic phosphate concentrations during experimental myocardial infarction. *Am. J. Cardiol.* 30:503-513 (1972).

Owen, P., Thomas, M., Young, V., and Opie, L., Comparison between metabolic changes in local venous and coronary sinus blood after acute experimental coronary artery occlusion. *Am. J. Cardiol.* 25:562-570 (1970).

Parker, J. O., Chiong, M. A., West, R. O. and Case, R. B.: The effects of ischemia and alterations of heart rate on myocardial potassium balance in man. *Circulation* 42:205-217 (1970).

Pitt, B., Mason, J., Conti, C. R.: Observations on the plasma kallikrein system during myocardial ischemia. *Trans. Assoc. Am. Physicians* 82:98-108 (1969).

Roberts, W. C., Buja, A. M., Bulkley, B. H., and Ferrand, V. J.: Congestive heart failure and angina pectoris. *Am. J. Cardiol.* 34:870-872 (1974).

Roe, C. R., and Starmer, C. F.: A sensitivity analysis of enzymatic estimation of infarct size. *Circulation* 52:1 (1975).

Scheuer, J., and Berry, M. N.: Effect of alkalosis on glycolysis in the isolated rat heart. *Am. J. Physiol.* 213:1143-1148 (1967).

Wollenberger, A.: The energy metabolism of the failing heart and the metabolic action of the cardiac glycosides. *Pharmacol. Rev.* 1:311-352 (1949).

Discussion

Jennings, Weissman and Brachfeld

DR. THOMAS M. GLENN (*University of South Alabama College of Medicine*): I would like to know what the mechanism of action of cobra venom factor is in inflammation. Is it depletion of complement or loss of platelets? Do platelets play any role in this phenomenon?

DR. NORMAN BRACHFELD (*Cornell University College of Medicine*): To my knowledge, the primary action is to reduce complement, which results in a decrease in the inflammatory response. I do not know of any specific platelet activity. I think Dr. Maroko has probably had more experience with that than I have.

DR. PETER R. MAROKO (*Harvard Medical School*): I do not know what the effect of cobra venom on platelet function is, but the platelet number remains the same.

DR. ALLAN M. LEFER (*Jefferson Medical College*): I think Dr. Weissmann has done a remarkable job of characterizing the anatomic and histochemical properties of the myocardial lysosome. Many of us have been classically oriented toward liver lysosomes. I should just like to ask Dr. Weissman if he has studied any lysosomal enzymes other than beta-glucuronidase and acid phosphatase. Some of the metabolic researchers are investigating myocardial cathepsins. Have you studied these in cardiac lysosomes?

DR. GERALD WEISSMAN (*NYU School of Medicine*):   No, we have not. We have limited ourselves to aryl sulfatase, acid (beta-glycerol) phosphatase and beta-glucuronidase. Of course, you know the studies of Bird in cardiac muscle, your own work, and that of Ricciutti. I think that as more chemical techniques become available, for demonstrating these enzymes in tissues, we will find whether they are indeed of lysosomal origin. I am certain that a number of proteases present in cells are by no means lysosomal. I do not know at this time what the subcellular distribution of cathepsin D is in the myocardium. I think that should be a very fascinating subject for study.

DR. D. EUGENE RANNELLS, JR. (*Hershey Medical Center*): Several groups have observed that when muscular tissue is homogenized in a sucrose medium, the precipitated myofibrils tend to trap lysosomal enzyme activity in lysosomes and other structures. I would like to ask you, first of all, what fraction of the total homogenate enzyme activity were you looking at in your sedimentable and non-sedimentable fraction in the 400 $\times$ g supernatant; and secondly, have you examined the activity that is sedimented at 400 $\times$ g?

DR. WEISSMAN: Yes, we have investigated these fractions by ultrastructural techniques and Dr. Hoffstein's and our studies indicate that in the microsomal myocardial fraction (i.e., the one that sediments at 100,000 $\times$ g), depending on how vigorously we fractionate, we can recover 15 to 40% of the total enzyme activity.

If we try to reach the point where we can obtain the debris fraction of the unbroken cells, to liberate their enzymes, the bulk of the enzyme activity is sedimentable, and so you are caught between inadequate homogenization, and rupturing and shearing the sarcoplasmic reticulum. I am much more personally impressed by our cytochemical than by our biochemical studies, because I do not know at present how to adequately homogenize mammalian myocardium so as to avoid shear liberation of these hydrolases, which, after all, are not present in granules. Consequently, I think the point you make is a real one.

DR. ROBERT B. JENNINGS (*Duke University Medical Center*): Could you speculate on the temporal relationship of plasma-membrane vs. lysosomal-membrane changes? In other words, do the plasma-membrane alterations result from this redistribution of acid hydrolase activity, or do they precede lysosomal changes?

DR. WEISSMANN: I think it is very difficult to establish in any damaged or solid tissue which organelle fails first before injury to the plasma membrane occurs. There are no techniques that I know of that will permit you to judge this. Before you can get an enzyme from an organelle into the surrounding medium, the plasma membrane has to break or markedly alter its properties. Thus, whatever the sequence of injury is, if one simply monitors the outside of cells, one cannot decide what the sequence of injury is within them.

Part IV

PHARMACOLOGIC MODIFICATIONS OF SIZE OF DEVELOPING INFARCT

18

Mechanisms of Glucocorticoid Protection in Experimental Myocardial Ischemia

ALLAN M. LEFER
MINORU OKUDA

Glucocorticoids have been recently found to be effective in preventing the spread of ischemic damage to myocardial tissue. This applies to the cat (Spath et al., 1974; Spath and Lefer, 1975), dog (Libby et al., 1973) and man (Morrison et al., 1975), and is purported to be one of the most efficacious means of reducing infarct size after acute myocardial ischemia. The concept of modifying the extent of the developing infarct is a new one, and its development is largely due to the availability of techniques capable of monitoring infarct size. The two major methods used are: (1) electrocardiographic and (2) biochemical. The first technique, developed by Maroko and coworkers (1971), involves the quantitation of the ST-segment elevation from multiple lead recording sites. There is a problem with quantitation and with reproductibility of recording sites, but this technique holds great promise. The second method, largely developed by Sobel and colleagues, is based on the serial determination of plasma creatine phosphokinase (CPK) activities (Sobel and Shell, 1973), and is becoming widely used. In the animal laboratory, one can obtain direct myocardial tissue samples to verify cardiac CPK loss. The primary problems are that isozymes of CPK that do not originate in myocardial tissue (e.g., skeletal muscle, brain) can contribute to the elevated plasma CPK activities.

The anesthetized open-chest cat has evolved into a reproducible model for the study of the early phases of infarct development. The left coronary artery is dissected free 13 to 15 mm from the coronary ostium and tied with a silk ligature. Recently we have cut the occluded coronary artery to prevent opening of collateral channels. Fig. 1 summarizes the anatomic features of this technique, indicating the extent of the ischemic area and the border zone. Within 30 min, mean arterial blood pressure (MABP), heart rate, and aortic flow (i.e., cardiac output) decrease significantly. Aortic flow gradually decreases over the next 4 hr, whereas MABP plateaus and heart rate increases slightly after 1 hr. The portion of myocardium supplied by the occluded left coronary artery becomes mottled and cyanotic in appearance. The ST-segment of the electrocardiogram increases within 30 to 60 min and usually remains significantly elevated over the 5-hr experimental period. This is additional evidence that direct ischemic damage occurs in the myocardium.

Other data indicating impairment of myocardial cell integrity are the marked rise in the plasma activity of the intramyocardial enzyme, creatine phosphokinase (CPK). The specific activity of this enzyme increases about 8-fold over the 5-hr observation period. The major increase appears to occur 2 hr after occlusion and increases progressively over the next 3 hr. These data *per se* do not prove that myocardial damage occurred, since CPK could have arisen from the brain or skeletal muscle. However, since sham-operated controls undergo only a doubling of plasma CPK activity, most of the increased plasma CPK is presumed to originate from the heart.

In order to specifically determine whether the ischemic portion of the myocardium does indeed undergo a loss in CPK, indicative of cellular damage, samples of normal and ischemic myocardial tissue were taken after 5 hr, and CPK activity was determined. This area exhibited a 42% reduction, compared with non-ischemic regions of the left ventricle of the same cats.

Since these indices of myocardial ischemia proved to be reproducible and sensitive, this model became useful for the study of the pharmacological modulation of infarct size. Glucocorticoids were selected for study because of their anti-inflammatory properties and their efficacy in circulatory shock states.

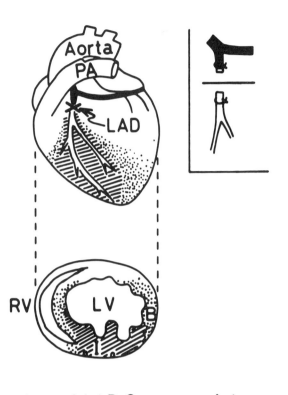

Occlusion of LAD Coronary Artery

I : Ischemic Myocardium (Hatched Area)
B : Border-zone Myocardium (Dotted Area)

1 Schematic diagram of method of induction of myocardial ischemia in cat heart. Inset shows proximal segment of left anterior descending (LAD) coronary artery (black) and distal segment (white) after ligation and cutting of vessel.

Methylprednisolone (MP), at a dose of 30 mg/kg, was administered intravenously to cats either at the time of coronary occlusion (pre-treatment) or 1 hr after occlusion (post-treatment). MP significantly retarded the increase in ST-segment elevation and plasma CPK activity (Spath et al., 1974). In addition, MP significantly prevents the loss of CPK from the ischemic area of the myocardium. Of the three indices of ischemic damage employed, myocardial CPK is perhaps the most reliable since it does not depend on subtle shifts in electrical properties of the heart nor is it confounded by isozymes of CPK, which are non-cardiac in origin.

Similar findings were obtained when 8 mg/kg of dexamethasone (Dexa) was employed rather than methylprednisolone. This glucocorticoid also prevented much of the increases in plasma CPK and in ST segment, observed after coronary artery occlusion. As with MP, Dexa (post-treatment) dramatically sustained myocardial CPK in ischemic myocardial tissue. However, pretreatment was only partially effective in this regard. Nevertheless, dexamethasone proved to be an effective agent in limiting the spread of ischemic damage (Spath and Lefer, 1975).

These findings, as well as those of Libby et al. (1973) in dogs and of Morrison et al. (1975) in humans, clearly indicate that pharmacological doses of glucocorticoids can be very effective in preventing the spread of ischemic damage in acute myocardial ischemia. The major unanswered questions regarding the protective action of glucocorticoids in this condition are: (1) Do the steroid molecules actually penetrate the ischemic area, and (2) What is the mechanism of the protective action of the glucocorticoids? Several mechanisms for the protective action of glucocorticoids in myocardial ischemia have been proposed. These are summarized in Table 1. Although the story is far from complete, some information concerning all of these mechanisms is available.

Regarding the possible anti-arrhythmic effect of glucocorticoids, neither MP nor Dexa prevented the incidence of premature ectopic beats after coronary artery ligation (Beardsley et al., 1976b). Also, these glucocorticoids did not appear to alter any of the arrhythmias occurring in myocardial ischemia (Spath et al., 1974; Spath and Lefer, 1975; Libby et al., 1973) despite the finding that corticosteroids are useful in a variety of atrioventricular conduction blocks, such as observed in Stokes-Adams attacks (Aber and Jones, 1960; Dall, 1964). The reduction in ST-segment elevation, observed in ischemic hearts after administration of glucocorticoid, can best be explained by an effect of these steroids on cellular integrity, elimi-

Table 1. Postulated mechanisms of action of glucocorticoids
in myocardial ischemia

1. Prevention of spontaneous arrhythmias
2. Augmentation of coronary perfusion
   a. increasing coronary blood flow
   b. opening collateral channels
3. Reduction of myocardial oxygen demand
   a. reducing metabolic rate
   b. decreasing cardiac work
4. Stabilization of myocardial cellular membranes
   a. lysosomal membranes
   b. plasma membranes

nating the consequences of myocardial ischemia which are responsible for ST-segment elevation (e.g., leakage of K^+ by the cell, acidosis, actions of released myocardial phospholipases, etc.). Thus, no convincing case has yet been made for an anti-arrhythmic effect of glucocorticoids in myocardial ischemia, which could explain the beneficial effect of these agents on infarct size.

Data obtained in several well-controlled cardiac preparations (i.e., isolated perfused hearts, isolated papillary muscle preparations) failed to show a significant positive inotropic effect in ischemic and nonischemic hearts. This is consistent with previous results in intact dogs (Jefferson et al., 1971) and cats (Glenn and Lefer, 1971), either in circulatory shock or in non-shocked animals. Fig. 2 illustrates this lack of an inotropic effect by dexamethasone in ischemic cat hearts isolated and perfused via the coronary arteries. Moreover, glucocorticoids added to a variety of isolated heart preparations, in concentrations equivalent to anti-shock doses, failed to augment the inotropic state of the heart (Lefer, 1975). This lack of inotropism exhibited by glucocorticoids in hypoxic or acidotic hearts, and in hearts of animals in severe shock when cardiac function is markedly depressed (Spath et al., 1973). In those few studies in which a positive inotropic effect was reported with large doses of glucocorticoids (Bouyard, 1965; Tecklenberg et al., 1973), the effect was quite small and transient (i.e., lasting only 20-30 min). Moreover, vehicle controls were lacking in these studies, so that the effect may have been due to the diluents or preservatives in the steroid

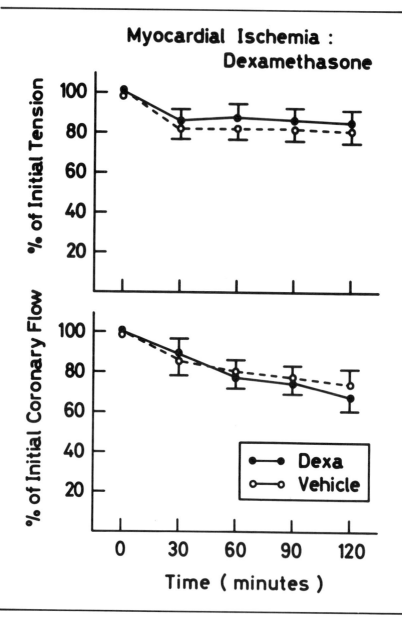

Myocardial Ischemia : Dexamethasone

2 Influence of dexamethasone on myocardial developed tension (upper panel) and coronary flow (lower panel) in isolated perfused cat hearts. Values are expressed as means ± SEM for 7 hearts in each group. (From Beardsley et al., 1976b.)

preparation. Only in chronic adrenal insufficiency do glucocorticoids improve myocardial contractility (Lefer et al., 1968), and then only to control levels—not to supranormal values. This cardiotonic effect requires several hours to develop and is exerted by replacement but not by massive doses of glucocorticoids. These replacement doses (i.e., on the order of 10 to 100 μg/kg) do not protect in circulatory shock or in myocardial ischemia. Finally, the potential value of a positive inotropic effect in the treatment of myocardial ischemia is limited since inotropic drugs raise myocardial oxygen demand, which would tend to increase ischemic damage to the myocardium (Maroko et al., 1971).

Although we observed no coronary vasodilation in response to glucocorticoids, such an effect would be desirable during myocardial ischemia. Coronary vasodilation would not be of direct value to an area supplied by a totally occluded coronary artery, but would benefit an area supplied by a partially occluded vessel, particularly if collaterals were opened to the ischemic region. In general, massive doses of glucocorticoids do not vasodilate most systemic beds (Lefer, 1975; Kadowitz and Yard, 1970). However, Vyden et al. (1974) recently reported that methylprednisolone increased coronary flow in the ischemic dog heart. This alleged dilator effect only occurred transiently 60-90 min after addition of the steroid and resulted in a coronary flow only slightly above control values. More critically, no vehicle controls were used, so that it is not known whether the reported coronary vasodilation was due to the methylprednisolone *per se*. In studies employing vehicle controls, no coronary vasodilation was observed with either MP or Dexa. Even if the coronary vasodilation were to be shown to be a true steroid effect, it would be difficult to explain the reduction in infarct size by such a transient action.

No evidence of an altered oxygen demand was obtained in ischemic perfused cat hearts, since heart rate, cardiac preload and afterload remained essentially unchanged. This lack of hemodynamic action during myocardial ischemia is consistent with previously published reports. Thus, glucocorticoids do not appear to have any significant acute effects on heart rate, blood pressure, or ventricular filling pressure. Only upon chronic administration of these steroids for periods of several weeks or months do significant hemodynamic effects occur in several types of circulatory shock (Lefer, 1974). Vyden et al. (1974), reported slight decreases in heart rate and mean arterial blood pressure in the dog during myocardial ischemia but these effects only lasted about 15 min. Again, no vehicle controls were used to verify that this action was due to the glucocorticoid. Thus, it is unlikely that these transient hemodynamic effects explain the preservation of myocardial integrity observed 5-24 hr later (Spath et al., 1974; Morrison et al., 1975).

Another major hemodynamic mechanism for explaining the protective effect of glucocorticoids on the infarction process would involve the opening of collateral vessels, improving the flow to ischemic regions. This remains an attractive hypothesis even though it is difficult to verify, since each heart has a different anatomical arrangement of coronary vessels, with differing stages of development of interarterial collateral channels.

Some years ago, Eckstein (1954) reported that glucocorticoids did not significantly modify the degree of coronary interarterial anastomoses in dogs. No differences in retrograde volume flow occurred in steroid-treated dogs for periods of 2 months after drug administration. It would be even more unlikely for such an effect to be manifested during the 5-hr observation period within which glucocorticoids protect the ischemic myocardium.

The mechanism of glucocorticoid action in myocardial ischemia for which evidence is thus far available is membrane stabilization, particularly, lysosomal membranes. The major evidence to support this contention is:

(1) Glucocorticoids prevent the loss of the myocardial lysosomal hydrolases, cathepsin D and β-glucuronidase, from ischemic myocardial tissue (Spath et al., 1974; Spath and Lefer, 1975) during myocardial ischemia. This action is consistent with a lysosomal or membrane effect but does not *per se* prove such a mechanism, since many non-lysosomal substances are also prevented from leaking out of the ischemic area. Thus, this may be a non-specific effect.

(2) Glucocorticoids stabilize myocardial lysosomes in the ischemic region of the myocardium after coronary artery ligation (Spath et al., 1974). Table 2 summarizes the effects of methylprednisolone on lysosomal stability and shows a significant stabilizing effect, with both β-glucuronidase and cathepsin D as marker enzymes. This finding coupled with the reduced loss of these enzymes constitute strong evidence for the lysosomal concept.

(3) Significant lysosomal membrane leakage in myocardial tissue occurs 1 to 2 hr after coronary artery ligation (Weissmann et al., 1975; Ricciutti, 1972), just prior to a time when CPK and other cell markers are appearing in the circulation.

(4) The myocardial plasma membrane marker, 5'-nucleotidase (5'ND) exhibits changes consistent with a membrane-stabilizing

Table 2. Bound lysoşomal hydrolase activities
in ischemic myocardial tissue in MI

| Group | % BOUND ACTIVITY | |
	β-Glucuronidase	Cathepsin D
Sham MI + MP	50.2 ± 3.7	47.8 ± 2.6
MI + vehicle	22.7 ± 1.5	26.1 ± 2.6
MI + MP-Pre	40.3 ± 1.7*	41.7 ± 2.7*
MI + MP-Post	49.2 ± 1.9*	46.7 ± 1.8*

All values are means ± SE for 4-5 hearts.
*p <0.01 from methylprednisolone + vehicle group.
MI = myocardial infarction
MP = methylpredninsolone

action of glucocorticoids. Fig. 3 summarizes these effects in isolated perfused cat hearts subjected to myocardial ischemia and, then, either not treated or treated with methylprednisolone or dexamethasone. Ischemia results in a significant ($p < 0.001$) decrease in 5'ND activity from about 15 to 5 units/mg protein. The 5'ND activity in border-zone tissue is midway between these two values (i.e., about 10 units/mg protein), being significantly different ($p < 0.001$) from both control and ischemic tissue. Each glucocorticoid was able to retard this decrease in 5'ND activity in the ischemic and border-zone tissue. Thus the border-zone 5'ND activity in steroid-treated hearts was not significantly different from control tissue, but was significantly higher than border-zone tissue in non-steroid treated hearts ($p < 0.025$). Similarly, ischemic tissue obtained from glucocorticoid-treated hearts exhibited significantly higher 5'ND activity than that from non-steroid treated hearts ($p < 0.025$). The 5'ND activity of the ischemic area in steroid-treated hearts was not significantly different from that of 5'ND in tissue obtained from the border-zone in non-steroid treated hearts. These data indicate that plasma membranes appear to disrupt early in acute myocardial ischemia, and that pharmacological concentrations of synthetic glucocorticoids can significantly retard this process.

In addition, the proportion of 5'ND activity in the supernatant and particulate fraction, for the three different cardiac areas and for the steroid-perfused and non-steroid perfused hearts, also indicates membrane stabilization by the glucocorticoids. Thus, in the

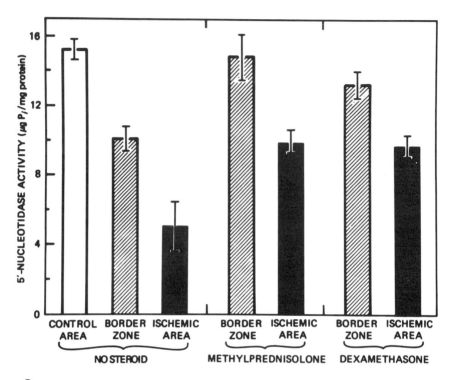

3 Action of methylprednisolone and dexamethasone on myocardial 5′-nucleotidase specific activity. Values are expressed as means ± SEM for 5 hearts in each group.

absence of glucocorticoids, 62% of the 5′ND activity is found in the soluble fraction of ischemic cardiac tissue, and 23% of the activity occurs in the border-zone supernatant. However, this activity was only 33-34% and 5-6% of the total in ischemic and border-zone tissue, respectively, in the presence of glucocorticoid. These data collectively strongly support the concept of membrane stabilization by glucocorticoids in myocardial ischemia. However, the second fundamental question remains regarding the ability of ischemic myocardial tissue to concentrate glucocorticoid, which could indicate a direct effect of the steroids on myocardial membranes.

The first experiments concerning cardiac uptake of glucocorticoids, in concentrations comparable to those used in the treatment of acute myocardial infarction, were studied in cardiac slices (0.5 mm thickness, incubated at 0° and 37°C) taken from cat myocardium (Beardsley et al., 1976a). Fig. 4 shows the uptake of DEXA

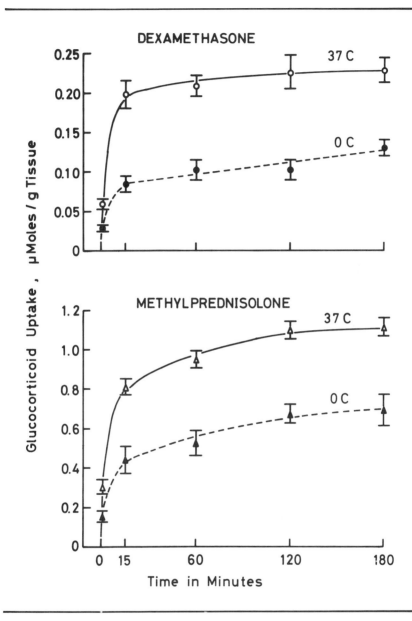

Uptake of tritiated dexamethasone (upper panel) and methylprednisolone (lower panel) over 3 hr in isolated cat heart slices at 0°C and at 37°C. Values are expressed as means $\pm$ SEM. (From Beardsley et al., 1976a.)

(upper panel) and MP (lower panel) by myocardial slices at temperatures of 0° and 37° over a period of 180 min. Both glucocorticoids showed a significant increase in uptake over this time. After 60 min of incubation, steroid uptake plateaued at 0.21 μmole of dexamethasone/g of tissue and 0.95 μmole of MP/g of tissue (Beardsley et al., 1976a).

With either steroid, the uptake rates and total amounts of glucocorticoids in the myocardial cell were significantly ($p < 0.001$) reduced at 0°, compared to 37°. Only about 50% of the 37° values were taken up at 0°. This occurred at every time point measured, indicating that the uptake process is temperature dependent. The pH optimum for the steroid uptake process was 7.3 to 7.4; it depended upon steroid concentration in the medium and was not blocked by metabolic or SH-inhibitors. This large degree of steroid incorporation does not appear to depend upon energy-requiring processes and is presumably a passive phenomenon. Since tissue slices unavoidably contain a certain amount of damaged cells which may favor steroid uptake, additional studies were performed in intact hearts, perfused under constant pressure, in order to further study this process. Similar results were obtained with these hearts, indicating that the steroid-uptake process does not depend on the presence of damaged or broken cells. Moreover, supernatant particulate ratios indicate that a large portion of the uptake is closely associated with cell membranes or other internal structures. Therefore, a cell-fractionation study was undertaken of the ischemic, border-zone and non-ischemic cardiac tissue in order to determine the localization of glucocorticoid uptake in isolated perfused cat hearts. These three regions were homogenized and subjected to density gradient ultracentrifugation, after perfusion for 1 hr with labeled glucocorticoid. The fractions corresponded to the following: F_1, plasma membranes; F_2, sarcoplasmic recticulum and light lysosomes; F_3, light mitochondria and light lysosomes; F_4, heavy mitochondria; and F_5, heavy lysosomes. Fig. 5 summarizes the results. The latter indicate that both glucocorticoids are taken up in very large quantities by the plasma membrane in all three areas of myocardium. This amounts to 66 to 82% of the total uptake. Secondly, there appears to be a gradient such that $F_1 > F_2 > F_3 > F_4 > F_5$. Finally, there seems to be a greater uptake of MP than DEXA in the F_3 and F_4 fractions containing light lysosomes and mitochondria. Nevertheless, these data indicate a significant degree of steroid uptake even in ischemic and border-zone tissue, which is apparently not much less than that in non-ischemic tissue.

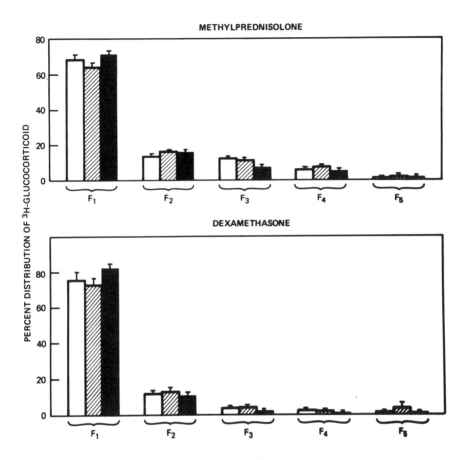

5 Subcellular distribution of ^{3}H-steroids in subcellular fractions of perfused cat heart. F_1 = plasma membranes; F_2 = sarcoplasmic reticulum and light lysosomes; F_3 = light mitochondria and light lysosomes; F_4 = heavy mitochondria; F_5 = heavy lysosomes. All values are means ± SEM for 6 hearts in each group.

Finally, in an effort to determine if significant glucocorticoid uptake occurs in blood-perfused *in situ* hearts, tritiated MP was injected intravenously in intact cats at the time of induction of myocardial ischemia, and followed for 2 hr.

Fig. 6 illustrates a typical example of one such experiment and also indicates the degree of metabolism by the label. We deal here with a sample of plasma, myocardium and liver chromatographed

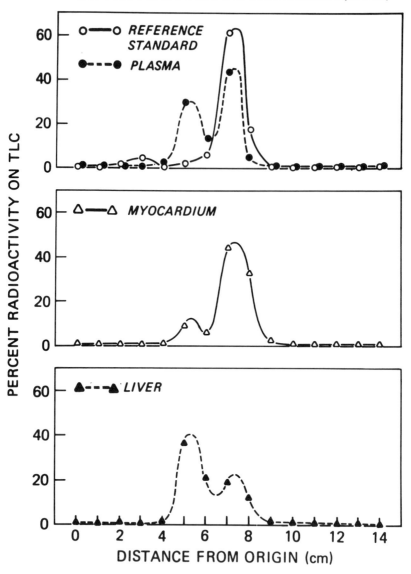

CAT NO. 14: MYOCARDIAL ISCHEMIA (2HRS)

REFERENCE STANDARD
PLASMA
MYOCARDIUM
LIVER

PERCENT RADIOACTIVITY ON TLC

DISTANCE FROM ORIGIN (cm)

6

Uptake and degradation of ^{3}H-methylprednisolone (MP) in myocardium, liver and plasma 2 hr after induction of myocardial ischemia in a typical intact cat. Reference standard is pure ^{3}H-MP. Graphs are thin-layer chromatographic patterns obtained by scraping each cm of plate and counting them separately.

on silica thin-layer plates. Most of the label appears to be identical to the MP reference standard and, thus, is intact MP. There is a small portion of myocardial label in a second peak, a moderate amount in plasma and a large amount in liver. Therefore, myocardial tissue, which concentrates ^{3}H-MP about 2.3 times plasma activities, maintains over 90% of the label as intact glucocorticoid 2 hr after injection, in acute myocardial ischemia. These findings indicate that the steroid-uptake process is an important one in the heart and is, therefore, consistent with a direct membrane-stabilizing effect in myocardial cellular membranes (i.e., lysosomal and plasma membranes).

In summary, the following conclusions can be drawn:

(a) High concentrations of glucocorticoids prevent spread of ischemic damage after coronary artery occlusion.

(b) The mechanism of their protective action does not involve an anti-arrhythmic effect, reduction of oxygen consumption, coronary vasodilation, alteration of the contractile machinery of the myocardium, or by opening of collateral vessels in the coronary circulation.

(c) The mechanism appears to be related to stabilization of myocardial plasma and lysosomal membranes.

(d) Large amounts of glucocorticoids are taken up passively by myocardial tissue, and they are metabolized to a very small extent during the first several hours after induction of myocardial ischemia.

ACKNOWLEDGMENTS

This work was supported in part by Research Grant No. HL-17688 from the National Heart, Lung and Blood Institute of the NIH.

We wish to thank Keith R. Young, Jr., Martin L. Ogletree and Dr. Anthony C. Beardsley, for their collaborative efforts during portions of these studies. We also wish to express our appreciation to Dr. Samuel S. Stubbs of the Upjohn Company, Kalamazoo, Mich., and Dr. Alexander Scriabine of the Merck Institute for Therapeutic Research, West Point, Pa. for their generous supplies of methylprednisolone and dexamethasone, respectively.

REFERENCES

Aber, C. P., and Jones E. W.: Complete heart block treated with corticotrophin and corticosteroid. *Br. Heart J.* 22:723 (1960).
Beardsley, A. C., Okuda, M., and Lefer, A. M.: Factors influencing non-

specific binding of glucocorticoids in myocardial tissue. *Proc. Soc. Exp. Biol. Med.* 151:457-461 (1976a).

Beardsley, A. C., Okuda, M., Lefer, A. M.: Absence of a cardiodynamic action of glucocorticoids in acute myocardial ischemia. *J. Surg. Res.* 20:17-24 (1976b).

Bouyard, P.: Actions cardiovascularies des derives stéroids. *Ann. Anesthesiol. Fr.* 6:37 (1965).

Dall, J. L. C.: The effect of steroid therapy on normal and abnormal atrio-ventricular conduction. *Br. Heart J.* 26:537 (1964).

Eckstein, R. W.: Ineffectiveness of cortisone on functional coronary inter-arterial anastomoses. *Circ. Res.* 2:466 (1954).

Glenn, T. M., and Lefer, A. M.: Anti-toxic action of methylprednisolone in hemorrhagic shock. *Eur. J. Pharmacol.* 13:230-238 (1971).

Jefferson, T. A., Glenn, T. M., Martin, J. B., and Lefer, A. M.: Cardiovascular and lysosomal actions of corticosteroids in the intact dog. *Proc. Soc. Exp. Biol. Med.* 136:276-280 (1971).

Kadowitz, P. J., and Yard, A. C.: Circulatory effects of hydrocortisone and protection against endotoxin shock in cats. *Eur. J. Pharmacol.* 9:311 (1970).

Lefer, A. M.: Myocardial actions of corticosteroids. In *Steroids and Shock*, T. M. Glenn, ed. University Park Press, Baltimore (1974), pp. 53-66.

Lefer, A. M.: Corticosteroids and circulatory function. In *Handbook of Physiology, The Adrenal Cortex*, H. Blashko, G. Sayers and A. D. Smith, eds., Williams & Wilkins, Baltimore (1975), pp. 191-207.

Lefer, A. M., Verrier, R. L., and Carson, W. W.: Cardiac performance in experimental adrenal insufficiency in cats. *Circ. Res.* 22:817 (1968).

Libby, P., Maroko, P. R., Bloor, C. M., Sobel, B. E., and Braunwald, E.: Reduction of experimental myocardial infarct size by corticosteroid administration. *J. Clin. Invest.* 52:599-607 (1973).

Maroko, P. R., Kjekshus, J. K., Sobel, B. E., Watanabe, T., Covell, J. W., Ross, J., Jr., and Braunwald, E.: Factors influencing infarct size following experimental coronary artery occlusions. *Circulation* 43:67-82 (1971).

Morrison, J., Maley, T., Reduto, L., Victa, C., Pyros, I., Brandon, J., and Gulotta, S.: Effect of methylprednisolone on predicted myocardial infarction size in man. *Crit. Care Med.* 3:94-102 (1975).

Ricciutti, M. A.: Lysosomes and myocardial cellular injury. *Am. J. Cardiol.* 30:498 (1972).

Sobel, B. E., and Shell, W. E.: Serum enzyme determinations in the diagnosis and assessment of myocardial infarction. *Circulation* 45:471-482 (1973).

Spath, J. A., Jr., Gorczynski, R. J., and Lefer, A. M.: Possible mechanisms of the beneficial action of glucocorticoids in circulatory shock. *Surg. Gynecol. Obstet.* 137:597-607 (1973).

Spath, J. A., Jr., Lane, D. L., Lefer, A. M.: Protective action of methylprednisolone on the myocardium during experimental myocardial ischemia in the cat. *Circ. Res.* 35:44-51 (1974).

Spath, J. A., Jr., Lane, D. L., Lefer, A. M.: Protective action of dexamethasone the early phase of acute myocardial infarction. *Am. Heart J.* 90:50-55 (1975).

Tecklenberg, P. J., Mullin, E. M., Stinson, E. B., and Morrow, A. G.: The effects of massive doses of methylprednisolone on myocardial contractility and peripheral vascular resistance. *Am. Heart J.* 85:216 (1973).

Vyden, J. K., Nagasawa, K., Rabinowitz, B., Parmley, W. W., Tomoda, H., Corday, E., and Swan, H. J. C.: Effects of methylprednisolone administration in acute myocardial infarction. *Am. J. Cardiol.* 34:677 (1974).

Weissmann, G., Hoffstein, S., Kaplan, H., Gennaro, D., Hirsch, J., and Fox, A. C.: Early lysosomal disruption in myocardial infarction and protection by methylprednisolone. *Clin. Res.* 23:383A (1975).

19

Modification of Myocardial Injury in Man: Glucocorticoids

JOHN MORRISON
ROY PIZZARELLO
LAWRENCE REDUTO
ALAN BINDER
STEPHEN GULOTTA

INTRODUCTION

Mortality following acute myocardial infarction has been diminished by Coronary Care Units, with their capacity for prompt treatment of potentially lethal dysrhythmias. However, mortality in these patients remains substantial (9-20%), primarily because of left ventricular power failure, the syndrome of decreased cardiac output and congestive heart failure (Weil and Shubin, 1968).

It is now well established that power failure, in the absence of complicating lesions such as ventricular septal defects or mitral regurgitation, occurs in proportion to the amount of myocardium damaged, i.e., power failure is directly related to infarct size (Hood et al., 1967). In experimental animal and in human clinical studies, it has been shown that signs of left ventricular failure exist when 20-25% of the left ventricular myocardium is damaged (Page et al., 1971). Lesions involving more than 40% of the left ventricular myocardium are often associated with the shock syndrome and a fatal outcome (Page et al., 1971). Presumably it is in this relatively narrow range of left ventricular damage, between 25-40%, that the entire spectrum of heart failure—from mild to severe—becomes clinically apparent. Accordingly, the sum total of heart-muscle damage is an important determinant of morbidity as well as mortality following acute myocardial infarction. Consequently, any measures capable of reducing the degree of left ventricular damage by a small percentage are likely to produce a considerable change in the clinical status of the patient and influence mortality to a significant degree.

Hence, the insult sustained by the heart itself rather than the impairment to peripheral circulation has become the focus of attention. An emerging hypothesis indicates that: (1) infarct size is a critical determinant of prognosis; (2) infarct size can be modified favorably by appropriate pharmacological interventions during the early evolution of infarction; and (3) such modifications also affect long-term prognosis favorably.

It has been postulated that pharmacological alteration of the biochemical environment of ischemic myocardial zones may modify ultimate myocardial infarction size. Abundant experimental evidence in animal models indicates that this is now possible (Maroko and Braunwald, 1973).

The results from several clinical investigations with glucocorticoids are conflicting in that some show a reduction in mortality in patients with acute myocardial infarction treated with steroids, while others have been unable to confirm this finding (Gerisch and Compeau, 1958; Dall and Peel, 1963; Barzilai et al., 1972). These apparent discrepancies may reflect, in part, a significant variation in the elapsed time between the onset of the acute myocardial infarction and glucocorticoid administration, the dosage of the drug, and the size of the myocardial infarction in the treated and untreated groups.

The present investigation was undertaken to assess the effect of glucocorticoid administration upon evolving myocardial infarction in man. Curve-fitting techniques (Shell et al., 1973) were applied to analysis of early serial serum CPK changes in patients with acute myocardial infarction in order to predict its ultimate extent. Predicted infarct size was compared with completed infarct size, following pharmacological intervention, and the extent of myocardial preservation was quantified. It was found that glucocorticoid administered early in the course of acute infarction, in certain patients, resulted in apparent salvage of myocardium. Furthermore, this intervention appeared to alter prognosis favorably. These data support the view that some myocardial tissue placed in jeopardy by coronary occlusion need not go on to become irreversibly damaged.

METHODS

Creatine phosphokinase activity in serial serum samples was assayed kinetically, at 30°C, with a CPK reagent kit (Calbiochem) on a dual-beam spectrophotometer. Samples were run in duplicate and the mean taken as the final value. One standard deviation of the CPK assay for 50 separate determinations of a sample with a known concentration of 254 mIU/ml was ± 8 mIU/ml. Duplicate assays on the same sample varied ± 2%

Determination of predicted and completed infarct size was accomplished with serial CPK analysis, using a computer algorithm (Shell et al., 1973) and assuming an enzyme clearance rate (kd) of 0.001 min^{-1}. Predicted infarct size was calculated from the initial 7-hourly CPK values, following the rise in enzyme from baseline, employing a standard nonlinear least squares curve-fitting system. Completed infarct size was calculated from all available serial CPK data (90-160 hr). In addition, the k_d for each patient was estimated (k_{d_1}) from a computerized mathematical inspection of CPK versus time plot (Morrison et al., 1976) at those times when myocardial enzyme release was zero (time intervals where f (t) = 0) and calculated (k_{d_2}) employing a least squares mathematical model (Norris et al., 1975). These individual k_d values were then used to recalculate predicted and completed infarct size data.

Comparison of data was accomplished utilizing paired and unpaired Student t-test, chi-square and covariance analysis.

CLINICAL DATA BASE

One-hundred-one patients who sustained an acute myocardial infarction as documented by clinical history, electrocardiographic criteria and central clinical laboratory enzyme elevations (SGOT, CPK, LDH) were studied. Inclusion in the study resulted if the first available CPK sample was normal (<80 mIU/ml).

The control group comprised 35 patients with documented acute myocardial infarction. The treated group included 66 patients, each of whom was given 2 g of methylprednisolone sodium succinate diluted with 5% dextrose and water to a total volume of 50 ml, and administered over 20 min, employing a controlled infusion system (Ivac Corporation), via a peripheral arm vein. This infusion was begun between 7 and 25 hr following the initial rise of CPK from baseline activity (mean = 8.9 hr). In 46 patients, a second 2-g dose of methylprednisolone was administered either 3, 6 or 12 hr after the initial dose. None of the patients was digitalized, received intramuscular injections, had DC cardioversion or was in cardiogenic shock during the study period.

RESULTS

Myocardial infarction size data in control and methylprednisolone-treated groups, together with acute myocardial infarction classification, location of infarction and presence or absence of prior infarction are presented in Table 1.

CPK Clearance

In each patient, calculation of infarct size was performed assuming a clearance of serum CPK activity (k_d) of 0.001 min^{-1}. In addition, in each patient where adequate data points were available, clearance was estimated by computerized mathematical inspection of CPK values at times when release of myocardial enzyme activity was assumed to be complete (k_{d_1}) and by a best fit least squares method (k_{d_2}). Linear estimates of predicted and completed infarction size, calculated from data employing k_d, k_{d_1} and k_{d_2} in 27 control patients and 61 methylprednisolone-treated patients, are shown in Figs. 1 and 2.

Control Group

Thirty-five patients with acute myocardial infarction constituted the control group. Employing a kit = 0.001 min^{-1}, mean predicted infarct size was 47.9 ± 6.8 (S.E.M.) creatine phosphokinase-gram-equivalents (CPK-g-eq) as compared to a mean completed infarct size of 66.9 ± 9.7 CPK-g-eq, (p = 0.001, paired t-test). In 27 of these patients where individually calculated k_{d_1} and k_{d_2} values were available, mean predicted infarct size was 38.0 ± 6.4 CPK-g-eq and 35.2 ± 5.7 CPK-g-eq, while mean completed infarct size was 51.5 ± 7.1 CPK-g-eq, and 48.7 ± 6.5 CPK-g-eq, respectively. (For k_{d_1} calculations p < 0.02, and for k_{d_2} calculations p < .009, paired t-test).

Methylprednisolone Group

The glucocorticoid-treated group comprised 66 patients with acute myocardial infarction. Utilizing a $k_d = 0.001$ min^{-1}, mean predicted infarct size was 102.3 ± 11.2 CPK-g-eq as compared to a mean completed infarct size of 84.3 ± 7.1 CPK-g-eq ($p < 0.004$, paired t-test). In 61 patients, it was possible to calculate k_{d1} and k_{d2} for each subject. Calculating infarct size with kd_1 resulted in a mean predicted infarct size of 96.2 ± 10.0 CPK-g-eq while mean completed infarct size was 84.6 ± 6.7 CPK-g-eq ($p < 0.04$, paired t-test). Recalculation, employing k_{d2}, yielded a mean predicted infarct size of 95.5 ± 10.5 CPK-g-eq and a mean completed infarct size of 82.2 ± 6.9 CPK-g-eq ($p < 0.02$, paired t-est).

Controls vs. Methylprednisolone Group

To compare the 35 controls and the 66 glucocorticoid-treated patients, regression lines were derived (predicted vs. completed infarct size) for each group and compared by covariance analysis (Fig. 3). Assuming a k_d of 0.001 min^{-1}, a regression line: completed infarct size $= 1.22 \times$ predicted infarct size $+ 8.66$ ($n = 35$, $r = 0.86$) was obtained for control patients. Similarly, a linear estimate, completed infarct size $= 0.56 \times$ predicted infarct size $+ 27.14$ ($n = 66$, $r = 0.89$) was derived for the glucocorticoid-treated group. A significant alteration in the linear relation of the predicted and completed infarct size determinations was found in comparing the two groups.

Predicted 50-150 CPK-g-eq Infarct Size

Since in small, non-transmural myocardial infarction, peak serum CPK activity may be relatively low, the fall in enzyme activity may not be large enough to accurately calculate individual enzyme clearance rates. Similarly, in patients with sudden and extreme increases in CPK levels and, therefore, extremely large predicted infarct size, the theoretical role of "wash-out" of enzyme from myocardium and subsequent overprediction of infarct size, though considered unlikely, could not be completely excluded. To obviate these potential problems with the mathematical model, data was analyzed in all control and treated patients who had a predicted infarct size ranging from 50-150 CPK-g-eq ($k_d = 0.001$ min^{-1}). In 13 control subjects, mean predicted infarct size was 91.3 ± 9.2 CPK-

Table 1. Clinical and "Infarct Size" Data

Pt. no.	Sex	Age	S.E.	T.M. Site	Prior M.I.	M.I. Class	Mortality	Time of Rx (min)*	$k_d \times 10^3$ (min^{-1}) (3)
								CONTROLS	
1	M	53		DMI	-	2	-		0.67
2	M	51		DMI	-	1	-		1.46
3	M	43	+		-	1	-		0.98
4	M	64		DMI	-	2	-		0.89
5	M	47	+		-	1	-		1.28
6	F	73		DMI	+	2	-		0.85
7	M	35	+		+	2	-		0.67
8	M	35		AMI	+	2	-		0.69
9	F	79		AMI	-	4	+		1.0
10	F	61		DMI	-	1	-		0.93
11	M	58		ASMI	+	2	-		0.59
12	M	60	+		-	1	-		1.4
13	F	58	+		-	1	-		1.0
14	M	44		ALMI	-	4	+		1.13
15	M	61		DMI	-	3	-		0.67
16	M	57		AMI	-	3	+		0.85
17	M	54		PMI	-	2	-		0.67
18	M	50		DMI	+	2	-		0.78
19	M	61		DMI	+	2	-		0.85
20	M	88	+		+	3	-		
21	M	55		PMI	-	2	+		0.57
22	M	57		AMI	+	2	-		1.50
23	M	51		DMI	-	1	-		1.05
24	M	61		DMI	-	2	-		0.76
25	F	50		DMI	-	1	-		1.48
26	M	61		PMI/DMI/ LMI	+	2	+		0.97
27	M	41		DMI	-	1	-		0.92
28	M	61		ASMI	+	1	-		1.25
29	M	61		DMI	-	2	-		0.76
30	M	70		PMI	+	2	-		0.90
31	M	58		PMI/DMI	-	2	-		0.81
32	M	64		DMI	-	2	-		0.84
33	M	63		ILMI	+	1	-		0.99
34	M	53		DMI	-	1	-		0.56
35	M	64		DMI	+	3	+		1.14
								Glucocorticoids I	
36	M	41		DMI	-	1	-	665	0.99
37	M	53		AMI	-	2	-	415	1.20
38	F	69		DMI	-	2	-	420	0.70
39	M	55		DMI	-	1	-	330	1.05
40	M	47		AMI	-	2	-	360	0.94
41	M	48		AMI	-	2	-	868	1.41
42	M	58		DMI	-	2	-	784	1.13

Myocardial "Infarct Size" (CPK-g-eq)					
Pred. I.S. (1, 2)	Comp. I.S. (2)	% Change (2)	Pred. I.S. (3)	Comp. I.S. (3)	% Change (3)
16.7	26.0	-55.7	11.2	19.9	-77.7
99.3	82.2	+17.2	144.6	101.1	+30.1
16.9	21.8	-29.0	16.6	21.5	-29.5
142.6	151.1	-6.0	127.0	136.7	-7.6
31.2	26.4	+15.4	39.9	30.2	+24.3
10.3	9.5	+7.8	8.7	8.6	+2.3
45.6	42.3	+7.2	30.6	35.1	-14.7
25.0	29.1	-16.4	17.3	24.1	-39.3
86.2	91.3	-5.9	86.2	91.3	-5.9
14.6	22.5	-54.1	13.6	21.7	-59.6
50.7	51.2	-1.0	30.1	41.6	-38.2
17.8	21.4	-20.0	24.8	26.4	-6.5
5.7	6.4	-12.3	5.7	6.4	-12.3
132.1	199.8	-51.2	149.1	212.9	-42.8
127.1	168.4	-32.5	85.5	129.5	-51.5
100.1	234.3	-134.1	85.3	215.3	-152.4
59.5	97.4	-63.7	40.0	77.6	-94.0
35.7	56.8	-59.1	28.0	49.6	-77.1
28.9	51.2	-77.2	24.6	46.3	-88.2
19.3	23.6	-22.3			
104.1	104.3	-0.2	59.6	73.9	-24.0
44.8	39.5	+11.8	66.9	49.4	+26.2
7.5	8.8	-17.3	7.9	9.0	-13.9
58.8	62.3	-6.0	44.7	52.0	-16.3
26.5	15.9	+40.0	39.0	18.0	+53.8
117.7	129.2	-9.8	114.1	126.6	-11.0
11.1	7.7	+30.6	10.2	7.6	+25.5
9.9	12.7	-28.3	12.4	14.6	-17.7
57.2	98.5	-72.2	43.6	84.1	-92.9
46.1	103.8	-125.2	41.5	97.3	-134.5
17.4	89.8	-416.1	14.1	80.8	-473.0
22.0	65.5	-197.7	18.5	59.8	-223.2
14.6	41.9	-187.0	14.4	41.7	-189.6
21.1	30.4	-44.1	11.9	23.6	-98.3
50.9	119.3	-134.4	57.9	129.3	-123.3
38.7	28.1	+27.4	38.3	53.5	-39.7
140.3	119.7	+14.7	168.1	130.4	+22.4
104.0	98.0	+5.8	73.0	82.3	-12.7
224.1	201.2	+10.2	211.7	205.5	+2.9
247.9	158.1	+36.2	233.5	154.0	+34.0
106.8	77.3	+27.6	150.4	93.1	+38.1
92.9	118.6	-27.7	104.9	128.2	-22.2

Table 1. Clinical and "Infarct Size" Data *(Continued)*

Pt. no.	Sex	Age	Type M.I. S.E.	Type M.I. T.M. Site	Prior M.I.	M.I. Class	Mortal-ity	Time of Rx (min)*	$k_d \times 10^3$ (min^{-1}) (3)
43	F	62		AMI	+	2	-	580	0.79
44	F	75		AMI	-	3	-	475	0.92
45	F	67		DMI	+	2	-	445	1.10
46	F	63		DMI	+	2	+	445	0.71
47	M	60		DMI	-	2	-	480	1.50
48	F	61		DMI	-	1	-	730	1.40
49	M	53		ASMI	-	2	-	598	1.38
50	M	65		ALMI	+	2	-	713	1.40
51	M	54		AMI/DMI	-	2	-	653	0.98
52	M	63	+		+	1	-	433	1.70
53	M	47		AMI	-	2	+	425	0.70
54	M	52		AMI	+	2	-	360	1.82
55	M	54		AMI	-	1		1140	
								Glucocorticoids II	
56	M	60		DMI		2	-	356	1.29
57	M	65		DMI		2	-	504	1.50
58	M	57		DMI	-	2	-	396	1.30
59	M	61		ALMI	+	2	-	315	1.46
60	M	52		AMI	+	2	-	480	0.87
61	M	56		AMI	-	3	-	360	1.07
62	M	40		AMI	-	1	-	480	0.50
63	M	61		AMI	-	3	-	445	0.82
64	M	48		AMI	+	2	-	360	0.73
65	M	58		ALMI	+	1	-	600	0.65
66	M	54		AMI	-	2	-	680	1.00
67	M	48		PMI	-	1	-	630	0.70
68	M	59		AMI	-	2	-	562	0.92
								Glucocorticoids III	
69	F	49		ALMI	-	2	-	510	0.78
70	M	58		PMI	-	2	-	478	1.24
71	M	46		AMI	+	2	-	480	1.47
72	F	54		DMI	-	1	-	519	1.43
73	M	47		DMI	-	2	-	510	1.51
74	M	38		DMI	-	2	-	360	1.79
75	M	60		DMI	-	2	-	647	0.64
76	F	59		AMI	-	2	-	573	1.29
77	M	46		DMI	-	1	-	360	0.77
78	M	65		ALMI	+	2	-	645	0.56
								Glucocorticoids IV	
79	F	62		ALMI	-	2	-	420	0.70
80	M	72		ALMI	-	2	-	435	0.58
81	M	28		PMI	-	2	-	420	1.37

		Myocardial "Infarct Size" (CPK-g-eq)			
Pred. I.S. (1,2)	Comp. I.S. (2)	% Change- (2)	Pred. I.S. (3)	Comp. I.S. (3)	% Change (3)
23.8	42.7	-79.4	18.8	33.2	-76.6
46.6	61.7	-32.4	42.9	58.6	-36.6
10.7	23.9	-123.4	11.7	24.4	-108.5
37.3	45.3	-21.4	26.6	37.4	-40.6
53.1	56.4	-6.2	79.4	72.6	+8.6
11.9	33.5	-181.5	16.7	42.0	-1.5
203.7	131.6	+35.4	280.7	162.9	+42.0
69.4	44.7	+35.6	96.8	54.3	+43.9
141.5	107.8	+23.8	138.7	106.7	+23.1
26.4	15.7	+40.5	44.8	19.3	+56.9
317.1	154.4	+51.3	222.6	134.4	+39.6
24.9	84.3	-238.6	45.1	124.7	-176.5
2.7	6.2	-129.6			
25.6	35.1	-37.1	32.9	39.6	-20.4
51.9	23.8	+54.1	77.6	29.4	+62.1
24.1	52.9	-119.5	31.3	61.3	-95.8
12.9	21.1	-63.6	18.8	26.6	-41.5
195.1	229.7	-17.7	170.1	214.6	-26.2
82.7	97.5	-17.9	88.4	102.1	-15.5
281.2	132.8	+52.8	140.9	92.9	+34.1
177.6	104.4	+41.2	146.1	95.2	+34.8
355.1	185.1	+47.9	259.8	159.8	+38.5
16.2	21.0	-29.6	10.6	17.5	-65.1
158.6	137.1	+13.6	158.6	137.1	+13.6
82.6	81.2	+1.7	58.1	65.9	-13.4
98.9	93.9	+5.1	91.1	89.7	+1.5
197.3	158.4	+19.7	154.2	142.9	+7.3
187.6	89.5	+52.3	232.2	102.1	+56.0
86.8	55.0	+36.6	127.2	71.0	+44.2
15.1	34.0	-125.2	21.6	45.9	-112.5
20.5	44.6	-117.6	31.0	63.1	-103.5
21.6	17.4	+19.4	38.6	25.6	+33.7
22.0	33.3	-51.4	14.1	27.0	-91.5
102.7	59.4	+42.2	132.0	65.9	+50.1
28.0	24.6	+12.1	21.6	20.9	+3.2
154.5	121.3	+21.5	86.6	86.2	+0.5
171.1	161.5	+5.6	120.2	129.7	-7.9
150.2	119.7	+20.3	87.7	89.4	-1.9
79.9	54.7	+31.5	109.2	68.3	+37.5

Table 1. Clinical and "Infarct Size" Data *(continued)*

Pt. no.	Sex	Age	Type M.I. S.E. T.M. Site	Prior M.I.	M.I. Class	Mortal-ity	Time of Rx (min)*	$k_d \times 10^3$ (min^{-1}) (3)
82	M	49	PMI	-	2	-	551	1.23
83	M	57	DMI	+	2	-	495	0.54
84	M	57	ALMI	+	3	-	225	0.98
85	M	58	AMI		2	-	435	0.54
86	M	79	AMI	-	3	-	522	1.31
87	M	66	AMI	-	3	-	540	0.65
88	M	54	ALMI	-	3	-	480	1.09
89	M	52	DMI	-	3	-	690	0.81
90	M	47	DMI	-	2	-	540	0.79
91	M	60	DMI	-	2	-	813	0.73
92	M	37	AMI	-	2	-	514	1.29
93	M	60	PMI	-	3	-	600	0.85
94	M	69	AMI	+	3	-	300	1.21
95	M	45	AMI/ALMI	+	3	-	580	0.65
96	M	78	AMI/DMI	+	4	+	610	1.07
97	F	50	DMI	-	1	-	1502	1.05
98	M	68	AMI	+	2	-	450	0.78
99	M	58	ALMI	-	3	-	540	1.21
100	M	57	DMI	-	2	-	680	1.30
101	F	61	DMI	-	1	-	510	1.12

Controls:
Mean ± SEM 57.2 ± 1.9

0.94
± 0.05

Glucocorticoids
Mean ± SEM 56.2 ± 12.

536.7 1.05
± 23.7 ± 0.04

Significance of
Difference (student
t-test)   n.s.   n.s.   n.s.

Abbreviations: TM = transmural; SE = subendocardial; MI = myocardial infarction;
    ALMI = anterolateral; MI Class = acute classification; I.S. = 'infarct size,"
*Time from rise in CPK from baseline to point of glucocorticoid administration (first dose).
(1) Predicted IS using CPK values over 7 hr after rise in CPK from baseline.
(2) CPK clearance rate (k_d) = 0.001 min^{-1},
(3) Individually calculated CPK clearance rate.
Glucocorticoids I   = patients who received 2 g of methylprednisolone (MP).
Glucocorticoids II   = patients who received 2 g of MP ql2h x 2.
Glucocorticoids III = patients who received 2 g of MP q6h x 2.
Glucocorticoids IV   = patients who received 2 g of MP q3h x 2.

Myocardial "Infarct Size" (CPK-g-eq)					
Pred. I.S. (1,2)	Comp. I.S. (2)	% Change (2)	Pred. I.S. (3)	Comp. I.S. (3)	% Change (3)
88.1	64.0	+27.4	108.2	70.7	+34.7
144.9	81.2	+44.0	78.5	53.1	+32.4
110.3	82.6	+25.1	108.2	81.3	+24.9
68.1	102.2	-50.1	37.0	67.2	-81.6
66.4	63.4	+4.5	86.8	72.1	+16.9
75.4	56.0	+25.7	31.1	47.1	-51.4
80.2	67.8	+15.5	87.4	72.7	+16.8
85.1	56.3	+33.8	69.0	64.0	+7.2
43.0	50.4	-17.2	21.7	43.3	-99.5
51.9	64.3	-23.9	37.9	52.9	-39.6
178.7	120.0	+32.8	230.3	140.0	+39.2
409.7	255.8	+37.6	348.5	233.7	+32.9
34.4	52.6	-52.9	41.6	59.8	-43.8
303.2	246.9	+18.6	197.7	200.0	-1.2
128.1	120.5	+5.9	136.8	124.9	+8.7
44.0	121.1	-175.2	45.7	125.9	-175.5
17.6	34.8	-97.7	13.7	29.0	-111.7
46.7	60.3	-29.1	56.5	70.5	-24.8
10.4	9.7	+6.7	13.5	10.9	+19.3
45.0	54.9	-22.0	50.4	59.7	+18.5
47.9 ± 6.8	66.9 ± 9.7	-50.0 ± 14.5	44.9 ± 6.9	63.6 ± 9.4	-60.4 ± 26.6
102.3 ± 11.2	84.3 ± 7.1	-12.5 ± 7.8	96.4 ± 9.5	84.1 ± 6.4	-11.7 ± 6.9
<0.001	n.s.	<0.03	<0.001	n.s.	<.01

DMI = inferior; ASMI = anteroseptal; AMI = anterior; PMI = posterior;
Pred = predicted; Comp = completed.

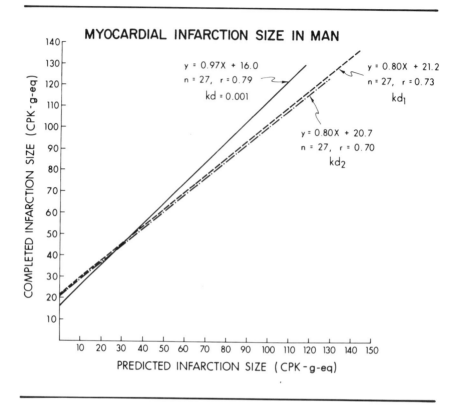

Regression lines developed from predicted and completed infarction-size data in 27 control patients. Solid line: derived from calculations employing a mean CPK clearance rate (k_d) of 0.001 min^{-1}. Broken lines: derived from calculations employing CPK clearance rates, as determined for each patient (k_{d1} and k_{d2}).

g-eq while in 23 glucocorticoid-treated patients mean predicted infarct size was 91.3 ± 5.8 CPK-g-eq ($p =$ n.s., unpaired t-test). Completed mean infarct size in the controls was 122.3 ± 14.8 CPK-g-eq ($n = 13$, $p < 0.02$, paired t-test) while completed mean infarct size in the steroid-treated group was 75.1 ± 5.2 CPK-g-eq ($n = 23$, $p < 0.002$, paired t-test (Fig. 4).

Mortality

Mortality was analyzed in the controls and glucocorticoid-treated patients who had a mean follow-up time of 18 months. Over-

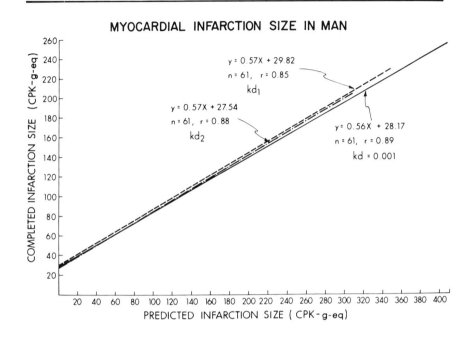

Regression lines developed from predicted and completed infarction-size data in 61 patients treated with glucocorticoid. Data depicted as in Fig. 1. Note that for a large group of patients, the slopes of the regression lines are virtually identical for data derived from a mean CPK clearance rate of 0.001 min^{-1} or individual calculated enzyme clearance rates (k_{d1} and k_{d2}).

all mortality in the control group was 17.1% (6/35) versus 4.5% (3/66) in the glucocorticoid-treated group (chi-square $= 4.47$, $p < .04$).

DISCUSSION

In just over a decade, the treatment of patients with acute myocardial infarction has changed dramatically. With the advent of Coronary Care Units in the early 1960s, and introduction of continuous computer algorithm electrocardiographic monitoring of arrhythmias, utilization of anti-arrhythmic agents, and liberalized use

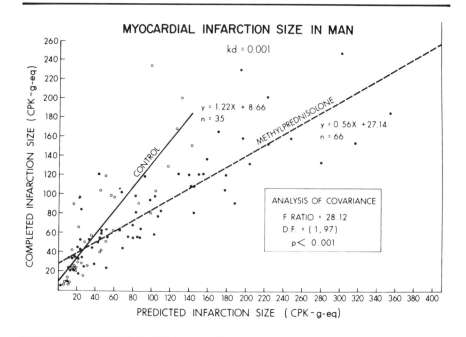

MYOCARDIAL INFARCTION SIZE IN MAN

kd = 0.001

y = 1.22X + 8.66
n = 35

CONTROL

METHYLPREDNISOLONE

y = 0.56X + 27.14
n = 66

ANALYSIS OF COVARIANCE

F RATIO = 28.12
D.F. = (1, 97)
p< 0.001

COMPLETED INFARCTION SIZE (CPK-g-eq)

PREDICTED INFARCTION SIZE (CPK-g-eq)

3   Regression lines developed from predicted and completed infarction-size data in 35 controls (open circles, solid line) and 66 patients treated with glucocorticoid (solid circles, broken line). The decreased slope in the methylprednisolone regression line implies conservation of myocardium.

of defibrillation and pacemaker techniques, mortality from electrical malfunction of the heart in acute myocardial infarction has been considerably reduced. However, mortality from power failure, following acute myocardial infarction, has been altered very little despite the additional availability of hemodynamic monitoring, increasing refinement of indications for the use of pressor and diuretic agents in the treatment of shock and pulmonary edema, availability of assisted circulation in the form of intra-aortic balloon counterpulsation, and the utilization of surgical approaches, including revascularization procedures, in early myocardial infarction. Recently, histological and biochemical data have demonstrated various gradations of ischemic injury throughout the infarcted regions of the myocardium. It has been postulated that pharmacological interven-

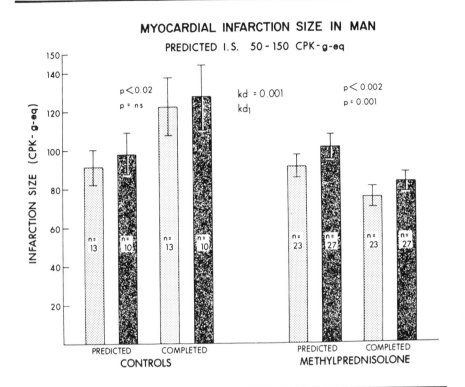

4 Mean predicted and completed infarction-size data for controls (columns at the left) and glucocorticoid-treated patients (columns at the right) with predicted infarction size between 50-150 CPK-g-eq. Light-shaded columns: Data derived employing a mean CPK clearance of 0.001 min^{-1}. Dark shaded columns: Data derived employing individual CPK clearance rates (k_{d_1}). The bars indicate the standard error of the mean. Note the reduction in mean predicted infarction size, following glucocorticoid administration.

tions which alter the biochemical environment of ischemic myocardial zones may modify ultimate infarct size (Maroko and Braunwald, 1973).

Glucocorticoids have been shown to reduce experimental infarct size when administered 30 min and 6 hr after coronary artery occlusion in the dog (Hepper et al., 1955; Libby et al., 1973). It is thought that glucocorticoids stabilize lysosomal and cellular membranes thereby limiting the spread of lysosomal hydrolases which are postulated to cause further myocardial destruction (Spath et al., 1974; Hoffstein et al., 1976). Furthermore, it has been shown that glucocorticoid administration, during experimental coronary occlusion, impedes ischemia and is additive to reperfusion in reversing ischemic myocardial dysfunction (DaLuz et al., 1976).

In addition to the biochemical and cellular mechanisms, there are several hemodynamic effects of glucocorticoids, which may serve to protect ischemic myocardium. It has been demonstrated that glucocorticoids reduce coronary vascular resistance in dogs with experimental acute myocardial infarction (Vyden et al., 1974). Furthermore, administration of glucocorticoids to dogs enhanced collateral blood flow to the infarcted area, with improvement of the metabolism of the ischemic tissue (Masters et al., 1976).

The results from several clinical investigations with glucocorticoids are conflicting in that some studies, indicating a reduction in mortality in patients with acute myocardial infarction treated with steroids (Barzilai et al., 1972), have not been confirmed by others. A recent investigation included 12 patients who received methylprednisolone 30mg/kg intravenously at 6-hr intervals for 48 hr (total dosage approximately 16 g). Five patients expired; at necropsy, two showed rupture of the ventricular septum (Roberts et al., 1976). Prolonged steroid administration in humans (Buckley and Roberts, 1974) and dogs (Green et al., 1974) has been associated with delayed healing of acute myocardial infarction.

These apparent discrepancies with the present study might reflect, in part, a significant variation in the elapsed time between the onset of myocardial infarction and glucocorticoid administration, the dosage and period of time over which the drug was employed, and the size of the myocardial infarction in the treated and untreated groups.

With the development of an enzyme "wash-out" method for predicting and quantitating infarct size in man (Shell et al., 1973), it seems possible to assess the effect of pharmacological intervention upon evolving myocardial infarction. However, the mathematical model of serum CPK activity, on which our study is based, has several theoretical limitations. Thus, small variations in the fractional disappearance rate of CPK (k_d) may impart error into individual estimation of infarct size if an average k_d is used. However, calculation of data in this study, employing the mean reported k_d of 0.001 min^{-1} (Shell et al., 1973) or using two methods (Norris et al., 1975; Morrison et al., 1976) to calculate individual k_d values, resulted in similar mean results. In addition, the pharmacological intervention employed appeared to have no effect upon the fractional disappearance rate of the enzyme (Morrison et al., 1976).

The present study was undertaken to assess the effect of methylprednisolone on evolving myocardial infarct size and subsequent prognosis in man. The data indicate that a pharmacological dose of the glucocorticoid given early in the course of acute myocardial infarction can, in some patients, significantly reduce predicted infarct size. This observation is of considerable theoretical importance, since it suggests that a significant percentage of myocardial injury is reversible in man even approximately 9 hr following the rise in CPK activity from baseline (10-14 hours after onset of coronary artery occlusion).

Although the results of this investigation are encouraging, it must be considered preliminary in nature. A larger series with a long-term follow-up, studied in a randomized double-blind manner, will be necessary to establish the clinical effectiveness of this specific pharmacological intervention.

SUMMARY

The effect of pharmacological doses of corticosteroids on the extent of acute myocardial infarction and upon subsequent mortality was assessed in 66 patients. After prediction of infarction size from analysis of early (7-hr) serum creatine phosphokinase (CPK) changes with a curve fitting procedure based upon nonlinear Gauss-Newton stepwise iterations, each patient received 2-g of methylprednisolone (MP) intravenously. In 46 patients, a second 2-g dose of MP was administered either 3, 6 or 12 hr after the initial dose. Completed infarction size (ISc) was calculated from all available CPK data (90-160 hr).

In 35 control patients with acute myocardial infarction, there was good correlation between predicted infarction size (ISp) and ISc (ISc = 1.22 ISp + 8.66, r = 0.86). In 66 treated patients, ISc was significantly less than ISp (predicted = 102.3 ± 11.2 (mean $\pm$ S.E.M.) CPK-gram-equivalents (CPK-g-eq), completed = 84.3 ± 7.1 CPK-g-eq, p < .004). In 50% of those patients treated, the actual CPK curve fell below the 95% confidence limit of the predicted CPK curve. The exponential clearance of CPK (k_d) was approximated in controls ($k_{d_1} = .00098 \pm .00005$ min^{-1}) and treated patients ($k_{d_1} = .00105 \pm .00004$ min^{-1}) and found to be similar. Mortality within 18 months after myocardial infarction in treated patients was less than 50% of that in controls (p < .04).

These data indicate that a pharmacological dose of methylprednisolone in certain patients with acute myocardial infarction results in salvage of ischemic myocardium. In addition, these observations suggest that a significant percentage of myocardial injury is reversible in man when pharmacological intervention is instituted 10-14 hr after onset of coronary artery occlusion.

ACKNOWLEDGMENTS

The authors wish to acknowledge the nurses and medical house officers in the Coronary Care Unit at North Shore University Hospital who generously provided time in order to make these studies possible.

Some of the data provided in this chapter was presented at the 24th Annual Scientific Session of the American College of Cardiology, held in Houston, Texas in February, 1975.

This study has been supported by the American Heart Association, Nassau Chapter, N. Y., Westchester Heart Association, The Foundation for Education in the Humanities, and the Board of Trustees Research Fund of the North Shore University Hospital.

REFERENCES

Barzilai, D., Plavnick, J., Hazani, A., Einath, R., Kleinhaus, N., and Kanter, Y.: Use of hydrocortisone in the treatment of myocardial infarction. *Chest* 61:488-491 (1972).

Buckley, B., and Roberts, W.: Steroid therapy during acute myocardial infarction. A cause of delayed healing and of ventricular aneurysm. *Am. J. Med.* 56:244-250 (1974).

Dall, J. L. C., and Peel, A. A.F.: A trial of hydrocortisone in acute myocardial infarction. *Lancet* 2:1097-1098 (1963).

DaLuz, P., Forrester, J., Wyatt, H., Diamond, G., Chag, M., and Swan, H.: Myocardial reperfusion in acute experimental ischemia. Beneficial effects of prior treatment with steroids. *Circulation* 58:847-852 (1976).

Gerisch, R. A., and Compeau, L.: Treatment of acute myocardial infarction in man with cortisone. *Am. J. Cardiol.* 1:535-540 (1958).

Green, R., Cohen, J., and DeWeese, J.: Short-term use of corticosteroids after experimental myocardial infarction: Effects of ventricular function and infarct healing. *Circulation* (Suppl. III) 49-50:103 (1974).

Hepper, N. G., Pruitt, R. D., Donald, D. E., and Edwards, J. E.: The effect of cortisone on experimentally produced myocardial infarcts. *Circulation* 11: 742-746 (1955).

Hoffstein, S., Weissman, G., and Fox A.: Lysosomes in myocardial infarction: Studies by means of cytochemistry and subcellular fractionation, with observations on the effects of methylprednisolone. *Circulation* (Suppl. I) 53:34-40 (1976).

Hood, W. B., Jr., McCarthy, B., and Lown, B.: Myocardial infarction following coronary ligation in dogs: Hemodynamic effects of isoproterenol and acetyl strophanthidin. *Circ. Res.* 21:191-199 (1967).

Libby, P., Maroko, P. R., Bloor, C. M., Sobel, B. E., and Braunwald, E.: Reduction of experimental myocardial infarct size by corticosteroid administration. *J. Clin. Invest.* 52:599-607 (1973).

Maroko, P. R., and Braunwald, E.: Modification of myocardial infarction size after coronary occlusion. *Ann. Intern. Med.* 79:720-733 (1973).

Masters, T., Harbold, N., Hall, D., Hackson, R., Mullen, D., Daugherty, H., and Robicsek, R.: Beneficial metabolic effects of methylprednisolone sodium succinate in acute myocardial ischemia. *Am. J. Cardiol.* 37:557-563 (1976).

Morrison, J., Reduto, L., Pizzarello, R., Geller, K., Maley, T., and Gulotta, S.: Modification of myocardial injury in man by corticosteroid administration. *Circulation* (Suppl. I) 53:200-203 (1976).

Norris, R. M., Whitlock, R. M. L., Barratt-Boyes, C., and Small, C. W.: Clinical measurement of myocardial infarct size: Modification of a method for the estimation of total creatine phosphokinase release after myocardial infarction. *Circulation* 51:614-620 (1975).

Page, D. L., Caulfield, J. B., and Kastor, J. A.: Myocardial changes associated with cardiogenic shock. *N. Engl. J. Med.* 285:133-137 (1971).

Roberts, R., DeMello, V., and Sobel, B.: Deleterious effects of methylprednisolone in patients with myocardial infarction. *Circulation* (Suppl. I) 53:203-206 (1976).

Shell, W. E., Lavell, J. F., Covell, J. W., and Sobel, B. E.: Early estimation of myocardial damage in conscious dogs and patients with evolving acute myocardial infarction. *J. Clin. Invest.* 52:2579-2590 (1973).

Spath A., Lane, D., and Lefer, A. M.: Protective action of methylprednisolone on the myocardium during experimental myocardial ischemia in the cat. *Circ. Res.* 35:44-51 (1974).

Vyden, J., Nagasawa, K., Rabinowitz, B., Parmley, W., Tomoda, H., Corday, E., and Swan, H.: Effects of methylprednisolone administration in acute myocardial infarction. *Am. J. Cardiol.* 34:677-686 (1974).

Weil, M. H., and Shubin, H.: Shock following acute myocardial infarction. *Prog. Cardiovasc. Dis.* 11:1-17 (1968).

20

Pharmacological Modification of the Response to Regional Left Ventricular Ischemia by Protease Inhibition

THOMAS M. GLENN
A. GARRETT MILLER
ROY D. GOLDFARB
S. JAMAL MUSTAFA

INTRODUCTION

Recent studies have already defined many of the hemodynamic and cellular consequences of myocardial ischemia. Certainly, it is now recognized that inadequate perfusion of cardiac tissue can result in metabolic alterations leading to irreversible changes in cardiac muscle fibers (Sommers and Jennings, 1964; Trump et al., 1976). Thus, the extent of cardiac cell damage determines the frequency and severity of pump failure following periods of cardiac ischemia. Since myocardial performance depends to a large degree upon the integrity of metabolic processes which generate, preserve and utilize energy (Olson, 1961; Olson et al., 1972), an inadequate

451

or discontinued supply of oxygen to cardiac tissue results in metabolic disturbances which lead to marked alterations in the ultrastructure of cardiac muscle fibers (Ekholm et al., 1968; Hall and Moravee, 1972; Heggtveit, 1972).

Among the more prominent metabolic disturbances associated with varying periods of cardiac ischemia are: a reduction of glycogen stores (Michael et al., 1959; Cornblath et al., 1963), breakdown of energy-rich compounds (Benson et al., 1961; Gudbjarnason, 1972; Olson et al., 1972), ion-balance disorders (Case, 1972), local release of catecholamines (Wollenberger, 1965), and accumulation of lactic acid (Wollenberger and Krause, 1968). Therefore, therapeutic modalities which might: (1) support metabolic activity, (2) interrupt progressive cell necrosis, or (3) maintain adequate coronary perfusion have all been suggested as exerting beneficial effects during or following cardiac ischemia.

PROTEASE ACTIVATION AND THE CELLULAR RESPONSE TO ISCHEMIA

Several investigators have established that cardiac ischemia is associated with activation of acid proteases of lysosomal origin (Ricciutti, 1972; Lefer and Spath, 1975; Ogletree and Lefer, 1976). Indeed, there is evidence that the primary or initiating defect under ischemic conditions, leading to widespread cell damage and eventual cell death, may well be the release of hydrolytic proteases. Hoffstein and coworkers (1964) found that lysosomes are among the first cellular organelles to exhibit damage early in the course of myocardial infarction. Thus, many of the irreversible morphological changes seen in cardiac ischemia (i.e., disruption of cellular components, such as plasma membrane, myozbrillar elements, and mitochondria) may result directly or indirectly from the proteolytic activity of released hydrolases.

There are several essential findings which support an important role for lysosomal protease activation in the development of irreversible cardiac cellular damage under ischemic conditions. First, lysosomal proteases are present in cardiac muscle; they can be isolated cytochemically and demonstrated morphologically (Canonico and Bird, 1976; Topping and Travis, 1976; Smith and Bird, 1976). Secondly, agents which disrupt the lipid membranes of lysosomes activate acid hydrolase activity, whereas, substances such as steroids, that stabilize lysosomal lipid membranes, decrease protease activation after varying periods of cardiac ischemia (Spath and Lefer, 1975; Hoffstein et al., 1976).

Since proteases may play a pivotal role in the sum total of pathophysiological events occuring in regional cardiac ischemia, it was decided to evaluate whether protease inhibition would alter the course of these cellular degenerative changes. The protease inhibitor, aprotinin, was selected as the agent for evaluation. Aprotinin (Trasylol®) is a polypeptide inhibitor of a variety of hydrolytic enzymes, including lysosomal proteases. Previously, it had been shown to exert protective effects in a variety of low-flow states where global ischemia and protease activation are the common denominators (Back et al., 1968; Glenn et al., 1973; Haberland, 1970).

PROTEASE INHIBITION AND HEMODYNAMIC CONSEQUENCES OF CARDIAC ISCHEMIA

Acute ligation of major branches of the left anterior descending (LAD) coronary artery produces marked hemodynamic changes, including decreases in cardiac output, external work (Shah et al., 1974; Skelton et al., 1974), and corresponding falls in arterial blood pressure and peripheral blood flow (Morita et al., 1974; Spath et al., 1975). Most of these alterations are secondary to a generalized decrease in the contractility of the left ventricle and overt pump failure.

Fig. 1 illustrates the changes in mean arterial blood pressure, heart rate and cardiac output in saline- and aprotinin-treated dogs in the 2-hr-period following LAD occlusion. No significant differences were observed between the two groups of animals. Alterations in LAD flow, LAD resistance and systemic vascular resistance are summarized in Fig. 2. Within 20 min of LAD occlusion, there were significant (p < 0.05) decreases in LAD flow and corresponding increases in LAD resistance. In saline-treated dogs, LAD flow continued to fall and LAD resistance to rise during the 20-100 min following occlusion, whereas, LAD flow remained significantly higher (< 0.05) in aprotinin-treated dogs. Systemic vascular resistance increased to 120% of control after a 120-min period following coronary occlusion in both groups of dogs.

Thus, aprotinin pretreatment acted to maintain LAD flow; it had no significant effects on the generalized systemic vasoconstriction secondary to coronary occlusion. Fig. 3 summarizes the values for both groups of dogs with coronary ligation for: left ventricular

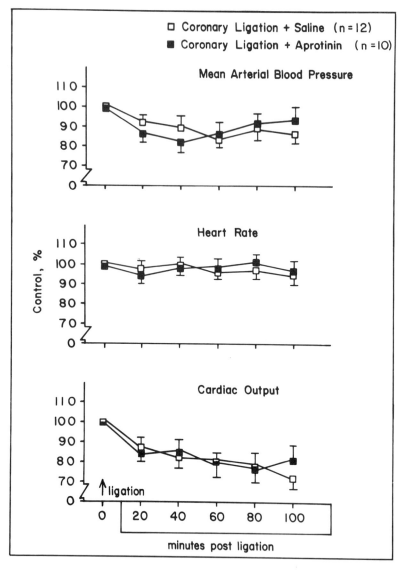

1 Alterations in mean arterial blood pressure (MABP), heart rate (HR) and cardiac output (CO) in saline- and aprotinin-treated dogs following coronary occlusion. Note that aprotinin-treated dogs exhibited a significantly higher ($p < 0.05$) MABP and CO 100 min after occlusion. Each point represents the mean value for the number of experiments indicated in parenthesis. Brackets give standard errors of the mean (SEM).

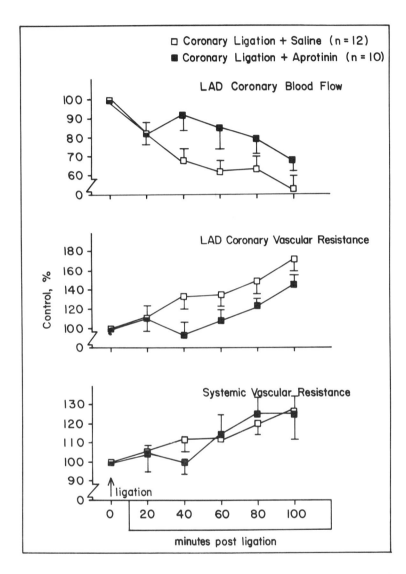

2 Alterations in left anterior descending (LAD) coronary blood flow, LAD coronary vascular resistance and systemic vascular resistance in dogs following coronary occlusion. Aprotinin-treated dogs exhibited a significantly higher value for LAD flow and lower (p < 0.05) compared to saline-treated animals.

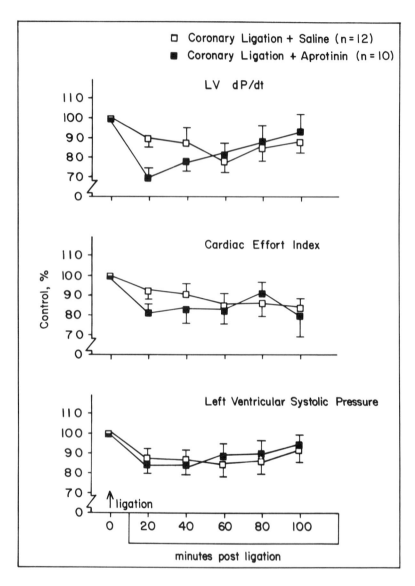

3 Alterations in left ventricular dp/dt, cardiac effort index (CEI) and left ventricular systolic pressure in saline- and aprotinin-treated dogs following coronary occlusion. There were significantly lower values for dp/dt and CEI 20 min after occlusion in both groups of animals.

dṖ/dt, cardiac effort index (CEI), and peak left ventricular systolic pressure (LVSP). After 20 min of coronary occlusion, values for dP/dt and CEI were significantly lower ($p < 0.05$) in saline-treated dogs, as compared to animals pretreated with aprotinin. However, during the next 100-min-period there were no significant differences in these parameters between the two groups. Peak LVSP fell promptly following occlusion in both groups; it then returned to a level slightly below the control values and remained there in both groups of dogs for the duration of the experiment.

The ability of aprotinin to improve cardiac function and, in particular, LAD flow following coronary occlusion does not appear to be related to a direct action of the drug on the myocardium or coronary vasculature. Aprotinin in sham-occluded dogs had no significant effects on arterial blood pressure, heart rate or cardiac output, compared to saline-treated, sham-occluded animals (Fig. 4); nor did the administration of 20,000 KIE/kg of aprotinin produce any changes in left ventricular minute work, left ventricular dP/dt, left ventricular contractile force, or left anterior descending coronary flow (Table 1). These findings are in agreement with previous studies (Glenn and Lefer, 1972; Lefer and Spath, 1974) in which aprotinin did not have any direct action on overall cardiac function, including ventricular contractile force and coronary blood flow.

In summary, the immediate response to ligation of the LAD coronary artery was a decrease in mean arterial blood pressure and cardiac output, and these parameters remained depressed throughout the entire experiment. Aprotinin-pretreated animals, 120 min post occlusion, had a significantly higher mean arterial blood pressure and cardiac output compared to saline-treated dogs. However, the most dramatic differences between these animals, following coronary ligation, were a higher LAD flow and a decreased LAD resistance. The more normalized coronary flow may well account for the observed beneficial effects of aprotinin on overall cardiac function. These findings are comparable to those obtained in several animal species subjected to various types of low-flow states and pretreated with aprotinin (Werde, 1963; Back et al., 1966; Massion and Erdos, 1966; Nagel et al., 1967; Lefer and Martin, 1970; Massion and Blumel, 1971; Glenn et al., 1973; Wilkens et al., 1975).

PROTEASE INHIBITION AND THE RELEASE OF CARDIAC ENZYMES DURING ISCHEMIA

Since progressive ischemic necrosis of the myocardium, following coronary ligation, has been previously related to cardiac cellular

Table 1. Left Ventricular Performance in Saline and Aprotinin Treated Dogs Following Sham Occlusion of the Left Anterior Descending Coronary Artery[1]

Parameter	Time After Administration (minutes)	Sham Occlusion + Vehicle (n=6)	Sham Occlusion + Aprotinin (n=5)
Left Ventribular Minute Work[2] (g-meter/sec/kg)	0	88 ± 7	88 ± 6
	15	87 ± 11	73 ± 11
	30	94 ± 8	89 ± 12
	60	92 ± 6	93 ± 7
	120	82 ± 9	86 ± 15
Left Ventricular dP/dt[2] (% control)	0	100	100
	15	103 ± 2	97 ± 5
	30	100 ± 9	94 ± 7
	60	111 ± 4	88 ± 10
	120	114 ± 6	88 ± 13
Left Ventricular Contractile Force[2] (% control)	0	100	100
	15	93 ± 8	94 ± 9
	30	86 ± 6	98 ± 10
	60	83 ± 7	85 ± 6
	120	83 ± 5	90 ± 5
Left Anterior Descending Coronary Flow (ml/min)	0	11.0 ± 1.2	12.1 ± 1.1
	15	10.6 ± 1.3	11.6 ± 0.9
	30	10.4 ± 1.2	11.6 ± 1.0
	60	9.8 ± 1.2	11.1 ± 1.1
	120	10.3 ± 1.6	9.4 ± 1.1

[1] All animals received aprotinin (20,000 KIE/kg, i.v.) or an equivalent volume of saline.
[2] All values are means (number of experiments in parenthesis) ± standard errors of the mean.

damage and the subsequent release of cardiac creatine phospho-kinase (CPK) activity, and activation of cardiac lysosomal protease (Kjekhus and Sobel, 1970; Lefer and Spath, 1975; Maroko and Braunwald, 1975), the release of cardiac CPK and beta-glucuro-nidase activity were determined in saline- and aprotinin-treated dogs following LAD occlusion. Fig. 5 illustrates the efflux of cardiac beta-glucuronidase activity in both groups of dogs following occlu-sion of the LAD. After 20-40 min of occlusion, there was a signif-icant comparable release of cardiac lysosomal enzyme activity. However, beta-glucuronidase release in aprotinin-treated dogs slowed, until 60 and 90 min post-ligation, the rate of release was

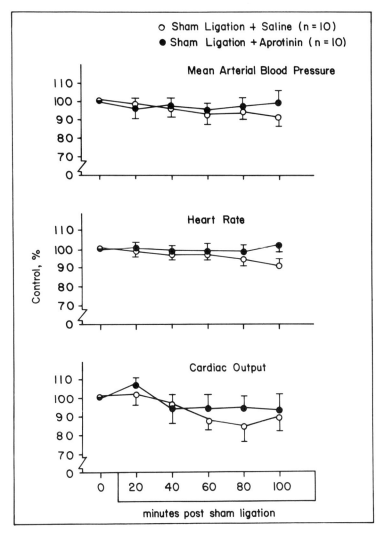

4 Alterations in mean arterial blood pressure (MABP), heart rate (HR), and cardiac output (CO) in aprotinin- and saline-treated dogs with sham occlusion. Aprotinin exerted no significant effects on any of these parameters when compared to animals receiving saline.

significantly lower $(p < 0.02)$ than that found in saline-treated animals.

The release of cardiac CPK following occlusion is summarized in Fig. 6. In the first 20 min of occlusion, there was a rapid release

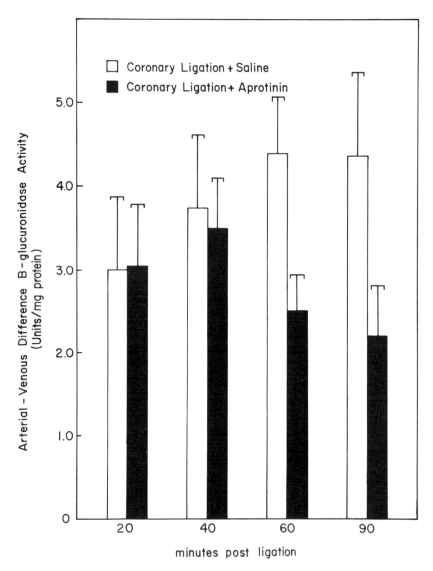

5 Bar graphs of coronary arteriovenous differences for lysosomal enzyme (beta-glucuronidase activity in saline- and aprotinin-treated dogs with occlusion of the LAD. Within 20 min of occlusion, there was a significant efflux of cardiac b-glucuronidase activity and the release continued throughout the 90-min period post occlusion. In aprotinin-pretreated dogs, there was a comparable release of cardiac lysosomal enzyme activity 20 and 40 min post occlusion, however, 60 and 90 min after occlusion, the rate of release fell and the total activity at these times was significantly ($p < 0.02$) lower than in saline-treated animals.

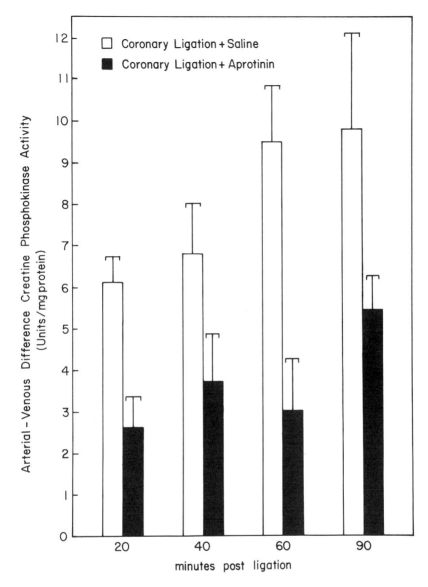

6

Bar graphs of coronary arteriovenous differences for creatine phosphokinase (CPK) activity in saline- and aprotinin-treated dogs with occlusion of the LAD. Release of cardiac CPK progressively increased during the 90 min following occlusion in saline-treated dogs; whereas, the release of cardiac CPK activity 20 min post occlusion was less than 50% of that of saline-treated dogs in animals pretreated with aprotinin. In these dogs, the rate of release of cardiac CPK remained constant over the 90-min experimental period post ligation and measured was significantly lower (p < 0.01) at all intervals than comparable activities obtained from saline-treated dogs.

of cardiac CPK activity, which continued to rise during the subsequent 90 min. However, the total amount of CPK released from the hearts of aprotinin-treated dogs was only 50% of that found in the saline-treated animals; in these dogs, the rate of CPK release remained constant throughout the remainder (20-120 min) of the experimental period. Thus, aprotinin pretreatment in some way altered lysosomal enzyme release, following LAD occlusion, and this decrease in hydrolytic enzyme activation was associated with a corresponding fall in cardiac CPK efflux. This suggested that, in aprotinin-treated dogs, there was a significant attenuation of ischemic necrosis and a reduction in the total tissue mass of the damaged left ventricle.

Numerous studies have hypothesized that the intracellular release of hydrolytic enzymes (i.e., lysosomal proteases) may represent one pathway by which regional myocardial ischemia can lead to widespread irreversible cellular injury and cell death (Ravens and Gudbjarnason, 1969; Haberland, 1970; Riciutti,1972a, 1972b; Gottwik, 1974; Lefer and Spath, 1974; Gottwik et al., 1975; Spath et al., 1975). Thus, as previously mentioned, activation of cardiac lysosomal proteases early in the course of infarction may well be responsible for the observed autolytic changes in the affected cells, involving such cellular constituents as the plasma membrane, myofibrillar elements and mitochondria.

In this connection, it should be noted that several biochemical and histochemical indices (Snitka and Nachlas, 1963; Jennings et al., 1969), have been employed in attempts to assess the degree of cellular damage in cardiac tissue. Kjekshus and Sobel (1970) have suggested that decreases in total cardiac CPK may quantitatively relate to the total mass of damaged tissue or—infarct size. In the present investigation, the continued release of large amounts of hydrolase activity from the myocardium of saline-treated dogs, following occlusion, was apparently associated with an extension of cellular damage and necrosis, as indicated by the progressive increases found in coronary sinus CPK activity. In contrast, aprotinin-treated animals had significantly lower rates of lysosomal enzyme release, 60-120 min post occlusion, and corresponding drops in the release of cardiac CPK, indicating, perhaps, a decrease in the total mass of cardiac cells suffering prominent damage. Similar protective responses of aprotinin have also been reported by Lefer and Spath (1974). Since this drug cannot be shown to exert a direct lysosomal stabilizing effect (Glenn and Lefer, 1972), its beneficial action is probably related to a direct inhibitory effect on proteases released in the affected myocardial cells. Thus, fewer cardiac cells which lie adjacent to those primarily damaged by ischemia may be subjected to the autolytic action of the released proteases in the presence of the protease inhibitor.

It is important to note that inhibition of the digestive activity of these proteases may protect the myocardium metabolically since in the studies of Lochner et al. (1975), mitochondrial phosphorylative reactions were damaged before the oxidative functions of ischemic cardiac tissue were affected. Moreover, Mellors et al. (1967) reported that the uncoupling of mitochondrial oxidative reactions, in the rat heart, by the addition of lysosomal enzymes resulted in a depression of phosphorylation but not of oxidation. Similar findings were reported by Mela et al. (1971) who demonstrated that changes in energy-linked mitochondrial function are related to a direct action of lysosomal proteases released from ischemic tissue on this function. Thus, aprotinin may preserve the ability of the ischemic myocardium to generate high-energy phosphate compounds.

PROTEASE INHIBITION AND METABOLIC ACTIVITY OF THE ISCHEMIC MYOCARDIUM

At the cellular level, adenine nucleotides normally act as an energy coupler between energy-yielding and energy-requiring events in the cell, and it is these aspects of energy metabolism that are markedly impaired under ischemic conditions (Jennings et al., 1969; Dhalla et al., 1972). Lochner et al. (1975) described the marked mitochondrial damage occurring in the heart of the baboon and dog subjected to coronary occlusion and found that oxidative phosphorylation mechanisms were depressed; they suggested that these changes were responsible for the marked alterations in the formation of high-energy compounds, manifest by depression of adenine nucleotide levels (Imai et al., 1964; Neely et al., 1972; Morita et al., 1974; Shah et al., 1974; Dewall et al., 1975; Sharma et al., 1975). Although ischemic changes in nucleoside levels have been less clearly defined, a fall in total adenine nucleotides is usually associated with increases in total nucleoside content (Imai et al., 1964; Mustafa et al., 1975), including increments in the levels of adenosine, a metabolic regulator of coronary blood flow (Mustafa et al., 1975).

Myocardial concentrations of adenine nucleotides, nucleosides

Table 2. Effect of Aprotinin (APT) Administration on Cardiac Adenine Nucleotides and Nucleoside Content Following Coronary Occlusion in Dogs

	ATP	ADP	AMP	ATP+ADP+AMP	HYPOXANTHINE	INOSINE (INO)	ADENOSINE (ADO)	HYPO+INO+ADO	TOTAL PURINES
Aprotinin (10,000 KIE/kg)									
Sham Occlusion + Saline	55.74 ±7.25	16.26+ ±.56	3.23 ±.72	75.23	0.64 ±.08	0.34 ±.08	0.012 ±.005	0.99	76.22
Occlusion + Saline	10.49 ±1.67	6.10 ±1.67	4.54 ±.28	21.13	5.57 ±.69	9.37 ±1.79	0.089 ±.047	15.02	36.15
Sham Occlusion + APT	47.22 ±6.26	15.92 ±.85	3.92 ±.77	67.66	0.48 ±.098	0.173 ±.052	.009 ±.002	0.66	67.72
Occlusion + APT	23.42 ±4.27	10.24 ±.67	2.55 ±.83	36.21	2.87 ±.37	3.10 ±.75	0.012 ±.003	5.98	42.19
Aprotinin (20,000 KIE/kg)									
Sham Occlusion + APT	52.90 ±5.95	10.99 ±1.98	3.17 ±.63	67.06	0.285 ±.047	0.146 ±.022	0.046 ±.007	0.477	67.53
Occlusion + APT	51.88 ±4.86	13.66 ±1.25	3.41 ±0.63	68.95	0.287 ±.080	0.283 ±.012	0.046 ±.001	0.616	69.56

Values expressed as n moles/mg protein ± SEM (mean of 4-6 experiments)

and their totals in sham-occluded and LAD-occluded ligated hearts, obtained from saline- or aprotinin-treated dogs, are summarized in Table 2. These data illustrate that aprotinin acted to preserve total concentrations of purine compounds. In saline-treated dogs, the levels of adenosine triphosphate (ATP) and adenosine diphosphate (ADP) fell 81 and 62%, respectively, following LAD occlusion; whereas, the adenosine monophosphate (AMP) levels increased 40%. The progressive degradation of nucleotides resulted in a 15-fold increase in total nucleoside content (including adenosine, inosine and hypoxanthine). Overall, there was a 47% reduction in total adenine nucleotides and nucleosides. With respect to the nucleosides, hypoxanthine and inosine exhibited the greatest increase, compared to adenosine which exhibited a 7-fold rise. This difference in regard to adenosine may be explained on the basis that adenosine released by hypoxia or ischemia is rapidly converted (Katori and Berne, 1966) to its metabolic products, inosine and hypoxanthine, due to the high tissue concentrations of adenosine deaminase. Finally, the ratios of ATP/ADP fell from 3.42 to 1.71, and ATP/AMP from 17.25 to 2.31 in the saline-treated ligated animals (Table 3). These changes in purine-base content were associated with significant alterations in the energy potential of the adenylate pool, which decreased 25% following coronary ligation.

Pretreatment of animals with 10,000 KIE/kg of aprotinin resulted in improved levels of myocardial high-energy phosphate compounds (Table 2). Although, the total adenine nucleotide value was 71% higher than the comparative value for saline-treated dogs, this figure was still significantly lower (48%) than that obtained from sham-ligated animals. The greater sum of adenine nucleotides in these dogs was primarily due to higher values for ATP (123%) and ADP (67%). With respect to total adenine nucleosides, the value was 60% lower following aprotinin treatment than that for saline-treated animals. However, values for the individual nucleosides, with the exception of adenosine, were not comparable to those obtained from sham-occluded dogs. Additionally, the total purine pool was found to be 16% higher compared to saline-treated dogs. Furthermore, animals pretreated with aprotinin also exhibited an overall improvement in the ratio for ATP/ADP and the calculated energy potential (Table 3). Thus, the administration of aprotinin (10,000 KIE/kg) provided a more favorable metabolic status with respect to nucleotide and nucleoside content, but significant imbalances still existed when compared to values obtained from sham-occluded animals.

Table 3. Percentile Representation of Adenine Nucleotides and their Ratios in Ischemic Myocardium of the Dog with Saline and Aprotinin (APT) Pretreatment

Group	%ATP	%ADP	%AMP	ATP/ADP	ATP/AMP	Energy Potential*
Sham Occlusion + Saline	74.09	21.61	4.19	3.42	17.25	0.848
Occlusion + Saline	49.64	29.15	21.48	1.71	2.31	0.640
Aprotinin (10,000 KIE/kg) Sham Occlusion + APT	70.41	23.73	5.84	2.96	12.04	0.822
Occlusion + APT	64.67	28.27	7.04	2.28	9.18	0.788
Aprotinin (20,000 KIE/kg) Sham Occlusion + APT	78.88	16.38	4.72	4.81	16.68	0.870
Occlusion + APT	75.24	19.81	4.94	3.79	15.21	0.851

$$*\text{Energy Potential} = \frac{0.5 \ (ADP) + (ATP)}{(ATP) + (ADP) + (AMP)}$$

For this reason, additional studies were performed using animals pretreated with 20,000 KIE/kg of aprotinin. This resulted in further normalization of the levels for adenine nucleotides and adenine nucleosides. The concentrations of ATP and ADP were 121% and 33% higher, respectively, and comparable to those obtained from sham-occluded animals. Moreover, the total content of adenine nucleosides was 10-fold less when the dose of aprotinin was increased from 10,000 KIE/kg to 20,000 KIE/kg in these dogs. Lower levels of hypoxanthine (10-fold) and inosine (10.9-fold) accounted for most of the decrease. The content of adenosine increased to levels approximating those measured in sham-occluded animals treated with 20,000 KIE/kg.

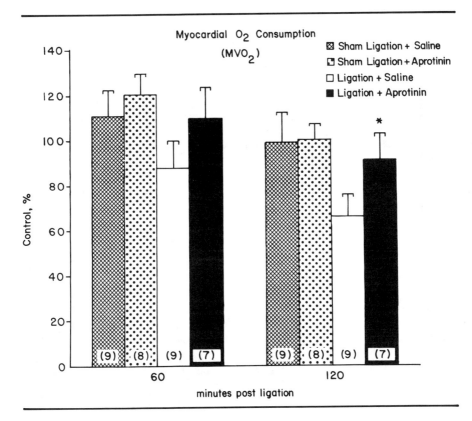

7 Effects of administration of aprotinin or saline on myocardial oxygen consumption (MVO_2) in sham-occluded and LAD-occluded dogs 60 and 120 min post occlusion. The data are expressed as percentage change from pre-occlusion or sham-occlusion values. Although saline-treated dogs with LAD occlusion had a lower MVO_2 60 min following occlusion, compared to sham-occluded and occluded dogs receiving aprotinin, this decrease was not significant. However, 120 min post occlusion, aprotinin-treated dogs had significantly ($p < 0.05$) higher values for MVO_2 than those obtained from saline-treated dogs.

The total sum of purines in the hearts of animals treated with 20,000 KIE/kg of aprotinin were equivalent to those found in sham occluded animals receiving 10,000 KIE/kg of aprotinin. The ratios of ATP/AMP and the energy potential compared favorably to the levels found in sham-ligated animals (Table 3).

Fig. 7 summarizes changes in myocardial oxygen consumption

60 and 120 min following coronary occlusion or sham occlusion in dogs treated with aprotinin or saline. There were no measurable alterations in myocardial oxygen consumption (MVO_2) in the first 60 min after occlusion; however, 120 min upon occlusion, there was a significant decrease in MVO_2 from preocclusion values in saline-treated dogs. Aprotinin-treated animals exhibited significantly higher values for MVO_2, 60 and 120 min post occlusion, compared to the values from saline-treated animals. Thus, a more normalized LAD flow following occlusion in aprotinin-pretreated animals was associated with a significantly higher myocardial oxygen consumption, and rather normal stores of high-energy phosphate compounds. A "sparing" action of aprotinin through inhibition of activated proteases on cardiac-cell mitochondria could well account for these changes.

Thus, the overall alterations in energy metabolism following occlusion of the LAD included: a lowering of ATP and ADP concentrations and an increase in the levels of AMP, with overall decreases in total adenine nucleotide content, accounted for by higher concentrations of adenine nucleosides. These changes in purine-base content are comparable to those previously reported by others (Imai et al., 1964; Tsubio and Buckley, 1965; Gerlach et al., 1966) in the ischemic heart. Aprotinin pretreatment completely reversed these alterations.

The release of adenosine into the interstitial space during ischemia is normally associated with changes in myocardial metabolism (Rubio et al., 1974). There is also evidence (Atkinson, 1968) that the different adenine nucleotides may have effects on several of the enzymes of the metabolic degradative pathway. Thus, the balance between the respective adenine nucleotides may serve as a major regulating factor, integrating metabolic activity and coronary flow. Since coronary occlusion results in marked changes in ATP, ADP and AMP, the overall effects of ischemia on metabolism can be described by a quantitative expression that takes into consideration their relative concentrations. Atkinson (1968) has proposed the term "energy charge (E) of the adenylate pool" in respect to relative concentrations of adenine nucleotides. The value of E normally ranges from 0.0 to 1.0 and represents that fraction of total adenosine moieties which exist in the form of high-energy phosphates.

Thus, aprotinin administration also resulted in a more normalized value for E (energy potential) and the quantity of total purines; whereas, the concentration of total purines in saline-treated dogs was markedly less, perhaps due to the movement of nucleosides through damaged cell membranes into the interstitial space, resulting in a washout of purines into the plasma and their conversion into other degradative products, such as inosine monophosphate and uric acid.

In addition, these data may suggest that aprotinin acted to preserve the nucleotide pool by blocking the further breakdown of adenine nucleotides, perhaps by inhibition of one of the enzymes of the purine metabolizing-pathway or by blocking the release of nucleosides from the cell, in which case the nucleosides would be more readily available for incorporation into the nucleotide pool. In this regard, Dewall et al., (1971) found significant improvements in cardiac contractile force and reversal of electrocardiographic changes in the ischemic myocardium when using allopurinol, a potent inhibitor of xanthine oxidase, an enzyme involved in the conversion of adenine nucleotide breakdown products to uric acid.

PROTEASE INHIBITION AND THE CORONARY DILATOR RESPONSE TO ADENOSINE

Since aprotinin was shown in the present study to exert significant effects on LAD flow and nucleoside metabolism, it was decided to investigate the possibility that the aprotinin-induced alterations in adenosine metabolism under ischemic conditions could account for the better maintenance of LAD flow following occlusion.

Changes in LAD coronary flow after the intraventricular administration of adenosine occurred in normal anesthetized dogs in the presence and absence of aprotinin. The data obtained are illustrated in Fig. 8. In augmenting doses (20-$60 \mu g$) adenosine produced progressive increments in excess coronary flow, peak coronary flow, and the duration of excess flow. Administration of aprotinin 10,000 KIE/kg, i.v., 30 min prior to that of adenosine (20-$60 ug$, intraventricularly) resulted in significant increases in excess flow. Since the latter is a product of peak response and the duration of response, the significant ($p < 0.05$) increases in excess flow, observed with all doses of adenosine after aprotinin pretreatment, could be accounted for by prolongation ($p < 0.05$) in the duration of response.

Interpretation of these findings centers on the increased duration of flow. Possible explanations include actions of aprotinin on the enzymes of adenosine metabolism or on the uptake of adenosine into the cardiac cell. However, the effects of aprotinin on two of

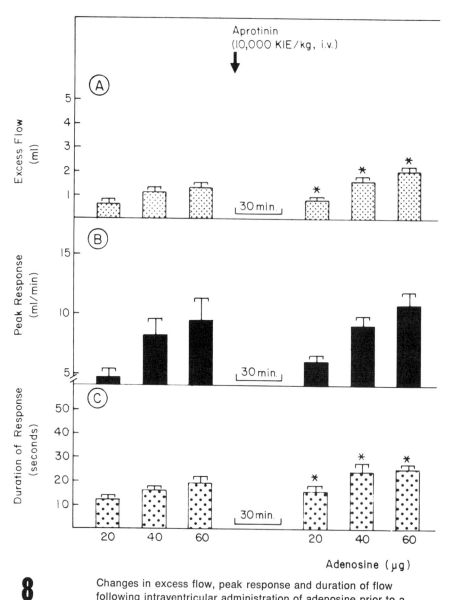

8

Changes in excess flow, peak response and duration of flow following intraventricular administration of adenosine prior to a 30-min period following the administration of aprotinin. Increasing doses of adenosine produced progressive increments in excess flow, peak response and the duration of response. Note that following aprotinin administration, although the peak response was unaltered, excess flow and the duration of response was potentiated at each dose level of adenosine. Each value represents the mean of at least 6 separate experiments. Brackets indicate SEM.

Table 4. Effect of Aprotinin on the Uptake of Adenosine into Cultured Cardiac Cell

Concentration of Adenosine (μm)	Adenosine Uptake* With Vehicle (n mole/mg protein)	Adenosine Uptake With Aprotinin** (n mole/mg protein)
1	0.066	0.049
3	0.198	0.153
5	0.380	0.264
10	0.821	0.370
20	0.859	0.469

*Each value represents the mean of 2-4 separate experiments.
**Concentration of aprotinin was 4,000 KIE/ml in the assay system. This concentration of aprotinin was determined from a dose response curve, wherein 4,000 KIE/ml resulted in the maximum inhibition of adenosine uptake.

the more important enzymes of adenylate metabolism, namely, adenosine deaminase and 5'-nucleotidase, were previously found not to be significant (Glenn, et al., 1973). Therefore, alteration of the mechanism for the uptake of adenosine into the cardiac cell becomes a prominent possibility.

In order to investigate the effect of aprotinin on adenosine uptake into cardiac tissue, cultured cardiac muscle cells were isolated, according to the methods of Mustafa et al. (1975), and placed for 2 days in growth media containing 40% N-16 Pucks, 45% modified Hanks solution and 15% Horse serum. Media and cells were separated and counted for radioactivity according to described procedures (Mustafa, et al., 1975).

A double reciprocal plot of the data obtained indicated that aprotinin produced a noncompetitive inhibition of adenosine uptake (Table 4). These findings suggest the possibilities that aprotinin may have an effect on the carrier-mediated protein involved in the transport of adenosine or on one or more of the enzymes active in the adenosine uptake into the cardiac cell. Furthermore, it is of interest to note that the percentage inhibition of adenosine uptake is greater at higher concentrations of extracellular adenosine.

Regardless of the exact mechanisms of this inhibitory action of aprotinin on uptake, it is clear that this drug does alter the uptake of adenosine into the myocardial cell. Such an action *in vivo* could result in higher extracellular levels of adenosine and, thus, in turn, greater concentrations of adenosine would reach coronary resistance vessels. This could cause a redistribution of coronary flow and an improved perfusion of the ischemic myocardium upon occlusion. These data are not inconsistent with the observed maintenance of high-energy phosphate levels and the normalization of coronary blood flow following aprotinin administration in animals with LAD occlusion.

SUMMARY

The improved coronary blood flow in aprotinin-pretreated dogs with LAD occlusion was associated with significant decreases in the activation of cardiac lysosomal enzymes and CPK activity, together with maintenance of high-energy phosphate pools. A resulting higher myocardial oxygen consumption probably reflects an overall cellular-sparing action of the drug. By inhibiting released lysosomal proteases, aprotinin may prevent the participation of these proteases in the autolytic phase of cell dysfunction and attenuate the progressive extension of the cellular damage that normally occurs secondary to acute ligation. These so-called sparing actions of aprotinin can account for the preservation of mitochondrial function, a more normalized high-energy phosphate pool, and a higher cellular energy potential, and associated normalized oxygen consumption.

Although more definitive cellular or subcellular mechanism(s) for the protective action of aprotinin in regional ischemia remain to be defined and requires further investigation, the metabolic data obtained in the present study correlate well with the overall improvement observed in left ventricular function, and support the concept that protease inhibition may be a successful therapeutic intervention under conditions of regional ventricular ischemia.

ACKNOWLEDGMENTS

Parts of this study were supported by grant GM-21235 from the National Institute of Health, and grants-in-aid from Bayer, AG and the University of South Alabama College of Medicine Research Advisory group.

The authors acknowledge the expert technical assistance of Mr. James Horan, Ms. Linda Kopaciewicz and Mr. Mark Tschudy. Dr. Gunther Schnells (Bayer AG, Leverkusen, German Federal Republic) graciously provided the aprotinin (Trasylol®).

REFERENCES

Atkinson, D. E.: Energy charge of the adenylate pool as a regulatory parameter: Interaction with feedback modifiers. *Biochemistry* 7:4030-4034 (1968).

Back, N., Jainchill, M., Wilkens, H. J., and Ambrus, J. E.: Effect of inhibitors on plasmin, kallikrein and kinin on mortality from scalding in mice. *Med. Pharmacol. Exp.* 15:597-602 (1966).

Benson, E. S., Evans, G. T., Hallway, B. E., Phibbs, C., and Fiver, F.: Myocardial creatine phosphate and nucleotides in anoxic cardiac arrest and recovery. *Am. J. Physiol.* 201:687-693 (1961).

Canonico, P. G., and Bird, J. W. C.: Lysosomes in skeletal muscle tissue, zonal centrifugation evidence for multiple cellular sources. In *Protection of the Ischemic Myocardium*, E. Braunwald, ed. American Heart Association, Inc., Dallas, Texas (1976), pp. 34-39.

Case, R. B.: Ion alterations during myocardial ischemia. *Cardiology* 56:245-262 (1972).

Cornblath, M., Randle, P. J., Parmeggiani, A., and Morgan, H. E.: Regulation of glycogenolysis in muscle. Effects of glucagon content, and phosphorylase activity in the isolated perfused rat heart. *J. Biol. Chem.* 238:1592-1597 (1963).

Dewall, R. A., Vasko, K. A., Stanley, E. L., and Kezdi, P.: Responses of ischemic myocardium to allopurinol. *Am. Heart J.* 83:362-366 (1971).

Dhalla, N. S., Yates, J. C., Walz, D. A., McDonald, V. A., and Olson, R. E.: Correlation between changes in endogenous energy stores and myocardial function due to hypoxia in the isolated, perfused rat heart. *Can. J. Physiol. Pharmacol* 50:333-345 (1972).

Ekholm, R., Kerstell, J., Olson, R., Rudenstam, C. M., and Svanborg, A.: Morphological and biochemical studies of dog heart mitochondria after short periods of ischemia. *Am. J. Cardiol.* 22:312-318 (1968).

Gerlach, E., Deuticke, B., and Dierkessmann, R.: Vergleichende Untersuchugen über die Bildung von Adenosin in Myokard verschiedener Tierspezies bei sauerstoffmangel. *Klin. Wochenshr.* 44:1307-1310 (1966).

Glenn, T. M., Herlihy, B. L., and Lefer, A. M.: Protective action of a protease inhibitor in hemorrhagic shock. *Arch. Int. Pharmacodyn. Ther.* 203:292 (1973).

Glenn, T. M., and Lefer, A. M.: Modification of the deleterious actions of lysosomal hydrolases in circulatory shock by Trasylol. In *New Aspects of of Trasylol Therapy: Protease Inhibition in Shock Therapy*, W. Brendel and G. Haberland, eds. Schattauer Verlag, Stuttgart (1972), pp. 53-72.

Gottwik, M. G., Kirk, E. S., Hoffstein, S., and Weglicki, W. B.: Early changes of lysosomal hydrolases following coronary occlusion: Effect of collateral blood flow. *Clin. Res.* 22:680A (1974).

Gottwig, M. G., Weglicko, W. B., and Kirk, E. S.: Collateral flow as a determining factor for lysosomal enzyme release and removal after 1 and 2 hours of myocardial ischemia. *Clin. Res.* 23:185 (1975).

Gudbjaranson, S.: Acute alterations in energenetics of ischemic heart muscle. *Cardiology* 56:232-244 (1972).

Haberland, G. L.: The effect of Trasylol in shock. In *Shock: Biochemical, Pharmacological and Clinical Aspects*, A. Bertelli and N. Back, eds. Plenum Publishing Corp., New York (1970), p. 273.

Hall, P. Y., and Moravee, J.: Acute hypoxia of the myocardium. Ultrastructural changes. *Cardiology* 56:73-84 (1972).

Heggtveit, H. A.: Morphological alterations in the ischemic heart. *Cardiology* 56:284-290 (1972).

Hoffstein, S., Gennaro, D. E., Weissman, G., Hirsch, J., Strenli, F., and Fox, A. C.: Cytochamical localization of lysosomal enzyme activity in normal and ischemic dog myocardium. *Am. J. Pathol.* 79:193-203 (1964).

Hoffstein, S. ,Weissman, G., and Fox, A. C.: Lysosomes in myocardial infarction: Studies by means of cytochemistry and subcellular fractionation, with observations on the effects of methylprednisolone. *Circulation* 53: 34-40 (1976).

Imai, S., Riley, A. L., and Berne, R. M.: Effect of ischemia on adenine nucletides in cardiac and skeletal muscle. *Circ. Res.* 15:443-450 (1964).

Jennings, R. B., Sommers, H. M., Hendson, P. B.: and Kaltenbagh, J. P.: Ischemic injury of myocardium. *Ann. N. Y. Acad. Sci.* 156:61-78 (1969).

Katori, M., and Berne, R. M.: Release of adenosine from anoxic heart-relationship to coronary flow. *Circ. Res.* 19:420-425 (1966).

Kjekshus, J. K., and Sobel, B. E., Depressed myocardial creatine phosphokinase activity following experimental myocardial infarction in rabbit. *Circ. Res.* 27:403-414 (1970).

Lefer, A. M., and Martin, J.: Relationship of plasma peptides to the myocardial depressant factor in hemorrhagic shock. *Circ. Res.* 26:59-69 (1970).

Lefer, A. M., and Spath, J. A.: Preservation of myocardial integrity by a protease inhibitor during acute myocardial ischemia. *Arch. Int. Pharmacodyn. Ther.* 211:225-236 (1974).

Lefer, A. M., and Spath, J. A.: Protective effect of protease inhibition in myocardial ischemia. In *New Aspects of Trasylol Therapy: Experimental Myocardial Infarction*, M. Cantin, G. L. Haberland, G. Schells, and H. Selye, eds. Schattauer Verlag, Stuttgart (1975), pp. 311-328.

Lochner, A., Opie, L. H., Owen, P., Kitze, J. C. N., Bruyneed, K., and Gevers, W.: Oxidation phosphorylation in infarcted baboon and dog myocardium: effects of mitochondrial isolation and incubation media. *J. Mol. Cell. Cardiol.* 7:203-217 (1975).

Maroko, P. R., and Braunwald, E.: Reduction of myocardial infarct size. In *New Aspects of Trasylol Therapy: Experimental Myocardial Infarction*, M. Cantin, G. L. Haberland, G. Schnells, H. Selye, eds. Schattauer Verlag, Stuttgart (1975), pp. 243-269.

Massion, W. H., and Blumel, G.: Irreversibility in shock: Role of vasoactive kinnins. *Anesth. Analg.* (Cleve.) 50:970:976 (1971).

Massion, W. H., and Erdos, E. G.: The effects of ATP and a proteolytic enzyme inhibitor in irreversible shock. *J. Okla. State Med. Assoc.* 59:467-471 (1966).

Mela, L.. Bacalzo, L. V., Jr., and Miller, L. D.: Defective oxidation metabolism of rat liver mitochondrial in hemorrhagic and endotoxin shock. *Am. J. Physiol.* 220:571-577 (1971).

Mellors, A., Tappel, A. L., Sawant, P. L., and Desai, I. O.: Mitochondrial swelling and uncoupling of oxidative phosphorylation by lysosomes. *Biochem. Biophys. Acta* 143:299-309 (1967).

Michael, G., Naegle, S., Danforth, W. H., Ballard, F. B., and Binjy, R. J.: Metabolic changes in heart muscle during anoxia. *Am. J. Physiol.* 197: 1147-1151 (1959).

Morita, Y., Ishiyama, T., Tsukamoto, N., and Yamamura, Y.: Effects of iso-proterenol and artificial pacing on hemodynamics and energy liberation of the infarcted heart in dogs. *Jap. Heart J.* 15:579-592 (1974).

Mustafa, S. J., Berne, R. M., and Rubio, R.: Adenosine metabolism in cultured chick embryo heart cells. *Am. J. Physiol.* 228:1474-1478 (1975).

Nagel, M., Karl-Schuch, W., and Rahmanzadeh, R.: Untersuchungen zur zusätzlichen Proteasen-inhibitor Therapie bei der septischen Peritonitis. In *New Aspects of Traysylol Therapy*, R. Marx, H. Imdahl, and G. L. Haberland, eds. Schattauer Verlag, Stuttgart (1967), p. 129.

Neely, J. R., Rovetto, M. J., and Oram, J. F.: Myocardial utilization of carbohydrates and lipids. *Prog.Cardiovasc. Dis.* 15:289-329 (1972).

Ogletree, M. L., and Lefer, A. M.: Influence of nonsteroidal anti-inflamatory agents on myocardial ischemia in the cat. *J. Pharmacol. Exp. Ther.* 197: 582-593 (1976).

Olson, R. E.: The contractile protein of heart muscle. *Am. J. Med.* 30:362-707 (1961).

Olson, R. E., Dhalla, N. S., and Sun, C. N.: Changes in energy stores in the hypoxic *Cardiology* 56:114-124 (1972).

Ravens, K. G., and Gudbjarnason, S.: Changes in the activities of lysosomal enzymes in infarcted canine heart muscle. *Circ. Res.* 24:851-856 (1969).

Ricciutti, M. A.: Myocardial lysosome stability in the early stages of acute ischemic injury. *Am. J. Cardiol.* 30:492-497 (1972a).

Ricciutti, M. A.: Lysosomes and myocardial cellular injury. *Am. J. Cardiol.* 30:498-502 (1972b).

Rubio, R., Wiedmeier, and Berne, R. M.: Relationship between coronary flow and adenosine production and release. *J. Mol. Cell. Cardiol.* 6:561-566 (1974).

Shah, A., Kechejian, S. J., Kavaler, F., and Fisher, V. J.: Effects of adenine nucleotides on contractility of normal and post-ischemic myocardium. *Am. Heart J.* 87:740-749 (1974).

Sharma, G. P., Varley, K. G., Kim, S. W., Borwinsdy, N., Cohen, J., and Dhalla, N. S.: Alterations in energy metabolism and ultrastructure upon reperfusion of the ischemic myocardium after coronory occlusion. *Am. S. Cardiol.* 36:234-243 (1975).

Skelton, C. L., Kirk, E. S., and Sonnenblick, E. H.: Influence of hypoxia and ischemia on myocardial contractile function. *Bull. N. Y. Acad. Med.* 50: 294-307 (1974).

Smith, A. L., and Bird, J. W. C.: Distribution and particle properties of the vacuolar apparatus of cardiac muscle tissue. In *Protection of the Ischemic Myocardium*, E. Braumwald, ed. American Heart Association, Inc., Dallas, Texas (1976), pp. 40-41.

Snitka, R. K., and Nachlas, M. M.: Histochemical alterations in ischemic heart muscle and early myocardial infarction. *Am. J. Path.* 42:507-527 (1963).

Sommers, H. M., and Jennings, R. B.: Experimental acute myocardial infarction. Histologic and histochemical studies of early myocardial infarcts induced by temporary or permanent occlusion of a coronary artery. *Lab. Invest.* 13:1491-1503 (1964).

Spath, J. A., Jr., and Lefer, A. M.: Effects of dexamethasone on myocardial cells in the early phase of acute myocardial infarction. *Am. Heart J.* 90: 50-55 (1975).

Spath, J. A., Reed, E. A., and Lefer, A. M.: Influence of increased circulating levels of splanchnic lysosomal enzymes on the response to myocardial ischemia *Ann. Surg* 181:813-818 (1975).

Topping, T. M., and Travis, D. F.: An electron cytochemical study of mechanisms of lysosomal activity in the left ventricular mural myocardium. In *Protection of the Ischemic Myocardium, E. Braumwald*, ed. American Heart Association, Inc., Dallas, Texas (1976), pp. 34-40.

Trump, B. F., Mergner, W. J., Kahng, M. W., and Saladino, A. J.: Studies on the subcellular pathophysiology of ischemia. In *Protection of the Ischemic Myocardium*, E. Braunwald, ed. American Heart Association, Inc., Dallas, Texas (1976), pp. 17-26.

Tsuboi, K. K., and Buckley, N. M.: Metabolism of perfused C[14] labeled nucleosides and bases by the isolated heart. *Circ. Res.* 16:343-352 (1965).

Werde, E.: Über Plasmakinine. *Nounyn Schmideberg's Arch Pharmacol.* 245: 254-262 (1963).

Wilkens, H. J., Steger, R., and Back, N.: Effect of the protease inhibitor Trasylol in acute coronary occlusion in dogs. In *New Aspects of Trasylol Therapy: Experimental Myocardial Infarction*, M. Catin, G. L. Haberland, G. Schnells, and H. Selye, eds. Schattauer Verlag, Stuttgart (1975), pp. 381-392.

Wollenberger, A.: Anoxia induced release of noradrenaline from the isolated perfused heart. Nature (Lond.) 207:88-89 (1965).

Wollenberger, A., and Krause, E. G.: Metabolic control characteristics of the acutely ischemic myocardium. *Am. J. Cardiol.* 22:349-3559 (1968).

Discussion

Lefer, Morrison and Glenn

DR. THADEUS PRUSS (*McNeil Laboratories*) : Dr. Morrison, it has been documented that steroids inhibit healing. It has also been demonstrated that they will inhibit the healing process after myocardial infarction has been induced experimentally. How much concern do you have for producing cardiac tamponade with steroids in patients after myocardial infarction?

DR. JOHN MORRISON (*North Shore University Hospital, Manhassett, N. Y.*) : I am concerned about this particular problem, although acute use eliminates most of the potential complications. I should like to point out several details that are important in this respect. Let us start on a basic level: in dogs, if up to 30 mg/kg of the glucocorticoid are given in acute myocardial infarction, no difficulty follows. Beyond 60 mg/kg, perhaps, problems can occur.

Several years ago, a case of Dressler's syndrome in man was reported on long-term steroids. This patient, who had been on a steroid preparation for 53 days, developed a left ventricular aneurysm and died during cardiac surgery to correct it.

There is no question that high doses of steroids given chronically can cause problems. Recently, Roberts and Sobel gave 12 patients a total, in divided doses, of 16 grams of glucocorticoid; 5 of those patients expired and 2 of them had a ruptured left ventricular septum. These data indicate that too much steroid is detrimental to healing, in general, and to healing of cardiac tissues, in particular.

DR. ALLAN M. LEFER (*Jefferson Medical College*) : I think that is an interesting problem and, as Dr. Morrison indicated, the answer is that chronic administration of high doses of glucocorticoids can cause complications in several ways. I do not think anybody here advocates chronic administration of glucocorticoids in acute myocardial infarction. Most of the data indicate that one dose is effective and I noticed in Dr. Morrison's slides, that his best results were achieved with 2 doses, 3 hr apart. Under these circumstances (i.e., one or two doses) one does not see a delay in wound healing or interference with the immune process, and I do not feel it is fair to compare acute with chronic administration continuing, for example, for 53 days.

DR. GERALD J. KELLIHER (*Medical College of Pennsylvania*) : Dr. Glenn, could you tell me what the cardiac effect of aprotinin is? Also, were you able to demonstrate that aprotinin actually exerted an action other than decreasing infarct size?

DR. THOMAS M. GLENN (*University of South Alabama, College of Medicine*) : Aprotinin does not appear to produce a positive inotropic effect either in the isolated heart or in the intact animal. Other than CPK determinations, we do not have mean ST elevations or any other index of that type. However, Dr. Lefer and Dr. Maroko have used aprotinin and they saw marked reductions in mean ST segment elevation, which indicated to them a decreased extension of infarct size.

DR. ALEXANDER SCRIABINE (*Merck Institute for Therapeutic Research*) : Dr. Glenn, the total ventricular performance, you said, was not altered by the aprotinin therapy. Did you have occasion to look at segmental performance, that is, ischemic segments?

DR. GLENN : No, we have not performed those types of studies. However, if you carry the protocol out for about 4 to 5 hr, you can then distinguish between the two groups of animals on a hemodynamic basis. But you cannot in the first 2 hr following the occlusion.

DR. ROBERT J. LEE (*Squibb Institute for Medical Research*): Dr. Lefer, how much of the glucocorticoid that is taken up by the heart is native glucocorticoid and, on the basis of the half-life of steroids, how soon after the first dose would you give a second dose of steroid?

DR. LEFER: About 85% of the glucocorticoid taken up by the heart remains as native steroid after 2 hr. The biological half-life of the glucocorticoids in our experiments was about 80 min. On the basis of these and other facts, I would recommend giving the first dose of steroid as soon as possible after myocardial ischemia occurs and the second dose about 4 hr later.

482

Modification of Developing Infarct Size by Beta-Adrenergic Blockade

ROBERT J. LEE

INTRODUCTION

There is considerable evidence that cardiac power failure, and thus mortality, following acute myocardial infarction is directly related to the ultimate size of the infarct, i.e., the amount of damaged myocardium (Cohn, 1974; Hood, 1975). Since blood flow to the region of the infarct is greatly reduced, the rate at which oxygen is consumed by the myocardium (MVO_2) becomes an important factor in the development of the infarct. Following experimental occlusion of a major coronary artery, evidence of myocardial ischemia is present within seconds (Hood, 1975). Available oxygen supplies are rapidly reduced in the central zone of the infarct and contractile function of myocardium in this area quickly ceases. If this is analogous to the clinical situation following acute myocardial infarction (AMI), therapeutic interventions that favorably alter the relationship between oxygen supply and demand in the ischemic area surrounding the central zone of the infarct should result in the salvage of viable myocardium and minimize final infarct size.

The pain and anxiety present after acute myocardial infarction

481

lead to an increase in circulating catecholamines (Gazes et al., 1959; Valori et al., 1967). In addition, Mueller (1976) has shown that, following coronary artery ligation, norepinephrine content in coronary venous blood increased, indicating catecholamine release by the ischemic myocardium. This high catecholamine milieu has positive chronotropic and inotropic effects that wastefully raise MVO_2 (Raab, 1968), leading to extension of infarct size. Furthermore, the potential for the induction of re-entrant ventricular arrhythmias is enhanced by increased catecholamine concentration (Wit et al., 1975). It seems reasonable, therefore, that blockade of beta-adrenergic receptors in the acutely infarcted heart would be beneficial from the point of view of decreasing MVO_2, as well as for the antiarrhythmic protection such intervention would confer.

EXPERIMENTAL FINDINGS

The major determinants of MVO_2 are heart rate, contractile state and wall tension (Sonnenblick and Skelton, 1971). Heart rate and myocardial contractile force are decreased by the administration of beta-adrenergic blocking doses of propranolol. These effects are, presumably, due to blockade of the stimulant action of the intrinsic catecholamine concentration. Higher doses of propranolol cause a further direct depression of myocardial contractility and increase in wall tension (Lee et al., 1975).

Intravenous administration of beta-adrenergic blocking doses of propranolol ($0.5 - 2$ mg/kg, i.v.) to anesthetized, open-chest dogs reduced the heart rate from 130 ± 6 to 111 ± 4 beats/min, and decreased the average S-T segment elevation, recorded from several epicardial sites, during coronary artery occlusion (Maroko et al., 1971). Average S-T segment elevation measured in this fashion is an indication of the degree of underlying myocardial ischemia, and its reduction during coronary artery occlusion must be due either to decreased MVO_2 or to redistribution of blood flow into the ischemic area (Fam and McGregor, 1968; Winbury et al., 1971). There is experimental evidence that the favorable action of propranolol on the oxygen supply/demand ratio may be due to both of these mechanisms (Sonnenblick and Skelton, 1971; Becker et al., 1971). The beneficial effects of decreasing heart rate and myocardial contractility would seem to outweigh the possible detrimental effect of increased wall tension, since MVO_2 diminishes after propranolol administration (Mueller, 1976). Furthermore, the prolongation of diastole provides more time for subendocardial perfusion to occur. This, plus the fact that propranolol may reverse ischemia-induced increases in ventricular diastolic compliance (Mueller, 1976), brings about a redistribution of coronary flow from subepicardial to more ischemic, subendocardial regions. The net result of the decrease in MVO_2 and redistribution of blood flow following propranolol is an increase in PO_2 in the ischemic region (Winbury et al., 1971). That these hemodynamic effects of propranolol have a practical application in acute myocardial infarction (AMI) was demonstrated experimentally by Sommers and Jennings (1972). They reported that intravenous administration of propranolol (5 mg/kg), prior to coronary artery occlusion lasting 20 or 25 min, markedly decreased the incidence of myocardial necrosis in surviving dogs.

CLINICAL FINDINGS

The usefulness of beta-adrenergic blockade in the therapy of angina pectoris has been well established (Gianelly and Harrison, 1970; Prichard and Gillam, 1971; Coltart, 1971). The major beneficial effect of such therapy is the reduction in cardiac work and, thus, MVO_2, both at rest and during activity. This decreases the incidence of stress-induced myocardial ischemia in susceptible areas, e.g., subendocardium, supplied by compromised coronary arteries. The potential of such therapeutic interventions in the salvage of viable ischemic myocardium in AMI is obvious from a theoretical point of view. When the hemodynamic state of the patient with AMI is taken into account, however, there are potential disadvantages to the administration of beta-adrenergic blocking drugs. A reduction in overall ventricular function exists, the extent of which is related to the size of the infarct. In this situation, maintenance of marginal cardiac performance may depend upon compensatory adrenergic stimulation (Harrison and Alderman, 1971). If this is removed by blockade of the beta receptors in the heart, congestive heart failure may result. In addition, beta-adrenergic blocking agents, such as propranolol, possess quinidine-like effects which directly depress myocardial contractility and represent further potential hazards.

Controversy exists as to whether or not its potential for inducing heart failure precludes the use of propranolol in AMI. The earliest reports of clinical trials of this drug in AMI indicated that propranolol treatment decreased mortality (Snow, 1965, 1966). Of particular interest in these studies was the fact that fewer patients in the propranolol-treated group developed heart failure than in the control group although this difference was not significant. Later studies failed to confirm a reduction in AMI mortality due to propranolol (Balcon et al., 1966; Clausen et al., 1966); in another investigation in which critically ill patients were not excluded, a greater tendency toward heart failure was observed in the treated group (Balcon et al., 1966). These studies demonstrate that propranolol does not increase mortality in AMI, nor does it raise the incidence of heart failure, except possibly in the critically-ill patient. They fail to show, however, whether or not propranolol diminishes the extent of myocardial damage in surviving patients.

Using a 35-lead serial precordial electrocardiographic technique (an extension of the epicardial-mapping technique mentioned above), Braunwald et al. (1974) reported that propranolol reduced the magnitude of S-T segment elevation in patients with uncomplicated infarcts, presumably reflecting a decrease in the degree of ischemia in the area of the infarct. The results of an extensive hemodynamic study of the effects of intravenous propranolol in AMI (Mueller, 1976) showed that the drug improved oxygenation of ischemic myocardium. Reduced heart rate and myocardial contractility, improvement of ventricular diastolic relaxation and, probably, a decrease in catecholamine release by ischemic myocardium were the main factors involved in this beneficial effect.

The specter of congestive heart failure due to direct myocardial depression, following propranolol administration in AMI, led to experimental studies with practolol, a cardioselective beta-adrenergic blocking agent with intrinsic sympathomimetic effects (Vaughn-Williams, et al, 1973). This agent decreased the extent and severity of myocardial ischemic injury, as manifest by epicardial S-T segment elevation, after acute coronary artery occlusion in dogs, without depressing ventricular function (Libby et al., 1973). Clinical studies utilizing practolol in AMI demonstrate a decrease in precordial S-T segment elevation (Thomas, 1976), a decrease in the occurrence of chest pain (Waagstein and Hjalmarson, 1976a) and a decrease in heart work, without signs of manifest heart failure (Waagstein and Hjalmarson, 1976b). Recent reports of serious side effects, after prolonged administration of practolol, make it unlikely that this agent will be available for future clinical use.

All beta-adrenergic receptor blocking agents that have been tested clinically in the treatment of angina pectoris have proven to be effective (Prichard, 1974). The compounds tested include representatives of all five groups classified by Fitzgerald (1969) on the basis of associated properties, such as selectivity, membrane stabilization and intrinsic sympathomimetic action. Thus, the antianginal efficacy of these agents is due primarily, if not solely, to their beta-adrenergic blocking properties. Presumably, the same mechanisms account for their efficacy in the treatment of AMI. The dilemma concerning their use in AMI is that the therapeutic goal is to reduce MVO_2 by decreasing myocardial demand for oxygen (i.e., decreasing cardiac work), but not to depress ventricular function to the point of causing congestive heart failure. Thus, it would seem that the ideal beta-adrenergic blocking agent for use in AMI is one with a high degree of potency and a lack of direct myocardial-depressant properties. Nadolol (SQ 11725, Corgard) is one such agent.

$$O-CH_2-CH-CH_2-NH-C(CH_3)_3$$

Nadolol

The beta-blocking potency of nadolol *in vivo* is 2-4 times that of propranolol, but it produces 20-40 times less direct myocardial depression than propranolol (Lee et al., 1975). A comparison of the direct myocardial-depressant properties of nadolol with those of several other beta-adrenergic blocking agents is seen in Fig. 1. The effect of increasing cumulative half-logarithmic concentrations of each agent on the contractile force of driven guinea pig left atria is shown. It is evident that propranolol caused a concentration-dependent depression of contractility at levels higher than 0.3 $\mu g/ml$, whereas nadolol produced no appreciable depression throughout the range of concentrations studied. Bunolol and pindolol were slightly less depressant than propranolol, whereas practolol had a slight positive inotropic effect, undoubtedly due to its sympathomimetic properties.

Increases in heart rate, mediated by increased sympathetic outflow, must be considered detrimental in AMI. Fig. 2 shows the effects of nadolol and propranolol on exercise-induced tachycardia in trained dogs. The experiment was a carefully controlled cross-

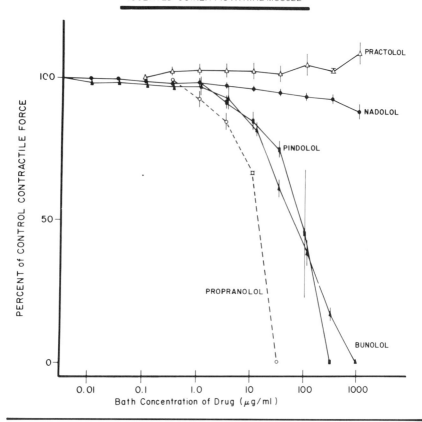

ISOLATED GUINEA PIG ATRIAL MUSCLE

1 The effect of increasing concentrations of several beta-adrenergic blocking agents on contractile force of electrically driven (60 beats/min) guinea pig left atrial muscle (3-9 tissues/compound). Nadolol was approximately 300 times less depressant than propranolol, in the absence of a sympathomimetic effect which is evident with practolol.

over study in which the magnitude and duration of inhibition of exercise-induced tachycardia, following administration by gavage of 0.5 mg/kg/day of either drug for 5 days, was studied. Nadolol inhibited the heart-rate response to exercise to a greater degree than did propranolol. The peak effect with either drug occurred at 4 hr

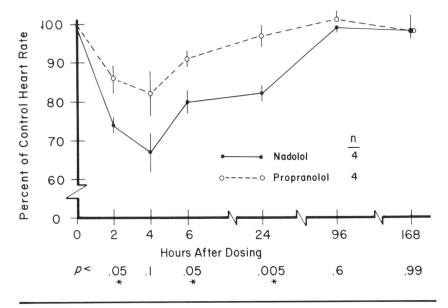

Effect of Nadolol and Propranolol on Maximum Heart Rate
Attained During Exercise

2 A comparison of the effect of nadolol and propranolol on maximum heart-rate response to treadmill exercise in trained dogs. The drugs were given orally for 5 days, at a dose of 0.5 mg/kg. Nadolol has a greater magnitude and a longer duration of effect than propranolol.

after drug administration, but the differences in their effects were not statistically significant at that time. The differences in effect at 2 and 6 hr were significant, however. After the administration of propranolol, heart-rate responses to exercise had returned to control values by 24 hr. In contrast, 24 hr after the administration of nadolol, heart rate responses were still inhibited. The prolonged duration of nadolol action is thought to be due to the fact that this drug is not extensively metabolized by animals (Wong et al., 1973) or man (Vukovich et al., 1976a).

Nadolol and propranolol were studied in respect to their ability to prevent epicardial S-T segment elevation in an area supplied by a branch of the left anterior descending coronary artery in the

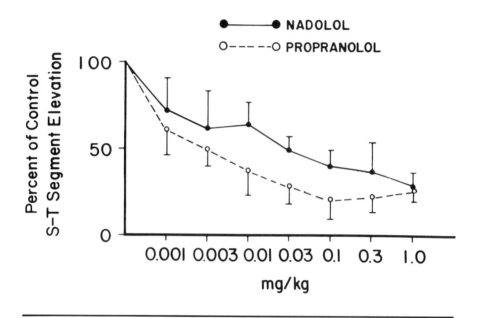

3   The effect of increasing doses of nadolol or propranolol on the degree of S-T segment elevation in the ischemic area during coronary occlusion. Both drugs inhibited the S-T segment elevation in response to occlusion in a dose-related fashion. There was no significant difference between the effects of the two drugs.

anesthetized dog during a 90-sec occlusion. Reproducible control occlusions were carried out and the S-T segment elevation at 90 sec was expressed as 100%. Occlusion was then repeated after injection of isoproterenol (3 μg/kg) and the S-T segment elevation at 90 sec was expressed as percentage of control. Subsequently, occlusions were performed in the absence and in the presence of isoproterenol, after each dose of either nadolol or propranolol. The magnitude of S-T segment elevation during occlusion in the presence of isoproterenol was double that seen during control occlusion. After the 0.03-mg/kg dose, significant inhibition of the S-T segment elevation due to occlusion alone was found with both compounds ($p < 0.05$) (Fig. 3). Propranolol appears to have a greater effect, but not significantly so. Both compounds inhibited the exacerbation of the S-T segment elevation by isoproterenol in a dose-related fashion and

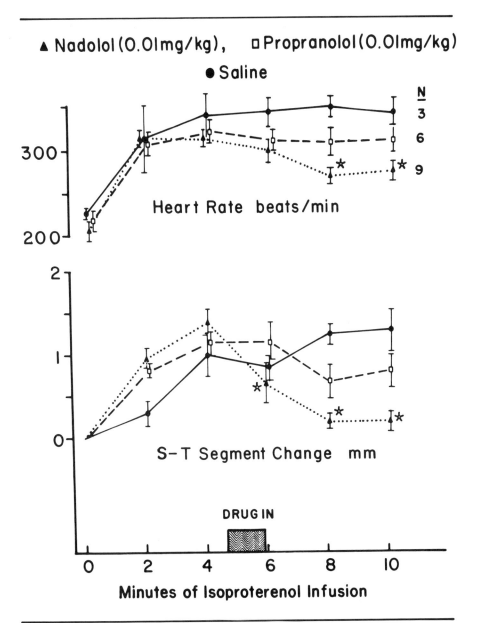

▲ Nadolol(0.01mg/kg),   □ Propranolol(0.01mg/kg)
● Saline

Heart Rate beats/min

S-T Segment Change   mm

DRUG IN

Minutes of Isoproterenol Infusion

4   A comparison of the effects of nadolol or propranolol (0.01 mg/kg) on the heart rate and S-T segment changes during a 10-min infusion of isoproterenol. Asterisks indicate significant differences, $p < 0.05$, when compared with the 4-min value. Nadolol, but not propranolol, is effective in reducing heart rate and S-T segment changes.

completely blocked the effects of the exogenous catecholamine after the 0.1-mg/kg dose.

Ischemic S-T segment changes (depression or elevation) can be elicited in unanesthetized, atherosclerotic rabbits by infusion of isoproterenol at rates of 1-3 μg/kg/min (Lee and Baky, 1976). The ability of nadolol and propranolol to reverse the heart rate and S-T segment changes during a 10-min infusion of isoproterenol was studied. Either nadolol or propranolol was injected into the marginal ear vein during the 5th min of the isoproterenol infusion. Both compounds caused a significant reversal of the heart rate and S-T segment changes, induced by isoproterenol at doses of 0.1 mg/kg and above. After a dose of 0.01 mg/kg, however, only nadolol had a significant effect (Fig. 4).

The antiarrhythmic activity of nadolol in experimental animal models (Evans et al., 1976) has proven to be predictive in that it has been effective against a variety of arrhythmias in man (Vukovich et al., 1976b). In preliminary clinical studies, nadolol has also been effective in the therapy of angina pectoris and has been shown to reduce arterial blood pressure in hypertensive patients (unpublished observations).

In conclusion, it seems clear that the decrease in MVO_2 and the favorable hemodynamic changes following beta-adrenergic blockade in AMI result in the salvage of ischemic myocardium and the reduction of ultimate infarct size. These agents should be used only with extreme caution (perhaps with digitalization) in patients with borderline congestive heart failure, who rely on adrenergic stimulation for adequate myocardial performance. Their use in patients with uncomplicated AMI, however, seems indicated on the basis of data available at this time.

REFERENCES

Balcon, R., Jewitt, D. E., Davies, J. P. H., and Oram, S.: A controlled trial of propranolol in acute myocardial infarction. *Lancet* 2: 917-920 (1966).

Becker, L. C., Fortuin, N. J., and Pitt, B.: Effect of ischemia and antianginal drugs on the distribution of radioactive microspheres in the canine left ventricle. *Circ. Res.* 28:263-269 (1971).

Braunwald, E., Maroko, P. R., and Libby, P.: Reduction of infarct size following coronary occlusion. *Circ. Res.* 34 and 35, Suppl. 3:192-201 (1974).

Clausen, J., Felsby, M., Jorgensen, F. S., Nielsen, B. L., Roin, J., and Strange, B.: Absence of prophylactic effect of propranolol in myocardial infarction. *Lancet* 2:920-924 (1966).

Cohn, J. N.: Pharmacological manipulation of myocardial metabolism. *Bull. N. Y. Acad. Med.* 50(3):328-340 (1974).

Coltart, D. J.: Comparison of the effects of propranolol and practolol on exercise tolerance in angina pectoris. *Br. Heart J.* 33:62-64 (1971).

Evans, D. B., Peschka, M. T., Lee, R. J., and Laffan, R. J.: Antiarrhythmic action of nadolol, a beta-adrenergic receptor blocking agent. *Eur. J. Pharmacol.* 35:17-27 (1976).

Fam, W. M., and McGregor, M.: Effect of nitroglycerin and dipyridamole on regional coronary resistance. *Circ. Res.* 22:649-659 (1968).

Fitzgerald, J. D.: Perspective in adrenergic beta-receptor blockade. *Clin. Pharmacol. Therap.* 10:292-306 (1969).

Gazes, P. C., Richardson, J. A., and Woods, E. F.: Plasma catecholamine concentrations in myocardial infarction and angina pectoris. *Circulation* 19:657-661 (1959).

Gianelly, R. E., and Harrison, D. C.: Propranolol in angina pectoris. *Clin. Med.* (Sept) 70:29-37 (1970).

Harrison, D. C., and Alderman, E. L.: Beta-adrenergic blockade in acute myocardial infarction. In *Circulatory Effects and Clinical Uses of Beta-Adrenergic Blocking Drugs*, D. C. Harrison, ed. Excerpta Medica, Amsterdam (1971), pp. 87-95.

Hood, W. B., Jr.: Modification of infarct size. In *Innovations in the Diagnosis and Management of Acute Myocardial Infarction*, A. N. Brest, L. Wiener, E. K. Chung and H. Kasparian, eds. F. A. Davis Company, Philadelphia (1975), pp. 259-278.

Lee, R. J., and Baky, S. H.: Effects of several antianginal agents in the isoproterenol stress test in atherosclerotic rabbits. *Fed. Proc.* 35(3):349 (1976).

Lee, R. J., Evans, D. B., Baky, S. H., and Laffan, R. J.: Pharmacology of nadolol (SQ 11725), a beta-adrenergic antagonist lacking direct myocardial depression. *Eur. J. Pharmacol.* 33:371-382 (1975).

Libby, P., Maroko, P. R., Covell, J. W., Malloch, C. I., Ross, J., Jr., and Braunwald, E.: Effect of practolol on the extent of myocardial ischemic injury after experimental coronary occlusion and its effects on ventricular function in the normal and ischemic heart. *Cardiovasc. Res.* 7:167-173 (1973).

Maroko, P. R., Kjekshus, J. K., Sobel, B. E., Watanabe, T., Covell, J. W., Ross, J., Jr., and Braunwald, E.: Factors influencing infarct size following experimental coronary artery occlusions. *Circulation* 43:67-82 (1971).

Mueller, H.: Propranolol in acute myocardial infarction in man. Effects of hemodynamics and myocardial oxygenation. *Acta Med. Scand.* Suppl. 587:177-183 (1976).

Pritchard, B. N. C.: Beta-adrenergic receptor blocking drugs in angina pectoris. *Drugs* 7:55-84 (1974).

Pritchard, B.N.C., and Gillam, P. M. S.: An assessment of propranolol in angina pectoris. A clinical dose response curve and the effect on the electrocardiogram at rest and during exercise. *Br. Heart J.* 33:473-480 (1971).

Raab, W.: Myocardial metabolic vulnerability. Key problem in pluricausal, coronary heart disease. *Cardiologia* (Basel) 52:305-317 (1968).

Snow, P. J. D.: Effect of propranolol in myocardial infarction. *Lancet* 2:551-553 (1965).

Snow, P. J. D.: Treatment of acute myocardial infarction with propranolol. *Am. J. Cardiol.* 18:458-459 (1966).

Sommers, H. M., and Jennings, R. B.: Ventricular fibrillation and myocardial necrosis after transient ischemia. Effect of treatment with oxygen, procainamide, reserpine and propranolol. *Arch. Intern Med.* 129:780-789 (1972).

Sonnenblick, E. H., and Skelton, C. L.: Oxygen consumption of the heart: physiologic principles and clinical implications. *Mod. Concepts Cardiovasc. Dis.* 40:9-16 (1971).

Thomas, M.: The effect of beta-blockade on S-T segment elevation after acute myocardial infarction in man with some experimental observations. *Acta Med. Scand.* (Suppl.) 587:185-188 (1976).

Valori, C., Thomas, M., and Shillingford, J.: Free noradrenaline and adrenaline excretion in relation to clinical syndromes following myocardial infarction. *Am. J. Cardiol.* 20:605-617 (1967).

Vaughan-Williams, E. M., Bagwell, E. E., and Singh, B. N.: Cardiospecificity of beta-receptor blockade. *Cardiovasc. Res.* 7:226-240 (1973).

Vukovich, R. A., Dreyfuss, J., Brannick, L. J., Herrera, J., and Willard, D.: Pharmacologic and metabolic studies with a new beta-adrenergic blocking agent, nadolol. *J. Clin. Pharmacol.* 16:631-637 (1976a).

Vukovich, R. A., Sasahara, A., Zombrano, P., Belko, J., Godin, P., and Brannick, L. J.: Antiarrhythmic effects of a new beta-adrenergic blocking agent, nadolol. *Clin. Pharmacol. Ther.* 19(1):118 (1976b).

Waagstein, F., and Hjalmarson, A. C.: Double-blind study of the effect of cardioselective beta-blockade on chest pain in acute myocardial infarction. *Acta. Med. Scand.* (Suppl.) 587:201-207 (1976a).

Waagstein, F., and Hjarlmarson, A. C.: Effect of cardioselective beta-blockade on heart function and chest pain in acute myocardial infarction. *Acta Med. Scand.* (Suppl.) 587:193-200 (1976b).

Winbury, M. M., Weiss, H. R., and Howe, B. B.: Effects of beta-adrenoreceptor blockade and nitroglycerin on myocardial oxygenation. *Eur. J. Pharmacol.* 16:271-277 (1971).

Wit, A. L., Hoffman, B. F., and Rosen, M. R.: Electrophysiology and pharmacology of cardiac arrhythmias IX. Cardiac electrophysiologic effects of beta adrenergic receptor stimulation and blockade. Part A. *Am. Heart J.* 90:521-533 (1975).

Wong, K. K., Drefuss, J., Shaw, J. M., Ross, J. J., and Schreiber, E. C.: A beta-blocking agent (SQ 11725) that is not metabolized extensively by dogs and monkeys. *Pharmacologist* 15:245 (1973).

22

Effect of Hyaluronidase on Infarct Size

PETER R. MAROKO

Death in hospitalized patients with acute myocardial infarction has two main causes: primary arrhythmias and cardiac pump failure (Lown et al., 1967; Scheidt et al., 1970). Death secondary to disturbances in rhythm has been markedly reduced through the use of modern monitoring techniques and by therapeutic measures, whereas death due to pump failure and cardiogenic shock, in particular, is still unacceptably high.

The classical approach to the treatment of the shock syndrome is to attempt to improve, either pharmacologically or mechanically, the associated adverse hemodynamic parameters. However, an alternative approach is to try to change the ischemic process itself at cell level so as to preserve as many viable myocardial cells as possible (Maroko et al., 1971; Maroko and Braunwald, 1976; Braunwald and Maroko, 1974).

Coronary artery occlusion triggers a sequence of events that eventually leads to myocardial cell death. These changes were once considered to occur very rapidly but they are now believed to take several hours (Maroko et al., 1971; Maroko et al., 1972b; Maroko and Braunwald, 1976). Cell death, which histopathologically constitutes an infarction, is, therefore, best considered as a dynamic sequence of complex changes. Analysis of this chain of biochemical and histological events is complicated not only by our fragmentary knowledge of the many reactions involved but also by certain special characteristics of the process itself. Thus, the necrobiosis should be considered not only from the point of view of each individual ischemic myocardial cell but also, and perhaps more importantly, from the point of view of the whole population of ischemic cells. The regional nature of ischemic heart disease compounds this difficulty, i.e., an acutely ischemic zone is surrounded by others, each of which may either be normal or have varying degrees of chronic ischemia, so that multifaceted, and not fully explored, interactions between the zones result. Thus, on the one hand, a nonischemic zone may be induced by ischemia in a neighboring zone to alter its flow, its contractility and its metabolic rate, while, on the other, metabolically or pharmacologically-induced changes in vascular tone in a nonischemic zone may cause redistribution of flow; the resulting augmentation or reduction in collateral flow to the ischemic zone itself will obviously have a major influence on the evolution of the necrotic process. Within an ischemic region, the consequences of the occlusion of a coronary artery are different for each cell. The effect may, in part, depend on the amount of collateral flow that reaches each cell and on the location of each cell within the ischemic zone (epicardium vs. endocardium, and periphery vs. center of the infarction). It is conceivable, for example, that metabolic substrates and pharmacological agents can reach the cells at the periphery of the infarct more easily than they can those in the center. Similarly, harmful metabolites can be more easily washed out from the periphery of the infarct. In addition, the response of the organism to the infarction may affect the subsequent course of the infarct more at its periphery than at its center. Thus, for example, the increased circulating level of catecholamines that follows infarction may adversely affect the oxygen balance in the border zone and so seal the fate of these cells.

Of the many interventions, acting through diverse mechanisms, that have been used in an attempt to reduce experimental infarct size, hyaluronidase is the most promising. In dogs with acute experimental coronary occlusion, this drug was shown to reduce epicardial ST-segment elevations, both when it was administered as a pretreatment and when given 30 min after occlusion (Maroko et al., 1972a). This was carried out in 14 dogs, and there was a reduction in both the sum of ST-segment elevations on the epicardium (ΣST) and in

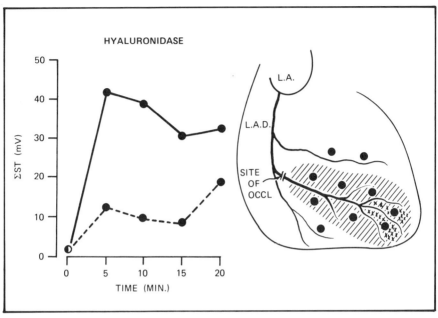

1 An example of the effect of hyaluronidase administration on the number of sites showing ST-segment elevation (NST), and on the sum of ST-segment elevations (ΣST). Right: schematic representation of the heart. Shaded area = area of ST-segment elevation 15 min following occlusion alone; cross-hatched area= area of ST-segment elevation 15 min following occlusion preceded by hyaluronidase administration. L.A. = left atrium; L.A.D. = left anterior descending coronary artery. Site of Occl. = site of occlusion; closed circles = sites where epicardial electrocardiograms were obtained. Left: comparison between the sum of ST-segment elevations (ΣST) in the same animal after the two occlusions. Continuous line = ΣST just before and after the control occlusion; broken line = ΣST just before and after the occlusion with hyaluronidase pretreatment; time = minutes after coronary occlusion. (From Maroko et al., 1972a; by permission of The American Heart Association, Inc.)

the number of sites showing ST-segment elevation over 2 mV (NST) ; therefore, by electrocardiographic criteria, ischemic injury was of smaller magnitude and of more limited extent when hyaluronidase had been given (Figs. 1 and 2). Further investigations were then carried out to ascertain the effects of hyaluronidase on the development of myocardial necrosis in the dog 24 hr after coro-

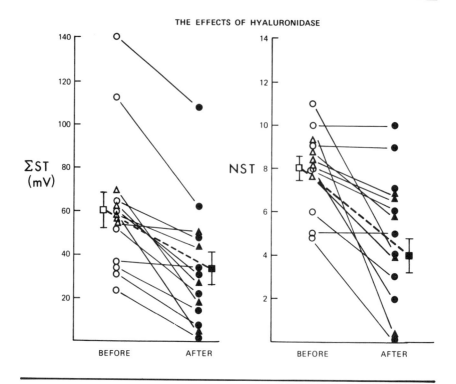

2   The effect of hyaluronidase on myocardial ischemic injury. Left: sum of ST-segment elevations (ΣST) before (open symbols) and after (closed symbols) hyaluronidase treatment. Each continuous line connecting two symbols represents one animal. Triangles = animals with permanent occlusions in which hyaluronidase was administered 30 min after occlusion; circles = animals with two 20-min occlusions in which hyaluronidase was administered prior to the second occlusion. Squares = mean ± standard error for all dogs. Right: number of sites showing ST-segment elevation over 2 mV (NST) before (open symbols) and after (closed symbols) hyaluronidase administration. (From Maroko et al., 1972a; by permission of The American Heart Association, Inc.)

nary occlusion. It was found that ST-segment elevations on the epicardium, 15 min after the occlusion, accurately predict necrotic changes 24 hr later, as assessed by myocardial creatine phosphokinase (CPK) depletion, severity of histological alterations and by epicardial QRS changes (Maroko et al., 1971; Maroko et al., 1972b;

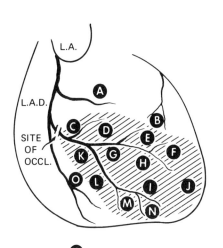

SITE	ST (mv)	CPK I.U./mg prot	HISTOLOGY
A	0	22.8	NORMAL
B	0	19.8	NORMAL
C	4	———	ABNORMAL
D	8	7.3	ABNORMAL
E	9	———	ABNORMAL
F	7	———	ABNORMAL
G	7	5.4	ABNORMAL
H	7	4.7	ABNORMAL
I	5	4.9	ABNORMAL
J	6	———	ABNORMAL
K	4	———	ABNORMAL
L	6	6.2	ABNORMAL
M	5	12.9	ABNORMAL
N	3	———	ABNORMAL
O	0	———	NORMAL

Ⓒ *SITE OF BIOPSY*
////*AREA OF ST SEGMENT ELEVATION*

3 The relationship of ST-segment elevations, 15 min after occlusion, to CPK activity and histological structure 24 hr later in an animal with occlusion alone. Left: schematic representation of the anterior surface of the heart and its arteries. Shaded region = area of ST-segment elevations 15 min after occlusion. Circles = sites where biopsies were taken. L.A. = left atrial appendage; L.A.D. = left anterior descending coronary artery; site of occl. = site of occlusion. Right: comparison between ST-segment elevation, CPK, and histological analysis 24 hr later in the same sites. (From Maroko et al., 1972a; by permission of The American Heart Association Inc.)

Maroko et al., 1972c; Hillis et al., 1976a) (Fig. 3). However, dogs that had received hyaluronidase (225 — 1,000 NF units/kg, i.v.), 30 min after the occlusion, showed that sites with ST-segment elevations similar to those in dogs with an occlusion alone had much less necrosis, as witnessed by less myocardial CPK depression, less histological damage and a smaller fall in R waves, with less Q wave development (Maroko et al., 1972b; Hillis et al., 1976a) (Fig. 4).

These studies, while demonstrating clearly that 24 hr after occlusion the extent of necrosis is smaller in animals treated with hyaluronidase, could not distinguish between a permanent preserva-

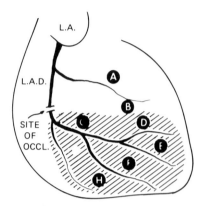

SITE	ST (mv)	CPK I.U./mg prot	HISTOLOGY
A	0	24.6	NORMAL
B	0	18.8	NORMAL
C	3	23.2	NORMAL
D	4	13.4	NORMAL
E	7	7.6	ABNORMAL
F	9	11.2	ABNORMAL
G	5	17.0	NORMAL
H	7	18.8	NORMAL

 BIOPSY SITES

/// AREA OF ST SEGMENT ELEVATION

4 The effect of hyaluronidase on the relationship of ST-segment elevation (prior to drug administration) to CPK activity and histological structure 24 hr later in an animal with a permanent occlusion. Left: schematic representation of the anterior surface of the heart and its arteries. L.A. = left atrial appendage; L.A.D. = left anterior descending coronary artery; site of occl. = site of occlusion; shaded area = area of ST-segment elevation 15 min after coronary occlusion (prior to hyaluronidase administration). Right: comparison between ST-segment elevation, 15 min after occlusion, i.e., prior to hyaluronidase administration, and CPK activity and histological structure 24 hr later. (From Maroko et al., 1972a; by permission of The American Heart Association, Inc.)

tion of jeopardized myocardium and a mere delay in the development of necrosis. Experiments were, therefore, carried out in rats in which the left main coronary artery was occluded (Maclean et al., 1976). These animals were either treated with hyaluronidase (1,500 NF units/kg i.v., 5 min after occlusion) or assigned to a control group. They were then sacrificed either after 2 or after 21 days in order to examine the effect of hyaluronidase at the peak of the necrotic changes (2 days) and when the infarct had completely healed (21 days). The extent of the necrosis was quantified by measuring planimetrically the histologic extent of the infarcted zone

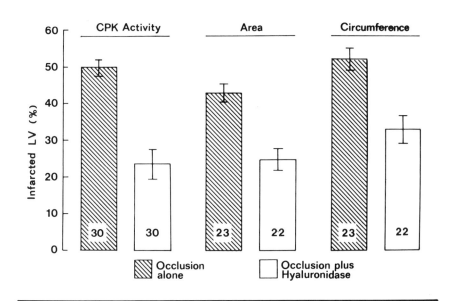

5 Percentage of the left ventricle which was infarcted 48 hr after occlusion of the main left coronary artery in the untreated (O) rats (shaded columns) and hyaluronidase-treated rats (OI) (open columns). The extent of the infarcts was assessed by left ventricular (LV) creatine phosphokinase activity (CPK) and by two histological methods based on the analysis of serial slices of the ventricle, i.e., the infarcted area and the circumference overlying it. Bars indicate $\pm$ 1 SEM. The number in parentheses is the number of rats studied in each group.

or by measuring the total left ventricular CPK (Fig. 5). The results of this study indicated that hyaluronidase significantly decreased necrosis at 2 days and resulted in smaller scars 21 days later. Thus, the effectiveness of hyaluronidase in reducing the electrocardiographic changes of acute ischemic injury (i.e., ST-segment elevations) and of myocardial necrosis at 1 or 2 days (QRS, CPK, and histological changes) is, finally, reflected in smaller scars and a larger area of viable and contracting myocardium.

Another question that still remained to be answered was, after what time delay following the occlusion did administering the drug still prove effective in protecting the jeopardized myocardial cells?

This issue is closely related to the problem of reversibility of injury. The irreversibility of myocardial ischemic injury has been studied extensively in recent years, but the transition from reversible to irreversible injury remains unclear. The mitochondria demonstrate striking changes in entering an irreversible stage of injury (Jennings and Ganote, 1976); more specifically, the appearance of amorphous matrix densities is believed to signal irreversible damage. Such densities are also a characteristic feature of irreversible injury in other tissues, such as the kidney (Ganote et al., 1974; Gritzka and Trump, 1968; Reimer et al., 1972) and liver (Smuckler and Arcasoy, 1969). Irreversible cell injury also coincides with defective mitochondrial function: pyruvate oxidation is severely impaired, even in the presence of generous amounts of cofactors (magnesium, NAD, reduced CoA, thiamine pyrophosphate): oxidation of succinate is maintained but at a reduced rate (Jennings et al., 1969); and there is little state 3 respiration and no respiratory control. It is not yet clear whether mitochondria that have progressed to this stage are capable of recovery if the ischemia is relieved.

Recently, loss of the cell-volume regulation and increased sarcolemmal permeability have been found to correlate more closely with irreversible injury than has mitochondrial failure (Jennings, 1976). The rapid accumulation of calcium phosphate within the mitochondria, following restoration of arterial flow, suggests that increased intracellular calcium is present, secondary either to increased sarcolemmal permeability to calcium (Kloner et al., 1974; Shen and Jennings, 1972; Jennings et al., 1975) or to defective sarcolemmal calcium transport (Jennings and Ganote, 1976). The primary event leading to irreversibility may, therefore, be a sarcolemmal defect which allows excess calcium to enter the injured cells (Jennings, 1976).

Several experimental studies have shown that when hyaluronidase is administered up to 6 hr after occlusion, it may reduce infarct size (Maroko et al., 1971; Maroko et al., 1972b; Libby et al., 1973). Accordingly, in a series of experimental dogs, the effectiveness of hyaluronidase on decreasing necrosis, 24 hr after occlusion, was examined using histological, CPK and QRS criteria (Hillis et al., 1976b). It was found that, when given 20 min after occlusion, the drug was most effective and its protective action decreased stepwise when given 3 or 6 hr later, and had disappeared completely when hyaluronidase was administered 9 hr after occlusion (Fig. 6). It was concluded that, while certain ischemic cells can be protected even after 6 hr of ischemia, this effect is not measurable after 9 hr have elapsed. This highlights the importance of early treatment.

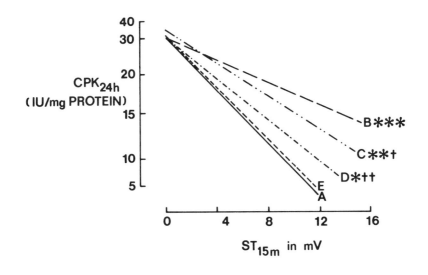

6

The relationship between ST-segment elevation, 15 min after coronary artery occlusion (ST_{15m}), and log CPK values of specimens obtained from the same sites 24 hr later. Group A (occlusion alone) (————): log CPK = $(-0.064 \pm 0.007)ST_{15m}$ + (1.49 ± 0.02); 14 dogs, r = -0.81 ± 0.03. Group B (hyaluronidase given 20 min after occlusion) (— — —): log CPK = $(-0.025 \pm 0.003)ST_{15m}$ + (1.48 ± 0.02); 12 dogs, r = -0.72 ± 0.04. Group C (hyaluronidase given 3 hr after occlusion) (·········): log CPK = $(-0.037 \pm 0.005)ST_{15m}$ + (1.53 ± 0.01); 8 dogs, r = -0.85 ± 0.02. Group D (hyaluronidase given 6 hr after occlusion (-··-··-··): log CPK = (-0.044 ± 0.003) ST_{15m} + (1.49 ± 0.01); 8 dogs, r = -0.78 ± 0.03. Group E (hyaluronidase given 9 hr after occlusion) (------): log CPK = $(-0.060 \pm 0.006)ST_{15m}$ + (1.50 ± 0.02); 6 dogs, r = -0.86 ± 0.06. Note that for any ST_{15m}, hyaluronidase given 20 min, 3 or 6 hr after occlusion results in significantly greater myocardial CPK activity; in contrast, hyaluronidase administered 9 hr after occlusion has no such effect (* = p<0.05, ** = p<0.025, *** = p<0.0005 in comparison to control; † = p<0.025, †† = p<0.0005 in comparison to hyaluronidase at 20 min).

The experimental evidence showing the favorable effect of hyaluronidase in reducing infarct size is now quite extensive, but the mechanism of action of the drug is still poorly understood. It is known that hyaluronidase depolymerizes hyaluronic acid and that it thereby facilitates the transport of a variety of substances through the interstitial spaces, and increases capillary permeability (Meyer, 1947; Hechter, 1950; Szabo and Magyar, 1958). This action may be particularly important in the presence of coronary occlusion in which these substances have to be transported through longer extravascular pathways than when the coronary arteries are patent. The transported substances may conceivably be nutrients, such as glucose necessary for the cells, and therefore transported into the infarct, or undesirable metabolites that have to be washed out. There is histochemical evidence showing the depolymerization of the mucopolysaccharides by hyaluronidase in the perivascular spaces in the infarcted zone (Maroko et al., 1972a), but direct proof of the facilitated transport of substrates in the ischemic heart is lacking. The electron-microscopic observation that glycogen is abundant in the ischemic myocardial zones of hyaluronidase-treated rats may lend indirect support to the theory of facilitated glucose transport (Kloner et al., 1976) (Fig. 7). Another possible mechanism is decrease in interstitial edema, with a consequent improvement in microvascular flow. The total water content of the heart is indeed reduced by hyaluronidase (Oliveira and Levy, 1960) but it is difficult to ascertain if this is the cause, or the effect, of smaller infarctions. More recently, it was found that the fall in collateral blood flow, which occurs usually between 15 min and 6 hr after coronary occlusion in dogs, can be prevented by hyaluronidase (Askenazi et al., 1976). It seems, therefore, that this drug does increase collateral flow but again it is difficult to ascertain if this effect is simply the consequence of smaller infarcts (smaller infarcts will permit better flow by the reduction in the amount of cell swelling) or whether hyaluronidase actually decreases edema, improves collateral flow and, thus, reduces myocardial damage. More studies are necessary to establish the mechanism of action of this drug.

After the usefulness of this drug had been shown in these animal experiments, two studies were carried out in patients with acute myocardial infarction. In both investigations, only patients whose pain started not more than 8 hr before the beginning of the study were admitted, since it was judged that the effectiveness of the drug, if given later, would be minimal. Furthermore, only patients with transmural anterior or lateral myocardial infarctions were admitted to the study since the method of evaluation of the effectiveness of treatment was based on the electrocardiographical criteria of injury (i.e., ST-segment elevation) and necrosis (QRS changes), which, by the method of 35 precordial electrode mapping, can be properly analyzed only in this group of patients (Fig. 8).

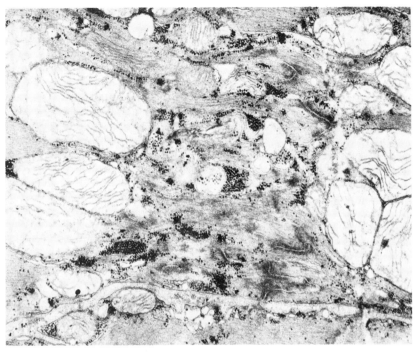

7   Hyaluronidase-treated ischemic myocardium, following 3 hr of coronary occlusion, shows a myocardial cell with severe ischemic changes. Despite these changes, glycogen is abundant.

Accordingly, the first pilot study (Maroko et al., 1975b) was carried out in 24 patients of whom 13 received hyaluronidase after the recording of the initial electrocardiographic map. The initial maps were similar in both groups in respect to the total sum of ST-segment elevations (ΣST) and the number of electrodes exhibiting ST-segment elevation equal to or over 1.5 mm (0.15 mV). However, after the administration of hyaluronidase (500 NF units/kg, i.v., every 6 hr for 48 hr), both ΣST and NST fell faster than in the patients that did not receive hyaluronidase. Thus, in the control patients, ΣST fell after 2 hr to an average of $93.5 \pm 17.3\%$ and after 24 hr to $89.6 \pm 7.5\%$ of the initial values, while NST dropped to $98.0 \pm 12.3\%$ and $94.3 \pm 10.4\%$, respectively. In contrast, in the hyaluronidase-treated group, at the same times, ΣST fell significantly more ($p < 0.05$) to $54.1 \pm 5.6\%$ and $51.3 \pm 11.8\%$ and NST was also more markedly reduced ($p < 0.05$) to $50.7 \pm 7.8\%$ and

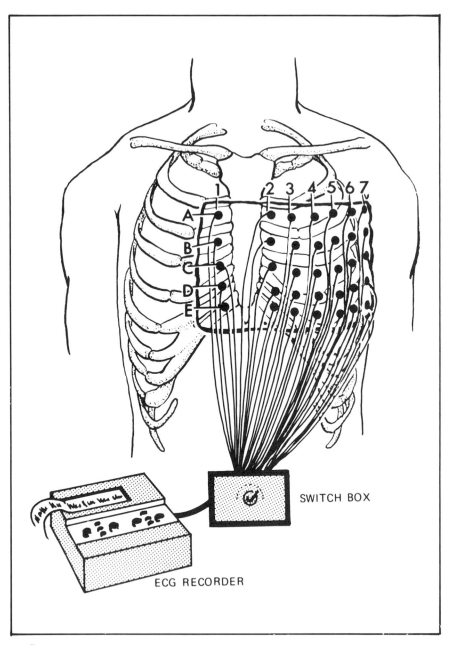

8 Schematic representation of the 35 electrode-set on a patient's chest. (From Maroko et al., 1972b; reproduced by permission.)

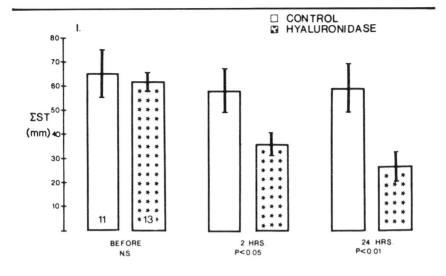

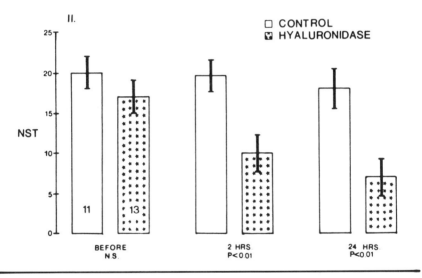

Panel I: The sum of ST-segment elevations (ΣST) in control and in hyaluronidase-treated patients at zero time (before treatment), and at 2 and 24 hr after treatment. Note that before treatment both groups had similar values of ΣST. However, in the treated group, ΣST dropped significantly more rapidly than in the control group. Panel II: Number of electrodes showing ST-segment elevations exceeding 1 mm (NST) in control patients and in hyaluronidase-treated patients at zero time, before treatment, and at 2 and 24 hr after treatment. Note that before treatment both groups had similar values of NST. However, in the treated group, NST dropped significantly more rapidly than in the control group. (From Maroko et al., 1975b; reproduced by permission.)

$50.1 \pm 12.4\%$ (Fig. 9). This study, therefore, indicated that hyaluronidase can reduce myocardial injury in patients with acute myocardial infarction.

The second investigation (Maroko et al., 1975a), which still continues, has as its primary aim examination of the effect of hyaluronidase on myocardial necrosis, as reflected by QRS changes in the 35-lead precordial map. The partial results indicate that hyaluronidase is, indeed, effective in minimizing necrosis in man. Thus, when the electrode sites with ST-segment elevations were analyzed in the 39 control patients, the sum of the R waves (ΣR), in these leads, decreased by $70.3 \pm 3.8\%$ and new pathologic Q waves developed in $58.6 \pm 5.2\%$. In contrast, in the 39 hyaluronidase-treated patients, ΣR fell by only $55.8 \pm 5.1\%$ ($p < 0.025$) and Q waves developed in only $46.0 \pm 5.4\%$ ($p < 0.05$). These interim results, therefore, strongly suggest that hyaluronidase not only resolves ischemic injury (as shown in the first study) but favorably influences the outcome of the ischemic process and results in a smaller infarction (as reflected by the smaller QRS changes). The administration of hyaluronidase in patients seems to have similar beneficial effects in reducing infarct size to those found experimentally. Moreover, hyaluronidase offers several advantages over other potential interventions that reduce infarct size: it (1) is simple to use and does not require special equipment; (2) does not depress cardiac contractility; (3) does not cause arterial hypotension; (4) has extremely low toxicity—in our own study, no severe adverse reactions were observed.

In conclusion, the effectiveness of hyaluronidase has been well established experimentally and its effect on infarct size is significantly better than that of other protective agents. Initial observations in patients concur favorably with these experimental results, but the impact of this intervention on the morbidity and mortality of patients with acute myocardial infarction has yet to be determined.

ACKNOWLEDGMENT

This study was supported, in part, by Contract No. N01-HV-53000 under the Cardiac Diseases Branch, Division of Heart and Vascular Diseases, National Heart, Lung and Blood Institute, NIH, Department of HEW.

REFERENCES

Askenazi, J., Hillis, L. D., Diaz, P. E., Davis, M. A., Braunwald, E., and Maroko, P. R.: Mechanism of reduction of myocardial injury by hyaluronidase. *Am. J. Cardiol.* 37:118 (Abstr.) 37:118 (1976).

Braunwald, E., and Maroko, P. R.: The reduction of infarct size—an idea whose time (for testing) has come. *Circulation* 50:206-208 (1974).

Ganote, C. E., Reimer, K. A., and Jennings, R. B.: Acute mercuric chloride nephrotoxicity. An electron microscopic and metabolic study. *Lab. Invest* 31:663-647 (1974).

Gritzka, T. L., and Trump, B. F.: Renal tubular lesions caused by mercuric chloride: Electron microscopic observations: Degeneration of the pars recta. *Am. J. Pathol.* 52:1225-1277 (1968).

Hechter, O.: Mechanisms of spreading factor action. *Ann. N. Y. Acad. Sci.* 52:1028-1040 (1950).

Hillis, L. D., Askenazi, J., Braunwald, E., Radvany, P., Muller, J. E., Fishbein, M. C., and Maroko, P. R.: Use of changes in the epicardial QRS complex to assess interventions which modify the extent of myocardial necrosis following coronary artery occlusion. *Circulation* 54:591-598, 1976. (October 1976a).

Hillis, L. D., Maroko, P. R., Braunwald, E., and Fishbein, M. C.: Influence of the time interval between coronary artery occlusion and the administration of hyaluronidase on myocardial salvage. *Circulation.* (Abstr.) 54:161, 1976 (October 1976b).

Jennings, R. B.: Relationship of acute ischemia to functional defects and irreversibility. *Circulation* (Suppl. I) 53:26-29 (1976).

Jennings, R. B., and Ganote, C. E.: Mitochondrial structure and function in acute myocardial ischemic injury. *Circ. Res.* 38 (Suppl. I): 80-89 (1976).

Jennings, R. B., Ganote, C. E., and Reimer, K. A.: Ischemic tissue injury. *Am. J. Pathol.* 81:179-198 (1975).

Jennings, R. B., Herdson, P. B., and Sommers, H. M.: Structural and functional abnormalities in mitochondria isolated from ischemic dog myocardium. *Lab. Invest.* 20:548-557 (1969).

Kloner, R. A., Fishbein, M. C., Maclean, D., Braunwald, E., and Makoro, P. R.: Effect of hyaluronidase on myocardial ultrastructure following coronary artery occlusion in the rat. *Circulation.* (Abstr.) 54:88, 1976. (October 1976).

Kloner, R. A., Ganote, C. E., Whalen, D. A. Jr., and Jennings, R. B.: Effect of a transient period of ischemia on myocardial cells. II. Fine structure during the first few minutes of reflow. *Am. J. Pathol.* 74:399-422 (1974).

Libby, P., Maroko, P. R., Bloor, C. M., Sobel, B. E., and Braunwald, E.: Reduction of experimental myocardial infarct size by corticosteroid administration. *J. Clin. Invest.* 52:599-607 (1973).

Lown, B., Vassaux, C., Hood, W. B. Jr., Fakhro, A. M., Kaplinsky, E., and Roberge, G.: Unresolved problems in coronary care. *Am. J. Cardiol.* 20: 494-508 (1967).

Maclean, D., Maroko, P. R., Fishbein, M. C., Carpenter, C. B., and Braunwald, E.: Reduction of infarct size up to 21 days after coronary occlusion in the rat. *Circulation.* (Abstr.) 54:161, 1976 (October 1976).

Maroko, P. R., Askenazi, J., Tavazzi, L., Muller, J. E., Distante, A., Salerno, J., Radvany, P., Libby, P., Luepker, R., Bobba, P., and Braunwald, E.: Effects of hyaluronidase on electrocardiographic evidence of necrosis in patients with acute myocardial infarction. *Circulation* (Suppl. III) 52: 106 (Abstr.) (1975a).

Maroko, P. R., and Braunwald, E.: Effects of metabolic and pharmacologic interventions on myocardial infarct size following coronary occlusion. *Circulation* 53 (Suppl. 1): 162-168 (1976).

Maroko, P. R., Davidson, D. M., Libby, P., Hagan, A. D., and Braunwald, E.: Effects of hyaluronidase administration on myocardial ischemic injury in acute infarction. A preliminary study in 24 patients. *Ann. Intern. Med.* 82:516-520 (1975b).

Maroko, P. R., Kjekshus, J. K., Sobel, B. E., Watanabe, T., Covell, J. W., Ross, J., Jr., and Braunwald, E.: Factors influencing infarct size following coronary artery occlusions. *Circulation* 43:67-82 (1971).

Maroko, P. R., Libby, P., Bloor, C. M., Sobel, B. E., and Braunwald, E.: Reduction by hyaluronidase of myocardial necrosis following coronary artery occlusion. *Circulation* 46:430-437 (1972a).

Maroko, P. R., Libby, P., Covell, J. W., Sobel, B. E., Ross, J., Jr., and Braunwald, E.: Precordial ST segment elevation mapping: An atraumatic method for assessing alterations in the extent of myocardial ischemic injury. The effects of pharmacologic and hemodynamic interventions. *Am. J. Cardiol.* 29:223-230 (1972b).

Maroko, P. R., Libby, P., Sobel, Bloor, C. M., Sybers, H. D., Shell, W. E., Covell, J. W., and Braunwald, E.: Effect of glucose-insulin-potassium infusion on myocardial infarction following experimental coronary artery occlusion. *Circulation* 45:1160-1175 (1972c).

Meyer, K.: Biological significance of hyaluronic acid and hyaluronidase. *Physiol. Rev.* 27:335-359 (1947).

Oliveira, J. M., and Levy, M. N.: Effect of hyaluronidase upon the water content of ischemic myocardium. *Am. Heart J.* 60:106-109 (1960).

Reimer, K. A., Ganote, C. E., Jennings, R. B.: Alterations in renal cortex following ischemic injury. III. Ultrastructure of proximal tubules after ischemia or autolysis. *Lab Invest.* 26:347-363 (1972).

Scheidt, S., Ascheim, R., and Killip, T., III.: Shock after acute myocardial infarction. A clinical and hemodynamic profile. *Am. J. Cardiol.* 26:556-564 (1970).

Shen, A. C., and Jennings, R. B.: Myocardial calcium and magnesium in acute ischemic injury. *Am. J. Pathol.* 67:417-440 (1972).

Smuckler, E. A., and Arcasoy, M.: Structural and functional changes of the endoplasmic reticulum of hepatic parenchymal cells. *Int. Rev. Exp. Pathol.* 7:305-418 (1969).

Szabo, G., and Magyar, S.: Effect of hyaluronidase on capillary permeability, lymph flow, and passage of dye-labeled protein from plasma to lymph. *Nature* (Lond.) 128. 377-379 (1958).

23

Effects of Vasodilator Therapy on Regional Myocardial Ischemia

LESLIE WIENER

INTRODUCTION

The systemic hemodynamic effects of vasodilators, such as nitroprusside and nitroglycerin, are well known. Nitroglycerin has long been considered an important antianginal drug (Murrell, 1879), while nitroprusside first received clinical attention as an antihypertensive agent (Page et al., 1955). More recently, these compounds have come under scrutiny because of their ability to favorably modify the hemodynamics of heart failure (daLuz et al., 1973; Gray et al., 1975; Taylor et al., 1975). The mechanisms responsible for this improvement in global cardiac hemodynamics include decreased peripheral resistance, increased left ventricular ejection fraction, diminished left ventricular filling pressure, and increased venous capacitance (daLuz and Forrester, 1976). The interaction between arterial and venous effects determines both the magnitude and variable direction of change in cardiac output and heart rate.

In the presence of left ventricular failure, vasodilator agents have had their pharmacological roles successfully extended for use in acute myocardial infarction, (Chatterjee et al., 1973; Walinsky

509

et al., 1974; Franciosa et al., 1972). However, following coronary occlusion, vasodilator-induced decrease in arterial pressure may be capable of upsetting the tenuous balance of factors controlling the extent of ischemic injury. Accordingly, their value in preserving ischemic myocardial tissue remains controversial.

The objective of this presentation is to examine and compare the effects of nitroprusside and nitroglycerin upon regional metabolic function in the acute ischemic left ventricular segment. In this context, an estimate of the effect of these interventions on the control of infarct size may be inferred.

METHODS

This study comprised three groups. The effect of nitroglycerin and nitroprusside on regional ischemia in the dog heart was examined in: (1) Group A experiments following total occlusion of direct coronary artery supply; (2) Group B experiments following partial occlusion; and (3) Group C experiments following partial coronary artery occlusion in addition to left ventricular volume loading. Group A consisted of 8 separate control experiments, 7 nitroglycerin experiments and 5 nitroprusside experiments. In Group B and C, each dog served as his own control. Group B comprised 5 nitroglycerin experiments and 5 nitroprusside experiments. Group C included 4 nitroglycerin experiments and 4 nitroprusside experiments. A total of 38 dogs, weighing 20 to 40 kg, were used in this investigation. All animals were intubated and ventilated with room air, using a mechanical respirator. After the induction of anesthesia (chloralose 100 mg/kg and morphine 1 mg/kg intravenously), the chest was opened, through a left lateral thoracotomy, and the anatomy of the left anterior descending artery and its accompanying vein was examined. A #20 teflon catheter needle was inserted into the vein draining the region supplied by the middle and distal third of the left anterior descending (LAD) coronary artery. In Group A experiments, a ligature was secured around the middle third of the LAD artery (Fig. 1). Group B and C experiments involved the introduction of a #16 or #14 gauge teflon catheter needle into the middle third of the LAD coronary artery (Fig. 2). Following catheter insertion into the coronary artery, 10,000 IU of heparin was administered intravenously, and a femoral artery to coronary artery shunt was immediately established via a specially designed silastic tube. The tube incorporated a 5 mm,

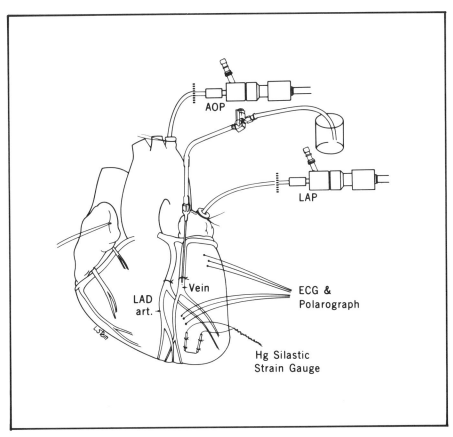

1

A diagrammatic display of the experimental design and monitoring systems for Group A experiments. The middle third of the left anterior descending (LAD) artery is ligated. AOP-aortic pressure; LAP-left atrial pressure. The regional coronary vein is noted to be cannulated.

Biotronex electromagnetic flow probe for measurement of distal left anterior descending flow. Cannulae were inserted into the descending aorta and left atrium. Pressures were obtained from these sites via a P-23 DB Statham strain gauge. Six platinum electrodes were inserted approximately 3 mm into the myocardial tissue, and used to monitor polarographic oxygen tension and local electrograms, as previously described (Wiener et al., 1976). Three of these

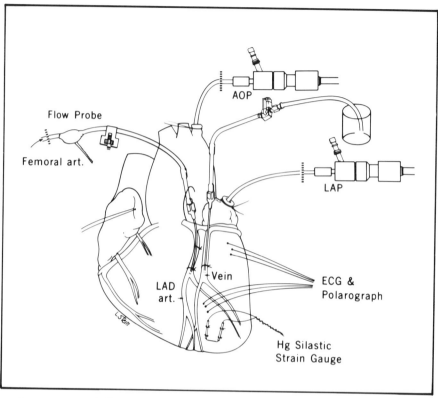

2   A diagrammatic presentation of Group B and C experiments. The experimental model was identical to Group A, except for the addition of a cannula in the left anterior descending artery. The cannula is connected to the femoral artery via a specially-designed silastic tube incorporating an electromagnetic flow probe and an adjustable screw used to control flow.

electrodes were placed in the region to be rendered ischemic and three were inserted in a remote location for control comparison. A mercury silastic strain gauge was sutured to the prospective ischemic segment, parallel to the direction of the superficial fibers. The strain gauge was then connected to a Wheatstone bridge. Aortic pressure, left atrial pressure, LAD coronary artery blood flow, wall motion, polarographic oxygen measurements and ECG were all monitored with the aid of a DR12 medical recorder (Electronics for Medicine). Blood samples obtained from the regional coronary venous drainage and femoral artery were analyzed for pH, PCO_2, PO_2, lactate, total CPK and CPK MB. Blood gas and pH analysis was obtained with the aid of an IL blood-gas analyzer. Lactate levels were analyzed by a rapid, enzymatic autoanalytic technique described by Antonis (Antonis et al., 1966). Total CPK and CPK MB measurements were performed with a method developed by Rao (Rao et al., 1975).

The experimental procedure in Group A called for baseline measurements followed by total occlusion of the LAD coronary artery. Thereafter, measurements were made at 15 intervals up to 45 min. Nitroglycerin (1.2 mg sublingually) or nitroprusside (100-150 μg/min intravenously) was administered at 30 min following occlusion in all treated animals. Nitroprusside dosage was adjusted to achieve a 20-25% reduction in aortic systolic pressure. The procedure for Group B animals involved baseline measurements, followed by two 15-min data sampling intervals (control). Partial occlusion was then performed and data was again collected at 15-min intervals. Nitroprusside and nitroglycerin were administered 15 min after occlusion, as described above. Group C animals differed from Group B in that all dogs were rapidly volume-loaded with approximately 1500 cc of blood and dextran infused intravenously at 15 min following left anterior descending coronary artery occlusion. In this experimental series, nitroprusside and nitroglycerin were administered 30 min after partial coronary artery occlusion and 15 min after volume loading.

All data were expressed as mean values ± standard error of the mean. Statistical significances were established through Student's t test.

RESULTS

Regional Lactate Concentration (Fig. 3)

Control experiments in Group A animals showed that regional lactate concentration increased from 4.48 mg/100 ml ± 1.11 to 17.42 ± 1.49 ($p < 0.001$) 15 min after complete occlusion of the LAD artery. At 30 min following occlusion, lactate concentration was 16.38 mg/100 ml ± 3.05, and at 45 min post-occlusion lactate concentration was 15.63 ± 2.26. At 30 min following complete occlusion of the LAD coronary artery, nitroprusside and nitroglycerin caused no significant change from control experiments (14.77 mg/100 ± 3.16 and 12.68 mg/100 ml ± 3.78, respectively).

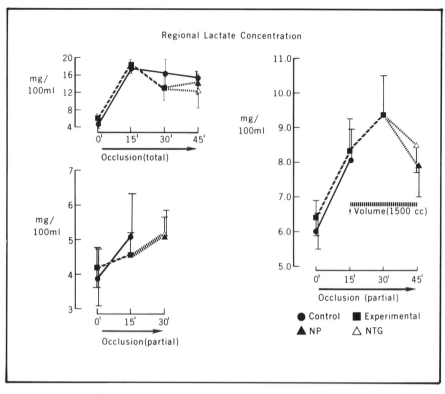

Regional Lactate Concentration

3

Regional lactate concentration is compared among Group A (top panel), Group B (middle panel) and Group C experiments (bottom panel). No significant difference in regional lactate concentration is evident, after total coronary artery occlusion, between control observations and the experimental group receiving either nitroprusside or nitroglycerin (Group A). Group B experiments (middle panel) show accentuated ischemia after nitroglycerin and nitroprusside, i.e., increased regional lactate build-up occurred following therapy. Group C experiments (bottom panel) indicate that volume loading increases regional lactate concentration. The addition of nitroprusside or nitroglycerin resulted in a reduction in regional lactate concentration to pre-volume-loading levels.

In Group B experiments, control data showed regional lactate concentration to increase from 3.87 mg/100 ml ± 0.78 to 5.10 ± 1.22 (p < 0.05) 15 min after partial occlusion of the left anterior descending coronary artery. Nitroglycerin and nitroprusside accentuated the ischemic effect of partial occlusion, since regional lactate concentration was observed to increase from 4.55 mg/100 ml ± 0.53 to 5.42 mg/100 ml ± 0.31 (p < 0.05) after nitroglycerin, and to 5.34 mg/100 ml ± 0.75 (p < 0.05) after nitroprusside.

In Group C animals, the addition of a 1500 cc volume load, 15 min after partial coronary occlusion, resulted in a more substantial rise in lactate concentration ($p < 0.01$) than did partial coronary artery occlusion alone (10.28 mg/100 ml $\pm$ 1.26 prior to nitroglycerin, and 8.58 mg/100 ml $\pm$ 0.84 prior to nitroprusside). Thereafter, nitroglycerin caused a significant reduction in lactate concentration to 8.54 mg/100 ml $\pm$ 0.84 ($p < 0.05$). Similarly, a decrease in lactate concentration was produced by nitroprusside administration (8.58 mg/100 ml $\pm$ 0.82 to 7.88 mg/100 ml $\pm$ 0.92, ($p < 0.05$).

Regional Blood Gas and pH (Fig. 4)

In Group A experiments, complete occlusion of the left anterior descending coronary artery progressively decreased regional pH (7.334 $\pm$ 0.006 to 7.199 $\pm$ 0.027), increased regional PCO_2 (46.05 $\pm$ 3.77 to 57.48 $\pm$ 3.51 and reduced regional PO_2 from 29.77 $\pm$ 3.41 to 23.70 $\pm$ 3.06 ($p < 0.001$). Regional blood gas and pH changes corresponded closely to the pattern of regional lactate release, i.e., as lactate augmented, pH and PO_2 fell, while PCO_2 increased. The effects of complete coronary artery occlusion were not significantly altered by either nitroprusside or nitroglycerin. In Group B experiments, nitroglycerin and nitroprusside augmented myocardial ischemia. Regional pH decreased 18.2% ($p < 0.05$) after nitroglycerin, and 3.5% (n.s.) after nitroprusside. Regional PCO_2 increased 10.1% ($p < 0.05$) after nitroglycerin, and 13.8% ($p < 0.05$) after nitroprusside. Regional PO_2 diminished by 3.9% (n.s.) after nitroglycerin and 12.4% ($p < 0.05$) after nitroprusside. Volume loading, in Group C experiments, accentuated myocardial ischemia by decreasing regional pH 10.4% ($p < 0.05$), increasing regional PCO_2 11.8% ($p < 0.05$) and reducing regional PO_2 12.1% ($p < 0.05$). In the presence of a volume-loaded state, vasodilator administration decreased myocardial ischemia, as manifested by a regional pH increase of 10.3% ($p < 0.05$), regional PCO_2 decrease of 11.4% ($p < 0.05$), and regional PO_2 rise of 6.2% (n.s.) following nitroprusside, and a regional pH increase of 26.8% ($p < 0.05$), regional PCO_2 decrease of 8.6% (n.s.), regional PO_2 rise of 11.4% ($p < 0.05$) following nitroglycerin.

Infarct Size as Reflected by Regional CPK and CPK MB Levels (Fig. 5)

Within 45 min, total occlusion of the left anterior descending coronary artery resulted in a predictable rise in regional CPK and

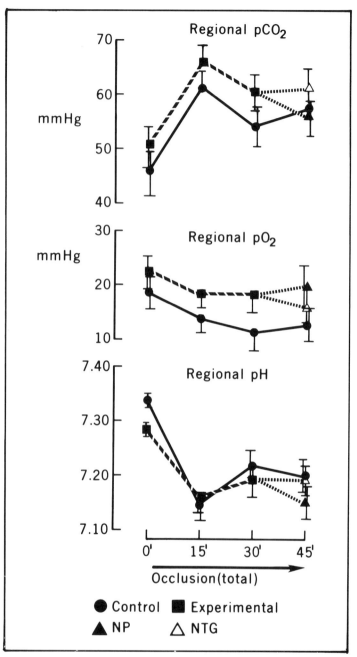

4 Following coronary artery occlusion, regional myocardial ischemia is demonstrated. Regional PCO_2 and pH are significantly altered in inverse fashion. Regional PO_2 is noted to steadily decline up to 30 min following occlusion. No significant changes are encountered following either nitroprusside or nitroglycerin administration in this experimental series (Group A).

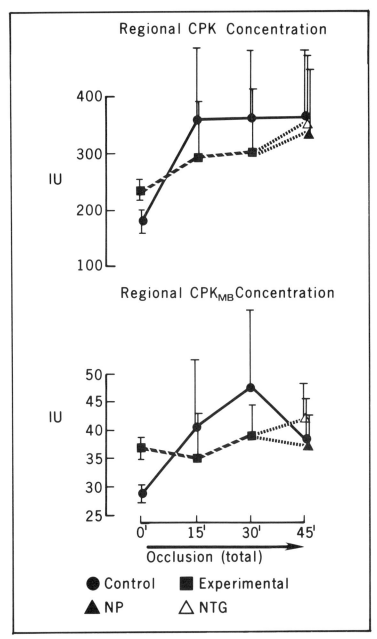

5 Estimation of myocardial infarct size, by regional CPK (total) and regional CPK MB efflux, shows that no significant changes resulted from nitroglycerin and nitroprusside administration in this experimental series (Group A).

CPK MB from 182.8 ± 20.84 and 29.4 ± 1.46 to 371.9 ± 136.72 and 38.4 ± 13.72, respectively. Among Group A dogs, nitroprusside and nitroglycerin showed no significant change in the rate of CPK increase, as compared with controlled studies.

Hemodynamic Responses

Heart rate averaged 116.9 beats/min $\pm$ 9.55 and did not vary significantly as a result of either total LAD coronary artery occlusion or partial coronary occlusion. Under the influence of nitroglycerin and nitroprusside, heart rate in Group A and Group B experiments increased 14% and 16%, respectively. However, following volume loading in Group C experiments, no significant changes in heart rate were affected by either nitroprusside or nitroglycerin.

Aortic systolic and diastolic pressures were not significantly altered by complete or partial occlusion of the left anterior descending coronary artery. Nitroglycerin decreased systolic aortic pressure from 163.86 ± 8.51 mm Hg to 146.5 mm Hg $\pm$ 7.57, while nitroprusside reduced systolic pressure from 163.9 ± 8.51 mm Hg to 130.0 ± 7.92 mm Hg. No significant change in left atrial pressure resulted from either partial or complete occlusion of the LAD coronary artery, and no alteration in pressure accompanied nitroprusside or nitroglycerin interventions, except in Group C experiments. In this group, volume loading produced a significant increase in left atrial pressure from 4.6 ± 0.75 mm Hg to 16.7 ± 2.31 mm Hg. Thereafter, nitroglycerin decreased left atrial pressure to 10.2 ± 2.63 mm Hg, and nitroprusside diminished left atrial pressure, in similar fashion, to 6.8 ± 0.48 mm Hg ($p < 0.01$).

ST Segment Elevation

Before coronary occlusion, ST segment elevation was 0.9 ± 0.39 mV. In the untreated Group A series, ST segment elevations increased to 3.6 ± 0.62 mV at 15 min, 3.5 ± 0.60 mV at 30 min, and 3.4 ± 0.64 mV at 45 min. Neither nitroglycerin nor nitroprusside altered ST segment elevation in this group. In Group B, the ST segment level did not change (1.0 ± 0.50 mV to 1.1 ± 0.46 mV) despite partial coronary artery occlusion. However, nitroglycerin and nitroprusside increased ST segment elevation when heart rate was increased by more than 30%. When nitroglycerin and nitroprusside failed to raise the heart rate above 30% of baseline level, there was no apparent ST segment change. The mean ST segment elevation went from 0.9 ± 0.46 to 1.9 ± 0.60 mV after nitroprusside, and to 1.8 ± 0.53 mV after nitroglycerin.

In Group C, volume loading increased ST segment elevation 173% to 3.0 ± 1.08 mV. After nitroprusside, ST segment elevation decreased 46% to 1.6 ± 0.63 mV (p < 0.05), while nitroglycerin reduced ST segment elevation by 17% to 2.5 ± 0.76 mV (p < 0.05).

Regional Coronary Blood Flow

In Group B and C experiments, left anterior descending coronary artery blood flow was decreased by intent to 24% of baseline value. Thereafter, nitroglycerin and nitroprusside failed to significantly change LAD coronary artery blood flow in the absence of volume loading. The response to volume loading was variable but, in general, resulted in an increase in LAD coronary artery blood flow from 22.0 ± 1.38 cc/min to 29.9 ± 2.390, despite partial coronary artery occlusion. Nitroprusside did not significantly change LAD coronary artery blood flow (32.3 ± 3.75 cc/min), after volume load, but nitroglycerin did result in a significant 21.1% (p < 0.05) rise to 36.1 ± 1.15 cc/min.

Regional Segment-Length Change

No attempt was made to quantify the segment length change since the stiffness characteristics of the mercury in silastic length gauge were not determined. Consequently, a linear relationship between length and electrical resistance change was not confirmed. For this reason, all assessments of segment shortening and lengthening were qualitative.

In Group A, total coronary artery occlusion resulted in prompt segment length increase, associated with evident paradoxical systolic expansion. Neither nitroprusside nor nitrogylcerin offset this abnormal wall motion change. In Group B experiments, the ischemic segment showed no significant abnormal changes from pre-occlusion observations. Nitroglycerin and nitroprusside did not alter the normal wall-motion pattern. By contrast, volume loading in Group C studies resulted in paradoxical systolic expansion. Both nitroprusside and nitroglycerin were effective in returning this abnormal wall motion change toward normal.

DISCUSSION

Published data on the effectiveness of vasodilators in acute myocardial ischemia have provided conflicting results. Using the epicardial electrocardiographic mapping technique, Smith (1973) observed a substantial reduction in the magnitude and distribution of ST segment elevations after short periods of nitroglycerin administration in conscious dogs. Similar results have been reported in studies involving ischemia of up to 5-hr duration (Hirshfeld et al., 1974). However, Myers and coworkers (1975), and others (Chiariello et al., 1976) have reported increased ischemic injury when experimental acute coronary occlusion was modified by nitroglycerin. Lang (1976) observed persisting metabolic and mechanical derangements in the ischemic region, which were not significantly different from those in untreated control series.

Clinical data on the influence of vasodilators in acute myocardial ischemia is sparse. Shell and Sobel (1974) observed that, in hypertensive patients experiencing myocardial infarction, estimated infarct size was 24% less than predicted by CPK-release technique when afterload-reducing vasodilators were used. Providing that arterial pressure is maintained, nitroglycerin has been reported to favorably decrease ST segment elevation in 6 of 12 patients undergoing acute myocardial infarction (daLuz and Forrester, 1976). Chiariello and coworkers (1976) compared the effects of nitroglycerin and nitroprusside in 5 patients with acute myocardial infarction. Although they observed both nitroglycerin and nitroprusside to improve overall hemodynamic function, they found that nitroprusside increased subepicardial injury while nitroglycerin reduced ischemic injury. Animal experiments performed by the same investigators showed that nitroglycerin improved flow to ischemic areas while nitroprusside decreased it.

6

The top panel shows the effect of partial coronary artery occlusion (Group B experiments) on distal left anterior descending blood flow (small arrow) and polarographically measured regional myocardial PO_2 tissue tension in the ischemic zone. Note that, as the blood flow decreases, a corresponding fall in myocardial tissue oxygen tension in the ischemic zone becomes apparent. Other polarographically measured myocardial oxygen tension sites, outside the ischemic zone, are not significantly affected (non-marked lines). Panel B shows the paradox of increasing regional coronary artery blood flow (small arrow) under the influence of rapid volume loading, while tissue oxygen tension is further reduced in the ischemic myocardium. The lower panel shows the effect of nitroglycerin in Group C experiments. Regional coronary blood flow increases slightly while myocardial tissue oxygen tension, in the ischemic region, does not change appreciably.

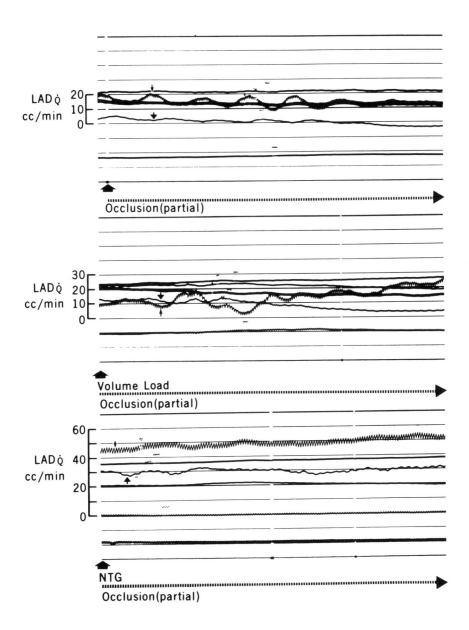

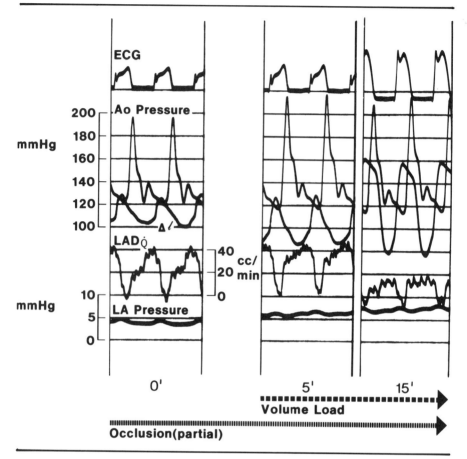

7 Volume loading of the mildly ischemic left ventricle (partial occlusion of the LAD artery) results in increased ST segment elevation (ECG), paradoxical ischemic muscle segment wall motion ($\triangle$ l) and a rise in left atrial (LA) pressure. Distal left anterior descending blood flow (LAD_Q) initially augments and then diminishes as ischemia worsens.

In this investigation, no significant differences in myocardial effects were apparent between nitroglycerin and nitroprusside. Both drugs failed to improve cardiac function of the regionally ischemic myocardium when the ischemia resulted from total occlusion of its direct vascular supply. When less intense myocardial ischemia was

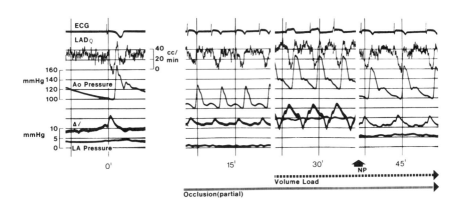

8

Nitroprusside intervention (large arrow NP) 30 min after volume loading achieves a reduction in ST segment (ECG), a decrease in aortic pressure (AO pressure), a return to normal wall motion in the ischemic segment ($\triangle$ I) and a marked drop in left atrial pressure (LA pressure). In this experiment, no significant change in distal left anterior descending artery blood flow (LAD_Q) is evident.

induced, by only partially obstructing direct coronary-artery supply, nitroglycerin and nitroprusside appeared to accentuate myocardial ischemic injury. This effect occurred despite the paradox of their augmenting coronary flow through the obstructed vessel. (Fig. 6) Increased ischemic injury invariably resulted when the heart rate rose 30% above control values. However, when left ventricular failure was induced by abrupt volume loading, an improvement in global hemodynamic function resulted in lessened ischemic injury. (Figs. 7 and 8) Under these circumstances, nitroglycerin and nitroprusside either reduced heart rate or did not change it significantly. The clinical implications of these experimental studies are that the two drugs do not favorably alter the extent of myocardial infarction resulting from complete coronary artery occlusion. In acute myocardial ischemic states, vasodilators may actually increase ischemic injury unless heart-rate responses are attenuated. When myocardial ischemia is accompanied by left ventricular failure, vasodilator therapy may reasonably be expected to reduce the extent of myocardial injury while improving left ventricular dysfunction.

REFERENCES

Antonis, A., Clark, M., and Pilkington, T. R. E.: A semi-automated method for the enzymatic determination of pyruvate, lactate, acetoacetate and B hydroxbutyrate levels in plasma. *J. Lab. Clin. Med.* 68:340-356 (1966).

Chatterjee, K., Parmley, W. W., Ganz, W., Forrester, J., Walinsky, P., Crexells, C., and Swan, H. J. C.: Hemodynamic and metabolic response to vasodilator therapy in acute myocardial infarction. *Circulation* 48:1183-1193 (1973).

Chiariello, M., Gold, H. K., Leinbach, R. C., Davis, M. A., and Maroko,, P. R.: Comparison between the effects of nitroglycerin and nitroprusside on ischemic injury during acute myocardial infarction. *Am. J. Cardiol.* 37:127 (Abstr.) (1976).

daLuz, P. L., and Forrester, J. S.: Influence of vasodilators upon function and metabolism of ischemic myocardium. *Am. J. Cardiol.* 37:581-587 (1976).

daLuz, P. L., Shubin, H., and Weil, M. H.: Effectiveness of phentolamine for reversal of circulatory failure (shock). *Crit. Care Med.* 1:135-140 (1973).

Franciosa, J. A., Guiha, N. H., Limas, C. J., Rodriguera, E., and Cohn, J. N.: Improved left ventricular function during nitroprusside infusion in acute infarction. *Lancet* 1:650-654 (1972).

Gray, R., Chatterjee, K., Vyden, J. K., Ganz, Forrester, J. S., and Swan, H. J. C.: Hemodynamic and metabolic effects of isosorbide dinitrate in chronic congestive heart failure. *Am. Heart J.* 90:346-352 (1975).

Hirshfeld, J. W., Jr., Borer, J. S., Goldstein, R. E., and Berrett, M. J.: Reduction in severity and extent of myocardial infarction when nitroglycerin and methoxamine are administered during coronary occlusion. *Circulation* 49:291-297 (1974).

Lang, T., Meerbaum, S., Corday, E., Davidson, R. M., Hashimoto, K., Farcot, J., and Osher, J.: Regional and global myocardial effects on intravenous and sublingual nitroglycerin treatment after experimental acute coronary occlusion. *Am. J. Cardiol.* 47:533-543 (1976).

Murrell, W.: Nitroglycerin as a remedy for angina pectoris. *Lancet* 1:80, 113, 151, 225 (1879).

Myers, R. W., Scherer, J. L., Goldstein, R. A., Goldstein, R. E., Kent, K. M., and Epstein, E. E.: Effects of nitroglycerin and nitroglycerin-methoxamine during acute myocardial ischemia in dogs with pre-existing multivessel coronary occlusive disease. *Circulation* 51:632-640 (1975).

Page, I. H., Corcoran, A. C., Dustan, H. P., and Koppanyi, I.: Cardiovascular actions of sodium nitroprusside in animals and hypertensive patients. *Circulation* 11:188-198 (1955).

Rao, P. S., Lukes, J. J., and Mueller, H. S.: A new chemical method for CPK-isoenzyme-MB determination by dithiothreitol. *Clin. Res.* 23:203A (Abstr.) (1975).

Shell, W. E., and Sobel, B. E.: Protection of jeopardized ischemic myocardium by reduction of ventricular afterload. *N. Engl. J. Med.* 291:481-496 (1974).

Smith, E. R., Redwood, D. R., McCarron, W. E., and Epstein, S. E.: Coronary occlusion in the conscious dog: effects of alterations in arterial pressure produced by nitroglycerin, hemorrhage, and alpha-adrenergic agonists on the degree of myocardial ischemia. *Circulation* 47:51-57 (1973).

Taylor, W. R., Forrester, J. S., Magnusson, P., Takano, T., Chatterjee, K., and Swan, H. J. C.: The hemodynamic effects of nitroglycerin ointment in congestive heart failure. *Circulation* 52:11-36 (Abstr.) (1975).

Walinsky, P., Chatterjee, K., Forrester, J., Parmley, W. W., and Swan, H. J. C.: Enhanced left ventricular performance with phentolamine in acute myocardial infarction. *Am. J. Cardiol.* 33:37-41 (1974).

Wiener, L., Feola, M., and Templeton, J. Y.: Monitoring tissue oxygenation of the heart following myocardial revascularization. *Am. J. Cardiol* 38: 38-45 (1976).

Discussion

Lee, Maroko, Wiener

DR. WILLIAM DAWES (University of Pennsylvania) : Since dead cardiac cells are not electrically active, how can the ECG distinguish production of infarct from progression of cell death?

DR. PETER R. MAROKO (*Harvard Medical School*) : Since the appearance of Q waves and the falling R wave correspond to tissue necrosis, they will show in a qualitative way if the infarct is larger or smaller. A lack of electrical forces as seen from the Q and R waves indicates how extensive the infarct is.

DR. DAWES: Does that mean that the amplitude of the Q waves is proportional to the number of healthy cells?

DR. MAROKO: Yes, it is proportional within limits. There are several investigations showing this, and the slide which I presented demonstrating the relationship of depth of Q waves to myocardial CPK activity constitutes one of these studies.

DR. DAWES: But this correlation would not apply to ST segment elevation or depression, would it?

DR. MAROKO: The ST segment elevations are completely different. ST segment elevation shows an injury to cells when it is still in the reversible stage, and this is the only reason why every time after an occlusion, the ST segment will go up. If you release the occlusion, the ST elevation disappears. So ST segment elevation just shows an injury in the reversible phase.

DR. JOHN K. VYDEN (*UCLA School of Medicine*):   I should like to ask Dr. Maroko two questions. My first question is, what was the hemodynamic status of the patients that received hyaluronidase and what effect, if any, did this agent have upon their hemodynamics?

DR. MAROKO: We did not exclude any patient from the hyaluronidase administration because of their hemodynamic status. We did not see any obvious hemodynamic changes when this enzyme was given. Also, experimentally, hyaluronidase did not change the hemodynamic status of the animals receiving this drug.

DR. VYDEN: Nitroprusside was detrimental in cases where there was no volume overload, but when the end-diastolic pressure increased, this drug seemed to produce a beneficial effect. The question I would ask you bears upon the work you presented in New Orleans earlier this year. When you gave nitroprusside, you apparently saw an increase in ST segment elevation. In respect to this last slide, then, it would be of critical importance to know what was the left ventricular end-diastolic pressure of the patients to whom you gave nitroprusside?

DR. MAROKO: Of the 10 patients that received nitroprusside, 9 had a left ventricular end-diastolic pressure of 15 mm Hg. In all cases, ST segment elevations increased. About one-third of the patients were hypertensive when they were given nitroprusside but after its administration, their systemic pressure returned to normal limits. Even in these patients, there was an increase in ST segment elevation. Some of them had a rise in heart rate and others did not. In patients that did not show an increase in heart rate, the ST segment elevation was augmented. Therefore, in this particular group of 10 patients, all had an increase in ST segment elevation. None in this group was in pulmonary edema or in shock.

DR. JOHN FLYNN (*Jefferson Medical College*):   Dr. Maroko, what was the dose of hyaluronidase, especially in the experimental animals? Do you have a dose-response curve, and if so, is there a maximum dose with which you can really eliminate these deleterious effects of coronary occlusion? And also, what dose would you use in humans?

DR. MAROKO: We do not have a dose-response curve. We are giving about 500 turbidity units per kilogram, every 6 hr for 2 days to patients; the dose in dogs is the same. In the first series, it was half of it, in the other series it was exactly the same.

DR. ALLAN M. LEFER (*Jefferson Medical College*): I should like to ask Dr. Wiener, in view of the fact that he saw beneficial effects with the nitrates in volume-loaded situations, under what circumstances would he recommend the use of these agents?

DR. LESLIE WIENER (*Thomas Jefferson University Hospital*): I would think the ideal clinical situation for nitroprusside or one of the nitrate preparations would be the acute myocardial infarction patient in left ventricular failure.

DR. ROBERT J. LEE (*Squibb Institute for Medical Research*): You would not use these agents in uncomplicated myocardial infarction?

DR. WIENER: Well, if I am to extrapolate the observations and the particular conditions of these experiments, I should say that the use of nitrates and nitroprusside in such circumstances would worsen the ischemia. I think the major aggravating factor seems to be an inappropriate increase in heart rate that results when the left ventricle is normally loaded and the left ventricular diastolic pressure is relatively normal.

DR. ROBERT REYNOLDS (*Medical College of Pennsylvania*): Dr. Wiener, when you produced ventricular overload with dextran, did this alter the coronary arterial hematocrit? And if so, could the effects that you might see with this procedure be in part due to additional ischemia resulting from anemia?

DR. WIENER: By and large, we used no more than 500 cc of dextran; the remainder was blood. This was roughly 1,000 cc of whole blood and 500 cc of dextran. I do not think that this would have rendered the animal anemic.

DR. JAMES SPATH (*Jefferson Medical College*): Dr. Lee, you have explored several beta-blocking agents. Which would be the most appropriate in a given situation? Would you rate them according to the least undesirable side effects or by relative potency? How would you classify these drugs in terms of myocardial ischemia?

DR. LEE: Well, as I have said, all of those agents that have been tested in angina have worked, and I do not think you can distinguish them on the basis of dose. If they have lower potencies, you have to use larger doses. I believe that, perhaps, compounds that have too much of a sympathomimetic effect and those that induce myocardial depression may be detrimental and, therefore, other drugs without these properties should be used.

DR. VYDEN: Dr. Lee, I was wondering if you could tell us what do you feel are the contraindications for the use of beta-blockers in acute myocardial infarction?

DR. LEE: Well, as I said in the conclusion, I think that in uncomplicated myocardial infarction, there appear to be no contraindications, and these agents have very definite beneficial effects, resulting from a decrease in oxygen demand probably due to beneficial hemodynamic changes.

Subject Index

531